Design Engineering of Biomaterials for Medical Devices

Wiley Series in Biomaterials Science and Engineering

Commissioned in the UK on behalf of John Wiley & Sons, Ltd by
Medi-Tech Publications, Storrington, West Sussex RH20 4HH, UK

Series Advisors
Robin N. Stephens
AVE (UK) Limited, Burgess Hill, UK

Julian H. Braybrook
Laboratory of the Government Chemist, London, UK

Patrick M. Maloney
CellPro Inc, Bothell, Washington, USA

Providing readers with comprehensive, authoritative and timely information in this
fast-developing area of research and biomedical technological advancement, this
series encompasses topics in biomaterials science and engineering including the
structure and function of materials and devices, their individual actions and
interactions, and practical and clinical applications.

Books in the *Wiley Series in Biomaterials Science and Engineering* are designed
to help stimulate further developments in biomaterials science and engineering
by disseminating up-to-the-minute, quality information to academic and industrial
research and development scientists employed in all areas of the medical,
biomedical and bioengineering sciences whether in medical device R&D,
pharmaceutical and pharmacological research or materials science, and to
clinical specialists in prosthetics and surgery.

RECENT TITLES IN THE SERIES

Biosensors in the Body: Continuous in vivo *Monitoring*
Edited by David M. Fraser (0 471 96707 6)

Biocompatibility Assessment of Medical Devices and Materials
Edited by Julian H. Braybrook (0 471 96597 9)

Design Engineering of Biomaterials for Medical Devices
David Hill (0 471 96708 4)

FORTHCOMING TITLES IN THE SERIES

Metals as Biomaterials
Edited by J. Helsen and J. Breme (0 471 96935 4)

Computer Technology in Biomaterials Science and Engineering
Edited by J. Vander Sloten (0 471 97602 4)

Design Engineering of Biomaterials for Medical Devices

David Hill

Rocket Medical Plc, Newcastle upon Tyne, UK

JOHN WILEY & SONS

Chichester · New York · Weinheim · Brisbane · Singapore · Toronto

This book aims to provide accurate and authoritative information on biomaterials and medical devices. Readers are, however, advised to familiarise themselves with the current regulations and standards applying to these areas of research. The author and publisher specifically disclaim any and all liability arising directly or indirectly from acting or failing to act on any information contained in the book. The views expressed herein are those of the author and should not be taken to represent the views of Rocket Medical Plc or any other company or official organisation referred to in the text.

Other Wiley Editorial Offices

John Wiley & Sons, Inc., 605 Third Avenue,
New York, NY 10158-0012, USA

WILEY-VCH Verlag GmbH, Pappelallee 3,
D-69469 Weinheim, Germany

Jacaranda Wiley Ltd, 33 Park Road, Milton,
Queensland 4064, Australia

John Wiley & Sons (Asia) Pte Ltd, 2 Clementi Loop #02-01,
Jin Xing Distripark, Singapore 129809

John Wiley & Sons (Canada) Ltd, 22 Worcester Road,
Rexdale, Ontario M9W 1LI, Canada

Library of Congress Cataloging-in-Publication Data

Hill, David
Design engineering of biomaterials for medical devices / David Hill.
    p. cm. – (Wiley series in biomaterials science and engineering)
    Includes index.
    ISBN 0-471-96708-4 (alk. paper)
    1. Biomedical materials. 2. Biomedical engineering. I. Title. II. Series.
R857.M3H55 1998
610'.28–dc21   97–17449
                                                                         CIP

British Library Cataloguing in Publication Data

A catalogue record for this book is available from the British Library

ISBN 0 471 96708 4

Typeset in 10/12pt Times by Florencetype Ltd, Stoodleigh, Devon.
Printed and bound in Great Britain by Biddles Ltd, Guildford and King's Lynn.
This book is printed on acid-free paper responsibly manufactured from sustainable forestry, in which at least two trees are planted for each one used for paper production.

Contents

Preface

The basic concept of this work is to provide a reference book of use to the professional design engineer and others within the medical device manufacturing industry. Managers, section heads and co-workers of the design and development department will derive benefit from the information contained.

During writing I have attempted to keep the text as informative as possible without becoming too immersed in unnecessary technical data which would prevent the reader from obtaining quick specific details for the job in progress. I do not claim that the book will turn anyone into a designer or a better engineer, nor solve all of their problems instantly, but it does offer the opportunity to have at hand information which is relevant, in a simple format and easy to find.

This same information is presently hidden away in separate books, journals and other publications buried in a library. The details contained, bar the anecdotes and practical examples, are already published or in the public domain; I have compiled, I hope, one easy to read volume. A book which will be retained by students, engineers and managers alike.

Dr John Coakley Lettsom (1744–1815) wrote, 'When people's ill, they comes to I \ I physics, bleeds and sweats 'em \ Sometimes they live, sometimes they die \ What's that to I ? I lets 'em.' This was fine for the gentlemen of the 18th century but in today's professional environment surgeons and all medical staff demand perfection from their equipment, be it a large magnetic resonance image scanner or a disposable suture. This is, of course, understandable since any fault or failure could result in death or permanent disability of the patient (not to mention the subsequent litigation). Hence, the function, method of use and construction of medical devices must be right first, last and every time. The design process and material selection are two crucial factors in ensuring that a correct product is finally manufactured.

Materials available to the designer are numerous, varied and complex; the first section of the book splits them up into generic groups with details of history, physical properties and applications. More specific information is given on PVC because of its uniqueness and dedicated uses. Other chapters in the first section cover subjects from material selection methods to biocompatibility, with a special chapter on battery specification.

The second section contains methods of design, with the restrictions and requirements placed on the designer explained and the actions the designer must undertake to ensure that the final product will be acceptable to the clinicians.

The penultimate section speculates on future trends of how medical devices will evolve. There is also a discussion about the effects of medical devices on the environment with regard to processes, manufacture and disposal.

This book does not and could not cover all the materials used within the medical field, nor does it delve into analysis of materials at a microstructural level. The book does not present all the information necessary to complete a final, functional, saleable design: it cannot since the disciplines involved are diverse and complex, but it was never intended to!

The book is intended as a tool for the thousands of engineers and students who are involved with medical product design, come into contact with or supply medical companies with materials or components, are ambitious to enter the arena of patient treatment and care or just wish to increase and improve their knowledge of materials and product design, thus providing a more comprehensive professional service for the welfare of patients.

David Hill
August 1998

About this Book

Part One of this book is about materials for medical devices.

In the first chapter the range of materials available to the designer is surveyed and the crucial nature of material selection in the design process is emphasised. Materials are categorised as an aid to understanding their properties and a prompt for open-minded selection.

Design requirements and the ways in which material selection can or should be undertaken are described in Chapter 2. Data sources to inform the selection process are reviewed.

Ferrous metals, their properties and uses, are the subject of Chapter 3. Stainless steel is often thought of as the material of choice for medical instruments but in this chapter five types of stainless steel are identified and suggestions made for their appropriate use, as well as other members of the family of irons and steels.

Elements and alloys that constitute the non-ferrous metals are considered in Chapter 4, concentrating on those with uses in medical devices. Practical examples illustrate the relation between material properties data and actual products.

In Chapter 5 the vast range of polymeric materials is presented. The complex world of polymers is classified into generic groups, with emphasis on the thermoplastic and thermosetting families. The text provides guidance to help the designer narrow down likely choices and have confidence in product development.

Chapter 6 is devoted to the special case of PVC, a widely used but somewhat controversial polymer about which the device designer needs to be well informed.

The seventh chapter consists of brief consideration of many other materials, less widely used but with particular properties that may make them the candidate of choice for specific applications. Notes are supplied on Bakelite, barium, cadmium, carbon, ceramics, diamond, latex, quartz, 'memory metal', Tufnol and biodegradable materials.

Adhesives are another class of materials with increasing applications in biomedical devices, and these are described and considered in Chapter 8.

In medical devices it is especially important that products continue to function as intended throughout their service life. In Chapter 9 the problems of corrosion and degradation are reviewed to assist the designer in both appropriate choice of material and sound understanding of the interaction between a device and the environment in which it exists.

This theme continues in Chapter 10 which is about biocompatibility. Requirements for testing and validation of materials for use as medical implants or devices are given, and relevance to design and construction is derived.

Chapter 11 is a survey of filters and membranes for medical applications; the use, construction and properties of filters are included as well as an account of substances to be filtered and methods of doing so.

Fibre optics is an expanding field of endeavour in the medical products industry, which is the subject of Chapter 12. The principles are explained, and examples given regarding information transfer and biological monitoring using fibre optic technology. New uses and potential developments are a feature of this chapter.

Many medical devices require an independent power source, so battery selection is an important aspect of the design. So many different types of power cells and batteries are available that the choice can be problematic: Chapter 13 includes information to assist. The potential consequences of misuse of batteries are particularly important in medical products, so this topic receives special attention.

The second part of this book is about the process of designing medical devices.

Chapter 14 is a personal view of the prerequisites for good design: the education and training of designers. Both junior and senior training requirements are considered, and the necessity of continuing technical education and professional development to company competitiveness is emphasised.

The process of design and factors that affect the outcome are the subject of Chapter 15. Practical steps to be followed by the designer and by the company as a whole are given. Before any design work is done, however, it is vital that the requirements of the application or the customer are researched in detail from both a marketing and a technical point of view. Otherwise a lot of effort can go into designing a product that does not optimally serve both manufacturer and user, which denies both commercial and humanitarian gain.

A feature of the medical device industry is the trend to miniaturisation. Chapter 16 is about microengineering, and includes descriptions of novel devices for minimally invasive surgery, minute mechanisms manufactured with state-of-the-art methods, and speculation about future developments in nanotechnology.

An important stage in the product design process is prototyping. The many traditional and new ways of making prototypes with varying levels of functionality are given and compared in Chapter 17.

Nearly all products for medical use need to be sterilised. In Chapter 18 different modes of sterilisation and their relevance to product design and material selection are discussed.

International, European and National Standards exist to regulate the design and manufacture of medical devices. The product designer needs to be aware of the implications of a vast amount of stipulation, and Chapter 19 is an overview of this topic with pointers to guide the design engineer.

Part of the product design process is the detailed specification of materials and processes to be used. There is no scope for uncertainty here, as made clear in Chapter 20.

Packaging has long been the last thing considered in product design. In Chapter 21 the advantages of integrating packaging into the product concept are set forth; this is relevant to all devices but especially disposable and sterile goods.

The design engineer does not work in isolation, but in a community of other company employees, clients, suppliers, regulators and so on. Team-work approaches are increasingly favoured by managers, and so communication becomes a core skill. Failure of communication can cost dearly in terms of time, money or even patient well-being, so the learning and development of communication skills is vital: these issues are the subject of Chapter 22.

In Chapter 23 the matter of manufacturers' liability for their products is explained. Designers need to understand the consequences of all their decisions and actions, so an awareness of product liability legislation is a necessary attribute for their work. Examples of actual cases illustrate how courts are interpreting the law.

In a competitive market innovative designs need to be protected. Sometimes keeping ahead of the game is the best policy, but patents and registration systems exist to preserve commercial advantage and protect the fruits of the design team's endeavour. Chapter 24 does not give legal advice, but indicates when to invoke patents or design registration, and offers guidance on the decisions to be taken.

Chapter 25 on Quality Assurance describes the audit of quality control as required in the latest Medical Device Directive and discusses the separate specific stipulations for a 'Design Dossier', as part of a corporate approach to quality engineering.

Part of the design function is not only to describe and specify a product, but also to decide an appropriate manufacturing and assembly route. Awareness of production engineering issues should be part of the design process from the outset. To assist this integrated approach, Chapter 26 consists of a wide-ranging survey of manufacturing methods.

Part Three of this book looks ahead to future trends.

Medical device design, far from standing still, is experiencing an increasing rate of change in terms of new clinical requirements, new materials, and new technologies applied to medicine. Chapter 27 is a personal view of the extension of existing engineering practices into the medical arena, and future developments in clinical techniques.

Another future trend is the increasing importance of environmental issues. Both the effect of the environment on a product, and the effect of the manufacture, use, and disposal of a product on the environment, are being analysed as never before. Chapter 28 examines these issues and offers pointers to a future where a competent and professional engineer will have to design the life-cycle of a product, not just its functional phase.

Part Four of this book deals with information and data.

Chapter 29 on Sourcing suggests how to find the data, information, suppliers, contacts and services that are required to enable the creation of a new product. For efficient operation of a design department, it is important to know what information, advice, funding and support is available externally, and to tap these sources to save time and effort before engaging in original work.

Finally a glossary of relevant words and phrases is supplied to ease the way of the reader through this book and other works about medical device engineering.

This book does not, nor could it, cover all materials ever used in the medical field; neither does it delve deeply into physics or materials science at a microstructural level. This was not the intention. The book is targeted at the engineers and students who are involved with medical product design and development, supply medical companies with components or materials, are ambitious to enter the arena of patient treatment and care, or wish to widen their knowledge of engineering materials and design.

Part One

Materials

1
Materials Available

The range of materials available to the medical device designer is vast, and includes unusual or unfamiliar materials. In this chapter I hope to inform, enlighten and provide advice which I believe you will find helpful and inspirational in both material selection and the design of new products.

Medical devices can be manufactured from many types of material. The choice is part of the designer's job. It is important that you are aware of the full range of materials available and new formulations being presented or you may compromise your design by not selecting the best option.

The successful engineer needs to be aware of more than just generic material groups. It is important to keep up with improvements and developments even if they do not appear relevant to existing work. Material updates and continuous reviews should be mandatory for all designers and engineers.

It is very easy to become complacent and insular regarding the materials used, but not selecting the correct type, make, or supplier, can prevent not only financial gains to the company but also therapeutic or health giving benefits to a patient. Many good ideas have to await the right technology for presentation, process or material. Twenty years ago magnetic resonance imaging was only an idea because no-one knew how to make or contain the magnets which were needed to enable images to be focused and recorded.

The materials available are constantly changing. There are now ceramics that mimic springs, paper laminates that can behave as a heat insulator, and plastics that have the properties of other generic groups but can be processed more easily and cheaper.

The best way of keeping up with this rapidly changing world is to maintain close contact with the material suppliers. They have the resources and commercial reasons to progress in this field, and the motivation to keep potential customers well informed. Suppliers will be your allies in validating material choices and providing written justification of their suitability.

The material selection process starts with the design brief and initially addresses the whole range of available materials. Design criteria limit this range, which will be further narrowed down by manufacturing considerations.

Classification of materials, whether for medical use or not, can act as a prompt when reviewing options or looking for the right material to start using for the prototype. Figure 1.1 shows how diverse the range is, and is the first step in your selection. The selection will evolve and may well end up with something completely different from the option you first thought of.

New materials can provide solutions to ideas put forward many years ago. An example is the treatment of constriction of the urethra when the prostate gland becomes enlarged. Surgery is the usual remedy but many have speculated 'why not just stick a tube in?'. The difficulty has been that a tube of adequate diameter would be difficult to insert and secure in place. With 'memory metal' a solution might be possible. These alloys undergo shape changes with changes in temperature. A coil of the material, suitably formed, sized and heat treated, could be cooled with water at about 5°C. This could be inserted in the urethra with ultrasound guidance and then made to expand by flushing with warm water via a catheter. Body heat (37°C) would maintain the coil in its open position and allow urine to pass freely. If the device later required removal, it could simply be flushed with cold water.

This example illustrates how new materials can enable new devices to be made or permit the redesign of existing devices with benefits to both patient and manufacturer. The difficulty is the unpredictability of future developments, but the better informed you are the more likely it is that you will be positioned to anticipate and exploit new materials.

Another example is the disposable scalpel. Traditionally, scalpel blades have been fitted to plated brass handles by theatre nurses and handed to the surgeon as required. Now there is the option of using a disposable scalpel consisting of a metal blade and a moulded plastic handle, prepacked and sterile. This has the advantages of not requiring assembly, disassembly, cleaning and resterilising. There is no danger of blades becoming detached and no worry of injury to the nurse preparing the scalpel before operations. The rationale behind this is that the nursing time required to dismantle, clean, pack, sterilise, sort, transport and store the reusable scalpel, and the other costs of this process, exceed the costs of the disposable version, thus giving a saving if disposables are used.

The option of the disposable scalpel came about because of changes in available materials and processing methods, allowing a stainless steel blade to be stud or heat welded to a plastic handle. Twenty or even ten years ago this concept would have been rejected but now it is viable. However, disposable scalpels are not yet universally used because the cost savings are not fully understood by senior medical staff.

The successful engineer must be aware of the generic material groups and of developments in materials technology, whether or not they seem directly relevant to the present work. It is very easy to become complacent regarding the materials used, but, not being aware of new or developing materials precludes not only financial benefits to your company but also therapeutic benefits to patients.

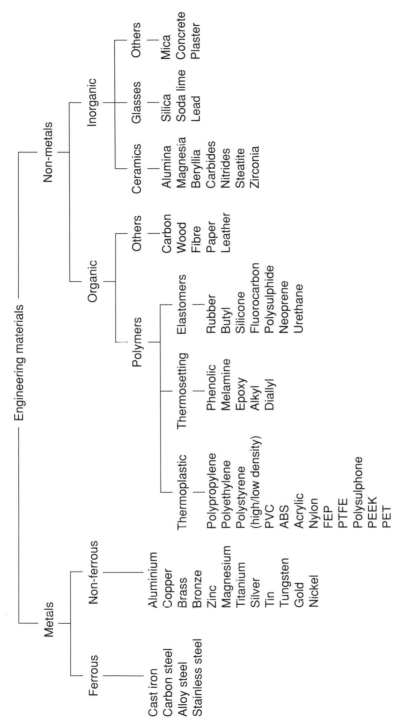

Figure 1.1 Choice and classification of engineering materials.

Table 1.1 Material density and shear strength

	Density (10^4 kg m^{-3})	Shear strength (MPa)
Aluminium (cast)	0.27	92.7
Aluminium (hardsheet)	0.28	193
Brass	0.85	278
Copper	0.89	193
Cast iron	0.72	185
Leather	0.094	54
Silver	1.08	230
Steel (cast)	0.79	463
Steel (stainless)	0.84	540
Tin	0.73	38.6
Paper	0.093	70 (Flat punch)
		23 (Hollow die)
Zinc	0.71	115
Bronze	0.88	310

One consideration to look at when assessing materials is the strength-to-weight ratio. You are, no doubt, aware of the oft-quoted example of steel and aluminium, but other materials need to be evaluated on their own merits. Table 1.1 shows density and shear strengths, not the complete range but enough to illustrate the point.

Economics is, of course, a major factor in picking the 'right' material for a product. There may be a material ideally suited for the task but it could be prohibitively expensive, so you would have to compromise on performance to achieve a saleable product. Material cost is not considered in isolation though, you must also evaluate the cost of manufacture.

An example is a radio frequency transmitting electrode (Figure 1.2) that I designed a few years ago. There were many materials that would have served the function and could be made into the product. Initially three models were made to check that the concept would function. Then it was necessary to assess the results of functional trials, the potential costs of manufacture, and the quantities that would be required for prototypes, pre-production trials and long-term manufacturing.

The product requirements included:

- a fixed electrical contact,
- a tip shape developed over protracted trials,
- a thermal safety trip, which linked with
- a surface temperature indicator.

The tip profile is shown in Figure 1.2.

I emphasise that all possible material choices should be considered. Here are the options considered for the r.f. electrode.

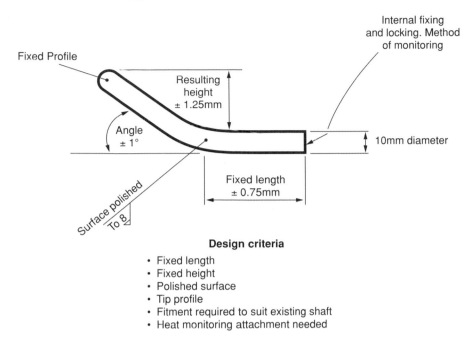

Figure 1.2 Design of radio frequency transmitting electrode. Reproduced by permission of Rocket Medical Plc.

- Stainless steel rod: machine, bend, re-machine and polish.
- Stainless steel: cast, machine bore, tap thread and polish.
- Zinc: investment cast, machine bore, tap thread and plate.
- Zinc: die cast, cut internal thread and plate.
- Aluminium: die cast, cut internal thread and anodise or plate.
- Aluminium rod: machine, bend, re-machine, polish and anodise or plate.
- Mild steel: machine, bend, re-machine, polish and plate.
- Copper: machine, bend, cut internal thread, polish and plate.
- Glass: mould with contact wire insert and fixing.
- ABS: injection mould, copper plate, press in thread insert and final plate.
- Conductive polymer: injection mould, press in thread insert, nickel plate or nickel and gold flash.

Some of these were discounted almost as they were written down, but they should still be examined. Others were put aside when rough costings were made.

The prototype was constructed by the first stainless steel option, and as it happened this was also the final manufacturing choice, primarily because of the production quantities involved. The costings had to be calculated, and this involves other departments, such as marketing and production engineering, and other considerations.

The design engineer should never fall into the habit of selecting a known material just because it is easier or safer. Each project should be examined from the start as a new challenge with a listing of requirements and a fresh start to material selection. Try new ideas and concepts, stretch options to the limit. The worst that can happen is that the tests on the prototypes prove that you did not make a good choice this time. Then you can revert to an older alternative or proven method.

I'm not advocating change just for change's sake, always use your judgement and all the available information that can be obtained. Use feedback from clients, both in-house staff and customers. If you are lucky enough to have access to clinical opinion, it is surprising how helpful the medical profession can be if you wish to discuss new ideas or methods of treatment, even at the concept stage.

Do not try to reinvent the wheel; you are not a materials engineer doing research into possible applications, you are there to design and develop medical devices for the benefit of both your company and the future patients. Keep an open mind and use all the information and support services available to you. Chapter 29 is about sourcing information and materials, it includes lists of contacts and specialists – use them.

2
Material Selection Processes

During this book I will refer to the material selection process but, to be honest, there is no rigid method for selecting materials, though there are good patterns which you should follow.

Do not restrict your options, and never just accept your first instinctive choice proceeding blindly without rechecking on the application. Question it over and over again; the previous chapter has shown there are vast numbers of materials, processes and combinations to influence your choice.

Medical devices have to work right first time. Material selection is a critical factor, and it is vital that you assess all the demands on a product: bone prostheses have to have good compressive strength of course, but they must also have good properties in bending and shear and tolerate any mis-use the patient might impose.

The ideal design, the technical best that can be achieved, is often a compromise between conflicting objectives and requirements. The optimal design is a concept that must contain elements from many disciplines and areas of expertise, Table 2.1 lays out some of these factors.

2.1 DESIGN FACTORS

Material selection is essentially in the hands of the product designer who, with the input at later stages from production and industrial engineers, will review and then justify the material finally specified. A simple illustration of the complexities which must be looked at can be seen in Figure 2.1. The figure shows the large number of possibilities or combinations which must first be considered just to manufacture a simple packing box.

It is surprising to realise that you must consider 256 possibilities to specify a folded box in white clad aluminium, presented in a shrink wrap. These same problems of eliminating possible combinations increase pro rata as the requirements and restrictions increase. In Chapter 1 I quoted the example of material and process advancements which permitted the combination of a metal scalpel blade with a moulded plastic handle, providing a disposable product. But even a simple device like this scalpel fulfils multiple mechanical and physical

Table 2.1 Factors to consider in material selection

Economic	Humidity	Finish
Material cost	Recyclable	Wear
Process introduction	Manufacturing waste	Friction
Strength	Pollution	Tactile
Tensile	Product life span	Heat
Compression	Cost/benefit analysis	Aesthetic
Dynamic	Corrosion resistance	Cosmetic appeal
Fracture	Safety	Ergonomics
Impact	Toxic contamination	Colours
Stress	Toxic interaction	Visual Clarity
Strain	Fire hazard	'Feel'
Electrical	Thermal	Semantics
Resistance	Shrinkage	Performance
Contact	Expansion	Does it meet the brief?
Power supply	Stability	Targets
Earthing	Insulation	Satisfied user
Tracking	Method of containment	Development
Insulation	Stiffness	Future use
Electromechanical	Non-linear	Changes in requirements
compatibility	Bending moments	New materials/processes
Environmental	Creep	
Weather	Surface	

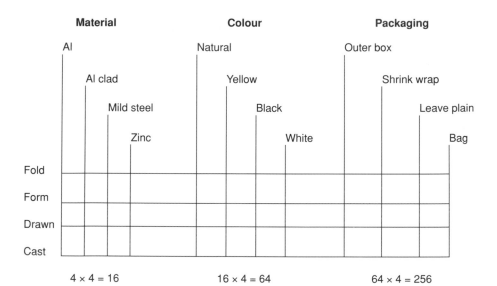

Figure 2.1 Combination of choices in material selection for a simple box. © 1993 Advanstar Communications Inc.: first published in *Proceedings of the Medical Design and Materials Conference*, 15 November 1993, Düsseldorf, Germany.

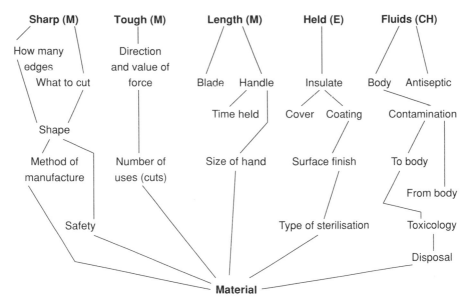

M = Mechanical, E = Electrical, CH = Chemical

Figure 2.2 Areas of influence on material selection for a scalpel blade.

criteria. The diagram in Figure 2.2 shows, somewhat simply, a method of cataloguing these parameters and progressively drawing out the requirements of
the blade. The diagram shows how all the qualities indicated have an influence
on the material selected; and this is not a fully comprehensive chart.

It is clear that no one discipline can cover the whole selection process;
interaction between departments is important and the product designer coordinates the various inputs from fields in which the designer is not fully
trained. It is not helpful for anyone to be protective of their own area of
expertise: collaboration is required to further the development of optimal
products.

Similarly, do not lose interest once your design work is completed, documented and handed over to the production engineers. You need to keep in
touch and follow the product through to ensure adherence to specification
and quality, and to learn from experience along the way.

A product I was involved with had problems when the stainless steel carefully specified to meet machining, cutting and polishing requirements was
changed by a buyer who could obtain a different grade at a cheaper price.
Material costs were reduced, certainly, but the machining time increased and
the impurities present showed themselves after sterilising. Three weeks later
tiny footprints of disaster over the surface made the item suitable only for

the scrap bin, not the customer. So ensure a good working relationship between the quality department and your own design group, then if they have queries about a product they will feel able to talk to the design team.

My own field of work is mainly in disposable devices, and this narrows the choice of materials, mainly because of the cost constraints but not always: single use need not always mean cheapest.

The plastics industry does very well out of their medical device involvement with something in excess of 60 000 tonnes of polymers used in the UK alone, giving an estimated market of £12 billion and increasing. Table 2.2 provides an insight into the more generally used polymers and examples of their applications plus a listing of properties which dictate their specific selection.

One of the most important factors influencing material selection is sterilisation. This is dealt with in detail in Chapter 18: at this stage it is sufficient to raise the topic and note that sterilisation can have effects on the materials used. Different sterilisation methods also have important cost implications.

A novel way of trying to narrow down material choices is to use a decision tree. Figure 2.3 illustrates the evolution of the scalpel problem again but shown as a problem-solving tree, which can highlight all possibilities and give scope for some lateral thinking.

2.2 ACCESSING MATERIAL DATA

The product design engineer is, of course, aware of the properties of engineering materials in general, but there is a huge amount of rapidly changing information about specific materials that cannot all be researched or remembered in detail. Accessing this data is made easier by the suppliers who provide databases, with updates, which I have found to be the best way of reaching the information.

You only need to keep enough information at your finger tips to act as a prompt for the correct direction to follow when selecting a material. Once you are on the right track you can contact material suppliers or manufacturers and use their expertise.

There are computer data bases available now which are free (in most cases) and easily obtained. Built into the majority is a basic selection program, suitable for the first step in the assessment of a suitable material. The information contained is not just a screen full of sterile figures and indigestible data, but may include details about standards, material selection and descriptive text. Such databases do not remove the necessity of carrying out further in-depth investigations but can give helpful reference data to enable you to progress a project. It is part of the narrowing down process, choosing options to speed up the final selection. Table 2.3 lists some of the free disks that can be obtained.

Table 2.2 Key properties and applications of polymers. © 1993 Advanstar Communications Inc. First published in Medical Design and Materials Conference Proceedings, 15 November 1993, Düsseldorf, Germany, and reproduced with permission

	Key properties	Key applications
Poly(vinyl chloride)	Low cost, processing versatility, clarity, easily sealed, low toxity	Disposable i.v. and blood bags, catheters, cannulaes, tubing, gloves, labware, moulded i.v. and blood parts, apparatus, packaging, trays, containers
Polypropylene	Cost processability, mechanical properties, inertness	Disposable syringes, hospital ware, fibres, equipment, components
Polystyrene (including high impact, HIP)	Optical clarity	Disposable labware, scalpels, packaging
Low density and high density polyethylene	Cost, processability, mechanical properties, inertness	Tubing, moulded containers
Polycarbonate	Optical clarify, strength, gamma radiation resistant	Equipment housings, sterile reservoirs and containers
Poly(ethylene terephthalate)	Odour barrier, clarity, strength, gamma radiation resistant	Vascular grafts, heat valves, sutures, packaging
Acrylonitrile–butadiene–styrene copolymer	Processability, inert, gamma radiation resistant	Equipment housings, instrument mouldings
Polyurethane	Resilience, biocompatibility	Catheters, mouldings
Poly(methyl methacrylate) (PMMA)	Low cost, good body tolerance, processability, aesthetic	Dentures, hearing aids, artificial eyes, bone cement, incubator covers
Polyamide (Nylon 6, Nylon 66, etc)	Strength, processability	Needle hubs, sutures, components
Silicone rubbers	Resilience, biocompatibility	Catheters, gloves, tubing, implants
Styrene–acrylonitrile copolymer	Processability, inertness	Syringes
High performance resins such as polysulphone (PSU), polyether sulphone (PES) and poly-etheretherketone (PEEK) etc.	Strength, durability, sterilisability, biocompatibility	Vessels, artificial joints, prostheses

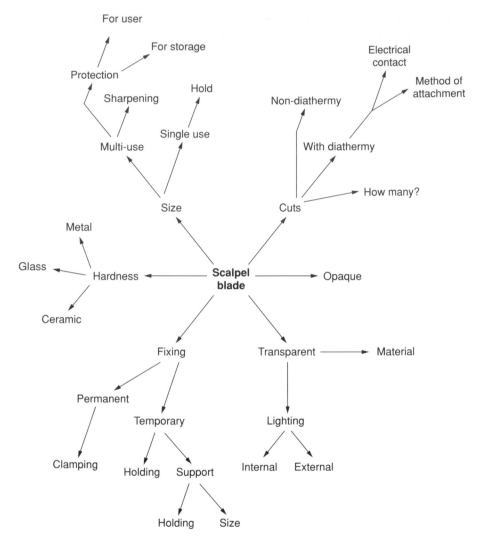

Figure 2.3 Tree structure of problem solving in selection of material for scalpel blade.

Once you get down to detailed specification of materials you will need specialised material selection and information programs. This becomes more costly as materials companies and research groups understand that we designers need to have up-to-date information and news of recent research. So they have now started to sell it. The cost is relative, as finding out by other means would take more of your time. If the details can be given early enough, or a new better option is open, then it will be money well spent. Table 2.4 lists some of the more popular systems like the excellent PLASCAMS from Rapra

Table 2.3 Free data and selection disks. From *Engineering Designer* Nov/Dec 1993: reproduced by permission of the Institution of Engineering Designers

Name	Company
Plastics	
CAMPUS	Bayer, BASF, Hoechst, Du Pont, Solvay,
Computer Aided Material Preselection	Dow, Huls,
By Uniform Standards	
ELASTOMER P & A	3M
Selection and design guide	
Metals	Trade groups, individual details from these
Copper alloys	01707 50711 Phone
	01707 42769 Fax
Aluminium bronze alloys	"
	"
Copper–Nickel alloys	"
Magnesium (+ alloys)	0161 794 2511 Phone
	0161 728 4842 Fax
Titanium (+ alloys)	01332 864900 Phone
	01332 864888 Fax

Table 2.4 Some PC databases available for purchase. From *Engineering Designer* Nov/Dec 1993: reproduced by permission of the Institution of Engineering Designers

	Available from
Plastics	
Cen BASE	
(Thermoplastics, thermosets elastomers	Info Dex Inc – USA
and composite engineering materials)	Tel: 00 1 714 893 2471
CHEMRES II	Rapra Technology
(Plastics and rubber chemical resistance	Tel: 01939 250383
selector)	
Adhesives	
PAL	Permabond Adhesives Ltd
(Permabond adhesives locator)	Tel: 01703 629628
Aluminium	
ALUSELECT	Aluminium Federation
	Tel: 0121 456 1103
General materials	Wolfson Cambridge Industrial Unit
Cambridge materials selector	Tel: 01223 334755

Table 2.5   Some on-line databases. From *Engineering Designer* Nov/Dec 1993: reproduced by permission of the Institution of Engineering Designers

	Database host
Data-Star	Tel: 0171 930 5503
	Fax: 0171 930 2581
Dialog Information Services	Tel: 01865 326226
	Fax: 01865 736354
Engineering Information Co Ltd	Tel: 0171 622 8155
	Fax: 0171 627 5076
IRS Dialtech	Tel: 0171 323 7951
	Fax: 0171 323 7954
ORBIT Search Service	Tel: 0181 992 3456
	Fax: 0181 993 7335
STN International	Tel: 01223 420066
	Fax: 01223 423623

Technologies, an independent knowledge-based selection system which contains a vast amount of data and is presented in an unbiased way.

An alternative to buying the disks and program is to use on-line databases: some are shown in Table 2.5.

2.3 SUMMARY

The essential aspects of this chapter about material selection are:

- never cling to set or tried and tested old formats, nor a popular easy choice of materials,
- always keep an open mind when considering materials, their application and uses,
- keep up-to-date on material advances, changes and processes,
- do not fix a design until the last option has been investigated, and
- do not let a deadline be the deciding factor for the selection.

3
Ferrous Metals

Materials used in medical devices, be they disposables or for continuous use, are seen to be the best available. The critical nature of many reusable instruments, requires the use of various iron and steel alloys: such demanding applications range from staples, via scalpels, to implants.

A ferrous metal is one which consists primarily of iron. The main body of engineering metals are in the ferrous group, mostly for commercial reasons since they are relatively cheap and easy to form. The difference between iron and steel is in carbon content: steels contain up to 1.7%C and irons have more. Other elements are added to modify properties and these will be explained in more detail later. Heat treatment also affects the properties, so it is essential that end use and methods of sterilisation are fully investigated before selection.

Ferrous metals are usually classified in four groups: cast iron, carbon steel, alloy steel and stainless steel. These groups are suitable for different uses, depending on their properties.

3.1 CAST IRON

Cast iron is important in engineering. It is versatile, including easily machinable grey iron, corrosion and heat resistant grades, and high wear resistant types. Specialist cast irons are produced in which the mechanical properties have been improved either by alloying or heat treatments. Spherical graphitic iron offers additional ductility and toughness, and may be used for load bearing applications within, say, an operating theatre. In SG iron, as it is known, the carbon precipitates in a spherical form, rather than as the usual weakening graphite flakes. This is achieved by adding small amounts of magnesium (not more than 0.1%), which causes the graphite to form in the desired shape. The resulting iron may have a tensile strength of 770 N mm^{-2}. Alloy cast iron uses the same elements as in alloys of steel. Chromium is used to increase hardness and wear resistance. Nickel promotes graphitisation and refines the grain during forming increasing the toughness. Vanadium adds to the heat resistance, while copper improves atmospheric corrosion

Table 3.1   British Standards for cast iron

BS 1452	Grey iron castings
BS 1591	Corrosion resisting high silicon iron castings
BS 310	Blackheart malleable iron castings
BS 3333	Pearlitic malleable iron castings
BS 309	Whiteheart malleable iron castings
BS 2789	Iron castings with spherical or nodular graphite
BS 3468	Austenitic cast iron

resistance. There are several British Standards covering cast iron as can be seen in Table 3.1.

3.2 CARBON STEELS

Carbon steel is the name given to an alloy of carbon and steel. These alloys also contain small amounts of manganese, phosphorus and silicon. The group can be divided into low-, medium-, and high-carbon steels. Those with a carbon content of 0.4% or less, cannot be hardened by heat treatment. Figure 3.1 shows the relationship between carbon content and heat treatability as well as other physical properties.

Dead mild steels, up to 0.15%C, have low tensile strength and are generally used for components where the main requirement is ductility, such as drawn parts. This material does not machine easily, although there are free cutting versions available with the addition of lead or sulphur.

Low-carbon, mild steels, 0.15–0.35%C, are common with the most popular being mild steel used as an easily machineable, easily worked, comparatively cheap grade of steel.

Steels in the range 0.4–0.7%C are called 'medium' and can be heat treated to a certain degree.

High-carbon steels 0.7–1.5%C, are used for components and products where wear and maintainable surface finish is a consideration. The surfaces of this group can be hardened by heat treatment and quenching, the level and ease dependent on the actual carbon content. Care is also necessary when heat treating to ensure the penetration is not too great, a soft ductile core is an essential requirement when shock loading may be applied.

Table 3.2 shows some properties and uses of steels.

3.3 ALLOY STEELS

Alloy steels are the family of steels specifically compounded and formulated to provide specialist materials that will suit specific needs and requirements. The alloying elements are added to carbon steels to improve and enhance

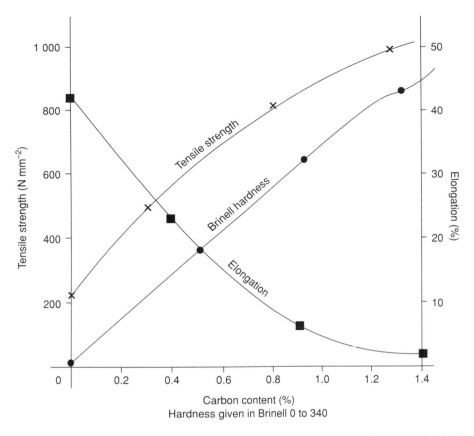

Figure 3.1 Relationship between carbon content, heat treatability and physical properties of carbon steels.

the existing properties. Alloy steels are the most expensive of the ferrous materials, because of the elements added, their compounding and accurate mixing, and the control process needed during their manufacture.

Normally alloys are produced by mixing the components and melting them together. Alloy steels have been around for more than 100 years, high-speed steel was produced in the USA in 1900 and the first form of modern stainless steel was made in 1913 in the UK, but they have only been made and used commercially in significant quantities since the middle of this century.

Table 3.3 shows the alloying elements commonly used, with examples of applications. Table 3.4 shows the mechanical properties of the nickel based alloys. The reasons for using the various alloying elements are described on page 23.

Table 3.2 Typical applications of carbon steels

Material	BS	Composition (%)	Elongation (%)	Impact (J cm^{-2})	Hardness (Brinell)	Application/use
Mild steel	BS 970	0.1 C 0.4 Mn	28	–	–	Low stress parts Pressed parts and deep drawn items
Casting steel	BS 1504	0.3 C	18	20	150	Medium strength with good machinability
Constructional steel	BS 970	0.4 C 0.8 Mn	20	55	200	Axles, crankshafts, medium stress
Tool steel	BS 4659 BW1A	0.9 C 0.35 Mn	–	–	800	Press tools, punches and dies, Minting and embossing dies
	BS 4659 BW1B	1.0 C 0.35 Mn	–	–	800	Taps, dies, twist drills, Reamers, blanking tools, knives and chisels
	BS 4659 BW1C	1.2 C 0.35 Mn	–	–	800	Engraving tools, files, surgical instruments, screwing dies

Table 3.3 Common elements used in alloy steels

Element	Composition examples (%)	Applications	Comments
Nickel (Ni)	1 + 0.9 Mn 3 + 1.0 Cr 4.25 + 1.25 Cr + 0.3 Mo	Crankshafts, axles, general engineering High stressed parts, shafts, high tension studs Air-hardened steel for aeroengine rods, valves, gears, ideal for surface hardening	Stabilises γ by raising a_4 and depressing a_3. Used in amounts up to 5% as a grain refiner in case hardening steels. In larger amounts used in stainless and heat-resisting steel
Manganese (Mn)	1.5 + 0.3 C 1.5 + 0.4 C + 0.5 Mo	Connecting rods on cars, cheap steel, low stress Cheap suitable for common nickel/chrome/molybdenum alloys	As nickel stabilises γ but unlike nickel forms stable carbides. Low manganese steels are not widely used but high content, above 12% is austenitic

Table 3.3 (continued)

Element	Composition examples (%)	Applications	Comments
Chromium (Cr)	0.5 + 0.7 Ni + 0.4 C + 1.4 Mn to 12.5 + 2.0 C + 0.3 Mn	Small percentages used for tool steels, larger amounts in stainless and heat resisting steels	Forms hard stable carbides. At above 13% classed as stainless but does increase grain growth
Cobalt (Co)	12 + 22 W + 4.7 Cr + 0.8 C + 1.5 V + 0.5 Mn	Varies from forming dies and cutters to turbine blades and ornamental metalwork. Lathe and shaping tools, gear cutters, reamers and drills	Sometimes called superhigh speed steel, permanent magnet alloys
Tungsten (W)	18 + 4. Cr + 1.2 V + 0.8 C to 22 + 12 Co + 4.8 Cr + 0.8 C	Used mainly for high speed steels and tools and dies. Very good for high temperature work. Bandsaws, reamers, broaches to lathe tools and millers	Similar to chromium for stabilising, forms a very hard carbide. Because it slows transformation, steels compounded resist tempering treatment
Molybdenum (Mo)	0.4 + 0.4 Cr + 3.6 V + 1.4 C + 0.4 Mn to 5 + 6.5 W + 4.3 Cr + 2.0 V + 0.9 C	Cold heading dies, severe machining requirements. Referred to as Moly 562, equivalent to standard high speed steel but tougher: drills, taps, reamers	Reduces temper brittleness in NiCr steel. Increases red hardness of tool steels: now replacing some tungsten high speed steels. Carbide stabilising
Silicon (Si)	1 + 0.4 C + 5 Cr + 1.5 Mo + 0.4 V + 1.35 W	Extrusion dies. Hot forming, piercing and heading tools. Brass forging	Imparts casting fluidity and improves oxidation resistance at high temperature. 0–0.3% for sand casting and up to 1% for heat resisting steels

Table 3.4 Comparative properties of nickel based alloys. Reproduced with permission from Inco Alloys Limited

Name	Comment	0.2% Stress* (MPa)	Tensile strength* (MPa)	Elonga- tion* (%)
INCONEL® 600	Used for furnace and heat treatment equipment. Good oxidation resistance at high temperature.	175	365	51
INCONEL® 617	An alloy with an exceptional combination of high temperature strength and oxidation resistance.	170	525	80
INCONEL® 718	High strength alloy with slow response to precipitation hardening that enables welding and annealing with no spontaneous hardening.	920	1150	20
INCONEL® X-750	Precipitation hardening non-magnetic alloy used for its corrosion resistance and strength up to 815°C.	830	965	5
INCOLOY® 800	Ni, Fe, Cr alloy that resists oxidation, carburisation and other harmful effects of high temperature exposure.	180	300	70
INCOLOY® DS	General purpose heat resisting alloy.	210	335	49
NIMONIC® 75	High temperature alloy with good mechanical properties and outstanding resistance to oxidation at high temperature.	200	420	57
NIMONIC® 81	High resistance to corrosion by NaCl, Na_2SO_4 and V_2O_5.	500	790	25
NIMONIC® 90	Precipitation hardening creep resisting alloy for service at temperatures up to 900°C.	680	970	12
NIMONIC® 91	Modified alloy 90 with increased chromium to improve corrosion resistance to salt and sulphur contaminanates.	580	945	28
NIMONIC® 115	Precipitation hardening creep resisting alloy for service at temperatures up to 980°C.	770	1060	16
NIMONIC® 263	Precipitation hardening creep resisting alloy for temperatures up to 850°C.	460	750	23

Table 3.4 *(continued)*

Name	Comment	0.2% Stress* (MPa)	Tensile strength* (MPa)	Elonga- tion* (%)
NIMONIC® PE13	High temperature matrix hardened sheet alloy similar to alloy 75, but with higher mechanical properties.	300	550	44
NIMONIC® PK33	Vacuum processed alloy providing sheet material with high ductility in welded assemblies and high creep strength (sheet).	710	1000	18

*At 700°C.

INCONEL, INCOLOY and NIMONIC are trademarks of the Inco family of companies.

3.3.1 ALUMINIUM

Al aids nitriding when approximately 1% is added; this is a surface harden-ing treatment at high temperature in a nitrogen rich environment.

3.3.2 BORON

B is used to enhance hardenability. It works well at low carbon levels but is affected detrimentally as the percentage of carbon increases.

3.3.3 CHROMIUM

Cr is added to increase hardness and enhance corrosion resistance. It gives heat-resisting properties and is essential in the manufacture of stainless steel. Cr gives excellent wear resistance because of the grain structure formed during cooling.

3.3.4 COBALT

Co is used for special high-speed steel applications as well as allowing perman-ent magnets to be produced.

3.3.5 MANGANESE

Mn increases hardness and increases the depth of case hardening.

3.3.6 MOLYBDENUM

Mo increases the hardenability of the finished alloy. It is not used by itself but rather as an enhancer to chromium and CrNi steels which are specifically corrosion-resistant, promoting better high temperature tensile and creep strengths.

3.3.7 NICKEL

Ni improves shock resistance and reduces the brittleness effect which occurs in most pearlite steels at low temperature. Not only does the nickel promote corrosion resistance but it also adds a larger degree of flexibility or tolerance, when heat treating a final product.

3.3.8 SILICON

Si is used in spring manufacture because of the increased resilience incorporated.

3.3.9 TITANIUM

In extremely small quantities, 0.02–0.05%, this element increases the alloy's yield point. Welded assemblies need not be normalised either and in austenitic stainless steel versions intergranular corrosion is retarded.

3.3.10 TUNGSTEN

W is used mainly for tool and die steels, it makes them particularly good for high temperature continuous work.

3.3.11 VANADIUM

Relatively small amounts are used, about 0.05%, giving a hard tough alloy with good shock resistance properties.

As with all alloys it is the correct composition and processing which will determine properties. The combined effect is greater than the sum of if each element had been used separately.

3.4 STAINLESS STEELS

Stainless steels are a family of alloys containing high proportions of chromium varying between 10 and 25%. Austenitic stainless steels contain both nickel and chromium (a stress-corrosion resistant type also has

2% silicon). Ferrous stainless steel cannot be hardened by heat treatment. Martensitic stainless steel can be hardened by the use of heat. Austenitic stainless steel is non-magnetic, a benefit sometimes overlooked.

The corrosion resistance of each type of stainless steel varies with the chemical composition, but it depends upon a tough self-perpetuating, non-porous, relatively insoluble chromium oxide film which protects and creates a 'rust proof' material. At least 10% chromium is needed for the formation of this oxide and up to 18% is necessary to withstand the most severe corrosion situations. There are many variations in the alloys to provide specialist steels. For example, an alloy with 18% chromium, 0.75% carbon, 0.5% silicon and 0.5% manganese keeps a fine cutting edge and retains a high polish, making it ideal for knives or surgical instruments. Diffused stainless is a sheet steel with a low carbon ductile core and a chromium alloy surface. It is produced by heat treating sheets in a retort containing a chromium compound, which diffuses into the steel surface at an elevated temperature of $\approx 1100°C$. The finished alloyed sheet has a surface containing as much as 40% chromium, providing a material to combat the majority of corrosive environments.

The discovery of stainless steel in 1912 by Harry Brearsley occurred when he added 12% chromium to a medium-carbon steel. This comparatively simple alloy has been developed ever since. Table 3.5 shows the more common grades available, their chemical composition and examples and descriptions of applications.

Stainless steels vary from basic 11% Cr stainless steel for general use, to multi-element alloys of chromium, molybdenum, nickel, titanium and iron like EN 58B for petrochemical pipework. A further example of specialist alloying is the ultrahigh Cr and Ni content of heat resisting stainless steels which can retain mechanical strength at temperatures as high as 1200°C. On the other hand there is an austenitic steel which can retain its mechanical properties at temperatures near to absolute zero.

Stainless steel presents no problems regarding manufacture since it can be fabricated, welded and heat treated all comparatively easily. Machining can be difficult, but if large-volume production is envisaged, you can use free-cutting stainless steel which incorporates 0.3% sulphur.

There are International Standards for stainless steel compositions, and some manufacturers will make custom alloys to suit specific needs, if your tonnage required is sufficient. If you are thinking of any high volume product or requirement, then use the manufacturer as your own research laboratory.

Table 3.6 shows examples of austenitic stainless steels.

Table 3.7 shows examples of ferritic stainless steels.

Table 3.8 shows examples of martensitic stainless steels.

Table 3.9 shows examples against standard and constituents with Figure 3.2 providing a visual representation of the examples listed.

The most significant problem when making medical instruments with stainless steel occurs when parts need to be brazed or welded together. For an

Table 3.5 The chemical composition and typical applications of some common stainless steels. ©1975 Ryton & Co Ltd. First published in Ryton Steels Databook

British Standard Specification	C	Cr	Ni	Mo	Ti
303 S21 (EN 58AM)	0.12	17.0/19.0	8.0/11.0	–	–
304 S12	0.03 max	17.5/19.0	9.0/12.0	–	–
304 S15 (EN 58E)	0.06 max	17.5/19.0	8.0/11.0	–	–
304 S16 (EN 58E)	0.06 max	17.5/19.0	9.0/11.0	–	–
316 S12	0.03 max	16.5/18.5	11.0/14.0	2.25/3.00	–
316 S16 (EN 58J)	0.07 max	16.5/18.5	10.0/13.0	2.25/3.00	–
316 S12 (EN 58B)	0.08 max	17.0/19.0	9.0/12.0	–	5 C/0.70
321 S20 (EN 58B)	0.12 max	17.0/19.0	8.0/11.0	–	5 C/0.90
325 S21 (EN 58BM)	0.12 max	17.0/19.0	8.0/11.0	–	5 C/0.90
416 S21 (EN 56AM)	0.09/0.15	11.5/13.5	1.00 max	0.60 max	–
430 S15 (EN 60)	0.10 max	16.0/18.0	0.50 max	–	–
431 S29 (EN 57)	0.12/0.20	15.0/18.0	2.0/3.0	–	–

	Mn	Si	Fe	S	P
303 S21 (EN 58AM)	1.0/2.0	0.20/1.00	REM	0.15/0.30	0.045 max
304 S12	0.5/2.0	0.20/1.00	REM	0.03 max	0.040 max
304 S15 (EN 58E)	0.5/2.0	0.20/1.00	REM	0.03 max	0.040 max
304 S16 (EN 58E)	0.5/2.0	0.20/1.00	REM	0.03 max	0.040 max
316 S12	0.5/2.0	0.20/1.00	REM	0.03 max	0.040 max
316 S16 (EN 58J)	0.5/2.0	0.20/1.00	REM	0.03 max	0.045 max
321 S12 (EN 58B)	0.5/2.0	0.20/1.00	REM	0.03 max	0.045 max
321 S20 (EN 58B)	0.5/2.0	0.20/1.00	REM	0.03 max	0.045 max
325 S21 (EN 58BM)	1.0/2.0	0.20/1.00	REM	0.15/0.30	0.045 max
416 S21 (EN 56AM)	1.50 max	1.00 max	REM	0.15/0.30	0.040 max
430 S15 (EN 60)	1.00 max	0.80 max	REM	0.03 max	0.040 max
431 S29 (EN 57)	1.00 max	0.80 max	REM	0.03 max	0.040 max

British Standard specification BS 970–Part 4 BS 1449–Part 4	Form and finish	Tensile Strength (MPa)	Hardness HB HV Rod/ Sheet/ bar plate	Description and application
303 S21 (EN 58AM)	Rod/Bar Softened	> 510	183 max	An austenitic steel, commonly described as 18/8. Contains additional sulphur to induce free machining properties and has high corrosion resistance. Non-magnetic.
304 S12	Plate HRSD	>495	192 max	Good corrosion resistant plate. Non-magnetic. The low carbon content prevents weld decay on fabrications therefore post weld heat treatment becomes unnecessary.

Table 3.5 *(continued)*

British Standard specification BS 970–Part 4 BS 1449–Part 4	Form and finish	Tensile strength (MPa)	Hardness HB HV Rod/ Sheet/ bar plate		Description and application
304 S15 (EN 58E)	Plate HRSD	> 510	192 max		A general purpose steel. Does not work harden to the extent of 321.
304 S16 (EN 58E)	Sheet, strip CRSD, HRSD, BA Polished	> 510	190 max		An excellent material for polishing, dull or mirror finish. Non-magnetic. Widely used for deep drawing in sink manufacture, kitchen utensils, hospital, restaurant, laundry and chemical industries. Has good spinning qualities. Excellent for welding.
316 S12	Plate HRSD	> 495	197 max		A highly corrosion resistant steel. This is weld decay immune, due to close control of carbon content, commonly used in chemical plant.
316 S16 (EN 58J)	Rods/nars Softened Sheet/ strip/ plate CRSD, HRSD, Polished	> 465 > 540	183 max 207 max		A very high corrosion resistant steel. Can be easily worked, welded and polished to all the standard finishes. Not normally accepted as weld decay immune. Used for cladding of buildings, tanks and vats, photographic and surgical equipment.
321 S12 (EN 58B)	Sheet/ strip/plate CRSD, HRSD, Polished	> 510	202 max		A titanium stabilised austenitic steel. It is an excellent welding quality being weld decay immune. Has a light resistance to corrosion with a maximum service temperature of 800°C. Work hardens fairly rapidly, very slightly magnetic. Used in general engineering, petrochemical, hospital and catering industries. Sheets can be polished to a dull or satin finish.
321 S20 (EN 58B)	Rods/bars softened	> 510	183 max		
325 S21 (EN 58BM)	Rods/bars softened	> 510	183 max		An austenitic, free cutting steel: used where easy machining and high corrosion resistant properties are required. Non-magnetic.

Table 3.5 *(continued)*

British Standard specification BS 970–Part 4 BS 1449–Part 4	Form and finish	Tensile strength (MPa)	Hardness HB HV Rod/ Sheet/ bar plate	Description and application
416 S21 (EN 56AM)	Rods/bars hardened and tempered	540–695	152–207	A 13% stainless iron with addition of sulphur to give free-machining properties. Fully magnetic. Normally used in general engineering for turned parts. Suitable for use on automatics.
431 S29 (EN 57)	Rods/bars hardened and tempered	850–1000	248–302	A high chrome, low nickel martensitic steel with a high tensile strength when hardened and tempered. It has reasonably good machining properties though subject to hard spots. Magnetic. Used for general engineering, spindles, shafts, bearings, HT nuts and bolts.

Table 3.6 Austenitic stainless steels

BS 1449	AISI	Form	Comments	Constituents (%)	Service temperature (°C)
301 S12	301	Plate, strip	High cold work hardening rate, moderate formability.	015 C 17 Cr 7 Ni	800
304 S15	304	Plate	Good weldability, formability and general corrosion resistance	0.06 C 18.3 Cr 10 Ni	800
304 S16	304	Strip	Excellent drawability, good weldability and general corrosion resistance.	0.06 C 18.2 Cr 10 Ni	800
316 S16	316	Plate, strip	Highly corrosion resistant, weldable.	0.07 C 17.5 Cu 10 Ni 1.5 Mo	800
317 S16	317	Plate	Extremely highly corrosion resistant, weldable.	0.06 C 18.5 Cr 13.5 Ni 3.5 Mo	800
320 S17	–	Plate, strip	Highly corrosion resistant, weldable, resistant to sensitisation.	0.08 C 17.5 Cr 12.5 Ni 4 × C 0.6 Ti 3.5 Mo	800

Table 3.6   *(continued)*

BS 1449 AISI	Form	Comments	Constituents (%)	Service temperature (°C)
321 S12 321	Plate, strip	Weldable and resistant to sensitisation, good corrosion and oxidation resistance.	0.08 C 18 Cr 10.5 Ni 5 × C 0.7 Ti	800
347 S17 347	Plate, strip	Weldable and resistant to sensitisation. Highly resistant to hot concentrated nitric acid.	0.08 C 18 Cr 10.5 Ni	800

Table 3.7   Ferritic stainless steels

BS 1449 AISI	Form	Comments	Constituents (%)	Service temperature (°C)
403 S17 403	Plate, strip	Weldable, heat resistance and moderate corrosion resistance.	0.08 C 13 Cr 0.5 Ni (max)	750
405 S17 405	Plate, strip	Weldable, heat resistance and moderate corrosion resistance.	0.08 C 13 Cr 0.5 Ni 0.3 Al	750
409 S17 409	Strip	Weldable, heat resistance and moderate corrosion resistance.	0.09 C 11.5 Cr 0.7 Ni 5 × C min 0.7 max Ti	750
430 S15 430	Plate, strip	Fairly good general corrosion resistance, formable.	0.1 C 17 Cr 0.5 Ni (max)	800
434 S19 434	Strip	Good resistance to atmospheric corrosion, formable.	0.1 C (max) 17 Cr 0.5 Ni max 1.1 Mo	800

*All above tensile strength of 425 N mm² (softened)

Table 3.8   Martensitic stainless steels

BS 1449 AISI	Form	Comments	Constituents (%)	Service temperature (°C)
410 S21 410	Strip	Heat resistant and moderate corrosion resistance.	1.0 C 11.8 Cr 1.0 Ni (max)	750
420 S45 420	Strip	Heat resistant and moderate corrosion resistance.	3 C 13 Cr 1.0 Ni (max)	750

Table 3.9 Examples of the use of various steels in medical applications. ©1994 AB Sandvik Steel, first published in product information

Surgical instruments
Cold rolled strip.

Sandvik Bioline 7C27Mo2 and 13C26
Hardened and tempered stainless martensitic steels with an optimal combination of ductility, hardness, strength and corrosion resistance. Used for bone saws and microsurgery blades.

Sandvik Bioline 12R11
Austenitic stainless steel corresponding to AISI/AMS 301, W.-Nr. 1.4310, BS 301S21 AFNOR Z12CN 17.07 and SS 2331. Used for blood lancets and syringe needles.

Sandvik Bioline 5R10
Austenitic stainless steel corresponding to AISI/AMS 304, UNS S30400/S30409, W.-Nr. 1.4301, BS 304S15, AFNOR Z6CN 18.0 and SS 2333.
Used for cannulas.

Dental instruments
Soft to hard drawn ground bar.

Sandvik Bioline 25T210P
Free cutting carbon steel with good hardenability, abrasion resistance and toughness.
Used for both drills and shafts.

Sandvik Bioline 4C27A
Hardenable stainless martensitic free-cutting steel with very good machinability.
Used for drill shafts.
Bright drawn wire in hard condition.

Sandvik Bioline 12R10 and 11R51
Austenitic stainless steels, also available vacuum remelted. The Mo-alloyed 11R51 is also available with extra high tensile strength.
The steels correspond to AISI/AMS 302, W.-Nr. 1.4310, BS 302S26, AFNOR Z10CN 18.09 and SS 2331. Used for nerve extractors and root canal reamers.

Cold rolled strip with close thickness tolerances.

Sandvik Bioline 5R60
Austenitic stainless Mo-alloyed steel with very good corrosion resistance

corresponding to AISI 316, W.-Nr. 1.4401, BS 316S42 AFNOR Z6CND 17.11 and SS 2343.
Used for braces.

Sandvik Bioline 7C27Mo2
Hardened and tempered stainless martensitic steels with an optimal combination of ductility, hardness, strength and corrosion resistance. Thin strip is used for separating strips, polishing discs and ribbon saws.

Implants
Bar, wire, profiles, tube, strip and billets for the manufacture of both reconstructive and internal fixation devices.

Sandvik Bioline 316LVM
Austenitic vacuum remelted stainless steel corresponding to ASTM F138/139, Grade 2, BS 7252/D, DIN 17443, W.-Nr. 1.4441, NF ISO 5832-1/D, ISO 5832-1/D and SNV 056506/B.

Sandvik Bioline High N
An austenitic Mo-alloyed high nitrogen electro-slag refined stainless steel for production of both temporary and permanent implants corresponding to BS 7252/9-90 & ISO 5832/9.

Surgical needles
Soft bright drawn wire.

Sandvik Bioline 4C27A
Hardenable stainless martensitic free-cutting steel corresponding to ASTM 420F.
Used for drilled suture needles.

Sandvik Bioline 7C27 and 7C27Mo2
Hardenable stainless martensitic steels corresponding to AISI 420 and '420Mo' resp. The Mo-alloyed steel, 7C27Mo2, has the highest corrosion resistance.
Used for channelled and eyed needles.

Sandvik Bioline 9X1R51, 11R51 and 1RK91
Austenitic stainless steels. 9XR51 and 11R51 correspond to AISI 302. Used for chanelled and drilled needles.

Table 3.9 *(continued)*

Catheters	Staples
Round or flat wire with bright surface in hard condition. Round wire also available with PTFE-coating.	*Bright drawn wire in half hard condition.*
Sandvik Bioline 12R10 and 11R51	**Sandvik Bioline 316LVM**
Austenitic stainless steels corresponding to AISI/AMS 302, W.-Nr, 1.4310, BS 302S26, AFNOR Z10CN 18.09 and SS 2331. The Mo-alloyed steel, 11R51, has the highest strength and best corrosion resistance.	Austenitic vacuum remelted stainless steel corresponding to ASTM F138 Grade 2, BS 7252/D, W.-Nr. 1.4441, NR ISO 5832-1/D, ISO 5832-1/D and SNV 056506/B.
Used for guide and safety wire, armour in tracheal tubes and stone extractors.	**Sandvik Bioline 5R60**
	Austenitic stainless Mo-alloyed steel with very good corrosion resistance corresponding to ASTM F55, Grade 1, W.-Nr. 1.4401, BS316S42, AFNOR Z6CND 17.12 and SS 2347.

effective joint, the brazing or welding metal has to diffuse into the stainless steel substrate. This will result in a loss of corrosion resistance at the weld, and heating effects on the surrounding material give rise to the possibility of stress-corrosion cracking. If this potential problem is recognised at the design stage then suitable steps can be taken to eliminate or reduce the problem. Appropriate selection of steel and welding material, and heat treatments, can minimize stress-corrosion cracking.

Many ferrous metals are used for orthopaedic purposes, particularly for joint replacement implants. Originally stainless steels were used, but increasingly stringent requirements for corrosion resistance and biocompatibility have led to the development of special cobalt–chrome and titanium alloys. These last better in the very hostile in vivo setting, which is warm, salty and even more corrosive than a tropical marine environment. Recently, requirements for longer-lasting prostheses have led to non-metallic materials such as polymers, ceramics, glasses and ceramic coatings being developed, and those can reduce rejection phenomena. It is therefore likely that the use of familiar metals will decline, but for the foreseeable future they will still be in the frame. Some advisable reading would be BS7252, ASTM F138-92 and DIN 17443, standards relating to metallic surgical implants.

An excellent information program which runs on the PC is the *Nickel Development Guide to Stainless Steel*. This is easy to install and use, full of detail, and includes a selection facility based on requirements: best of all it is free! For more information see Chapter 29 on sourcing.

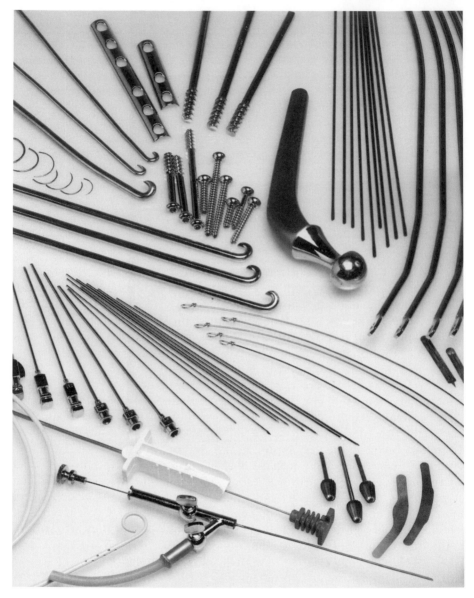

Figure 3.2 Examples of medical instruments made of various steels. © 1994 AB Sandvik Steel: first published in product information.

4
Non-ferrous Metals

There are many non-ferrous metals and alloys but not all are suitable for use in medical devices. Others are not worth considering because of their limited physical properties, e.g. lead. In this chapter, therefore, I shall include those metals that I consider relevant to a medical device design engineer. Figure 1.1 shows the more common non-ferrous metals. Table 4.1 is a comparison of the properties of some non-ferrous metals with mild and stainless steels.

Also worth mentioning at this stage are the solders, alloys of tin and lead, which are too soft for structural purposes but can be very useful for model or prototype making, exactly because of their softness and ease of manipulation. If you require a model to show the size and shape of your concept, solder could be your choice.

4.1 ALUMINIUM

In its pure state aluminium is very resistant to most forms of corrosion, but it is not a strong metal and must be modified by alloying with other elements such as copper, zinc, silicon, magnesium, manganese or combinations of them all, to enhance its properties. The important fact to remember about alloys is that some properties are improved at the expense of others. With aluminium strength or stiffness may be improved at the cost of corrosion resistance, so you need to take care with selection.

Aluminium is protected by a transparent oxide film, immediately propagated on exposure to air. Aluminium is easily machined or formed, it is suitable for light weight fabrications and components, and limited-production mould tooling. The hard oxide film can be increased in thickness by anodising, a process which adds to the original protection ensuring a hard, wear and corrosion resistant surface. The oxide layer can be coloured to act as a decorative coating, see Chapter 9, section 9.2.1.

A commercially developed lithium and aluminium alloy has been developed in recent years which is 10% lighter and 10% stronger than conventional aluminium aircraft alloys, improving even further the high strength-to-weight ratio.

Table 4.1 Comparison of some metal properties. Reproduced by permission of Arnold from *Properties of Engineering Materials*, 2nd edn, R.A. Higgins, 1997

Metal or alloy	Specific gravity	Melting range (°C)	Yield point (N mm⁻²)	Modulus of elasticity (kN mm⁻²)	Ultimate tensile strength (N mm⁻²)	Elongation % on $\sqrt{(5.65)}\,s_o$	Hardness (Brinell unless marked)	Izod impact strength (J cm⁻²)	Electrical resistivity (μΩ.cm)	Thermal conductivity (W m⁻¹K⁻¹)	Coefficient of linear expansion (×10⁻⁶ K)
Aluminium (castings)	2.57–2.81	477–649	90–240	69	240–310	2–8	65–90	–	8	138–151	21
Aluminium (wrought)	2.66–2.84	449–649	70–270	69	112–375	6–40	20–70	–	4	109–201	23
Brass (60 Cu–40 Zn)	8.47	932	108	103	151–324	4–55	65–185 (Vickers)	–	7	125	19
Copper	8.9	1082	108–324	117	96–172	4–60	45–115 (Vickers)	–	1.7	408	17
Iron, ductile	7.2	1149	–	172	–	–	–	–	60	34	13
Lead	11.35	327	–	14	–	–	–	–	21	36	30
Magnesium	1.8	650	77–154	41	69–255	1–15	35–70 VPN	0.26–1.37 (Charpy)	4	89	29
Nickel	8.89	1441	–	207	–	–	50–80 (110 Rockwell)	–	10	63	12
Phosphor-bronze Cu–Sn–P	8.98	–	–	–	180	15	–	–	–	91	32
Solder (63 Pb –37 Sn)	8.89	183	–	–	–	–	–	–	15	48	24
Steel (0.4% carbon)	7.85	1515	–	207	228	28	135	3.42	10	55	11
Steel (cast carbon)	–	–	185–587	207	193–310	8–22	170–300	5.26–10.5	17	–	11
Steel (mild 0.6% carbon)	7.87	–	–	207	207	45	92	24.2	18	70	13
Steel (stainless)	8.02	1427	–	193	–	–	–	–	72	19	17
Tin	5.77	232	–	–	6.9	–	–	–	12	36	36
Zinc	7.14	418	–	–	–	–	–	–	6	113	32

Aluminium alloys can be classified into four groups: wrought, cast, heat treated and non-heat treatable. Table 4.2 compares these alloys and gives their compositions. Table 4.3 shows the common aluminium casting alloys.

Aluminium alloys are divided into two main groups: those which can be strengthened by heat treatment, and the work-hardening types. Final heat treatment is designated by a suffix on the material grade or classification and these notations are given in Table 4.4.

4.2 COPPER

Copper is a very ductile metal in its pure state. It is an excellent conductor of electricity, being the second most conductive after silver with a value of 1.7×10^{-8} Ω m. When exposed to the atmosphere copper forms a distinctive green layer of corrosion products.

Copper is normally considered a malleable material owing to its low tensile and shear strengths; it can elongate up to 60%. Copper can be modified to suit particular applications. By adding only 1% cadmium and cold drawing to work harden the surface, the tensile strength can be increased from the normal value of < 215 N mm^{-2} to nearer 460 N mm^{-2}; it can then be used, for example, in telephone wires. A more recent development is oxide-dispersion strengthened copper; this gives a material with high strength and conductivity which is able to stand up to high temperatures. It is produced by dispersing inorganic oxides in copper powder, compressing into a mould and sintering. Another recent development is copper–zinc–aluminium alloys which have a shape-memory effect. In the low-temperature martensitic condition these alloys can be formed into shapes that are retained at ambient temperatures; on heating the original form is recovered. Presently only 6–8% deformation can be recovered, which limits the usefulness of this material.

Copper is used for electrical wires, switches, plumbing and heating pipes, chemical and pharmaceutical machinery. The best known medical application is for its chemical effect in contraceptive intrauterine devices.

Copper can be electroplated onto other metals to provide a protective coating; alternatively it serves as a key or undercoat for nickel, chrome, zinc etc. Copper plates readily onto specific plastics like ABS, allowing other metals to be applied on top. It is widely used as a method of making polymers conductive.

Copper alloys with other base metals to form more widely used engineering metals like brass, bronze, Monel metal, beryllium-copper and nickel-silver. Table 4.5 shows some copper alloys and their chemical composition. Table 4.6 shows some casting alloys, their processes and properties.

Copper is also used as an additive in insecticides, as a catalyst in chemical reactions, and as an ingredient in antifouling paints.

Table 4.2 Some important aluminium-based alloys.

	Relevant specifications	Composition (%)	Condition	Typical mechanical properties			Characteristics and uses
				0.1% Proof stress (N mm⁻²)	Tensile strength (N mm⁻²)	Elongation (%)	
Wrought alloys not heat-treated	BS 1470 5:N3	1.2 Mn	Soft Hard	45 170	110 200	34 4	Metal boxes, milk bottle caps, food containers, cooking utensils, roofing sheets, panelling of transport vehicles.
	BS 1470 5:N4	2.5 Mg	Soft ½ hard	75 215	185 265	24 4	Marine superstructures, life boats, panelling for marine atmospheres, chemical plant, panelling for land-transport vehicles.
	BS 1473:NR6	5.0 Mg	Soft ½ hard	125 215	265 295	18 8	Used mainly for rivets.
Cast alloys not heat-treated	BS 1490:LM4	5.0 Si 3.0 Cu	Sand cast Chill cast	70 80	150 170	2 3	Sand castings: gravity and pressure die-castings. General purpose alloy where mechanical properties are of secondary importance.
	BS 1490:LM6	11.5 Si	Sand cast Pressure die cast	55 85	170 215	7 4	Sand castings: gravity and pressure die-castings. Excellent foundry properties. One of the most widely useful aluminium alloys ('modified'). Radiators, sumps, gear boxes and large castings.
Wrought alloys heat-treated	BS 3L70* BS 3L77*	4.0 Cu 0.8 Mg 0.5 Si 0.7 Mn	Solution treated at 480°C, quenched and aged at room temperature for 4 days	280	400	10	General purposes stressed parts in aircraft and other structures. The original 'duralumin'.
	BS 1470 5:H30	1.0 Mg 1.0 Si 0.7 Mn	Solution treated at 510°C, quenched and precipitation hardened at 175°C for 10 hours	150	250	20	Structural members for road, rail and sea transport vehicles: architectural work; ladders and scaffold tubes. High electrical conductivity hence used in overhead lines.

Table 4.2 (continued)

	Relevant specifications	Composition (%)	Condition	Typical mechanical properties			Characteristics and uses
				0.1% Proof stress (N mm^{-2})	Tensile strength (N mm^{-2})	Elongation (%)	
	BS 2L88* BS 2L95*	1.6 Cu 2.5 Mg 6.2 Zn 0.3 Ti	Solution treated at 465°C: quenched and precipitation hardened at 120°C for 24 hours	590	650	11	Highly stressed aircraft parts such as booms. Other military equipment requiring a high strength mass ratio. The strongest aluminium alloy produced commercially.
Cast alloys heat-treated	BS 1490:LM9	11.5 Si 0.5 Mn 0.4 Mg	Solution treated at 530°C for 3 hours; quenched in warm water; precipitation hardened at 160°C for 16 hours	–	290	2	Good corrosion resistance. High fluidity imparted by silicon – hence suitable for intricate castings.
	BS 4L35*	4.0 Cu 0.3 Si 1.5 Mg 2.0 Ni 0.2 Ti	Solution treated at 510°C: precipitation hardened in boiling water for 2 hours or aged at room temperature for 5 days	215	280	–	Pistons and cylinder heads for liquid and air-cooled engines. General purposes. The original 'Y alloy'. Heavy duty pistons for diesel engines.

*BS Aerospace Series, Section L (aluminium and light alloys).

Publisher's note: British Standards are continually being updated. Readers are advised to contact British Standards Institution from whom complete editions of the standards can be obtained by post from BSI Customer Services, 389 Chiswick High Road, London W4 4AL, UK.

Table 4.3 Aluminium casting alloys and their properties.

Alloy	Process	Properties	Applications
LM0	Sand	99.5% aluminium. Very soft, difficult to machine	Main uses in electrical and food industries
LM2	Die	Has a high silicon content and is essentially a diecasting alloy	Wide range of applications in all types of industries except where more corrosion resistance is required
LM4	Sand and die	Can be used in both processes, can be heat treated to improve mechanical properties	General engineering applications where moderate strength is required
LM6	Die	Excellent corrosion resistance and medium strength	Especially suitable for marine and other corrosion prone applications also good for large castings
LM20	Sand	Normally used as a substitute for LM6 in sand casting (which is more difficult to cast)	Similar applications to LM6 with high resistance to corrosion. Suitable for thin wall castings.
LM24	Die	Pressure diecasting alloy	Suitable for most engineering applications, good for thin sections but would need painting in corrosive environments
LM25	Sand and die	General purpose high strength alloy with good corrosion resistance	Favoured for vehicle castings such as wheels, cylinder heads etc.
LM27	Sands and die	Good castability and pressure tightness	Moderate strength applications such as general engineering, domestic and office equipment
LM31	Sand	Age hardening alloy particularly useful for large castings, good shock resistance	Large general engineering sand castings
ZA12	Sand and die	Non-sparking alloy	Used in hazardous areas where sparks could cause explosions e.g. mines.

Publisher's note: the information in this table has been compiled from BS 1490 (Al based alloys).

4.3 BRASS

Brasses are alloys of copper and zinc with other elements, giving a wide range of properties.

With 15% zinc a highly corrosion resistant grade sometimes called 'red brass' is formed.

With a zinc content up to 20%, a stress-corrosion cracking resistant brass is formed.

Table 4.4 Heat treatment classification for aluminium alloys

Heat treatment designation	Definition
	Non-heat treatable materials or treatable materials
M	As manufactured. Materials which acquire some temper from shaping processes in which there is no special control over the thermal treatment or amount of strain hardening.
O	Annealed: material which is fully annealed to obtain the lowest strength condition.
	Non-heat treatable materials
H2	Strain hardened: material subjected to the application of cold work
H4	after annealing (or hot forming) or to a combination of cold work
H6	and partial annealing or stabilising in order to secure the specified
H8	mechanical properties. The designation is in ascending order of tensile strength.
	Heat-treatable alloys
TB	Solution heat-treated and naturally aged: materials which receive no cold work after solution heat treatment except as may be required to flatten or straighten it, properties of some alloys in this temper are unstable.
TE	Cooled from an elevated-temperature shaping process and precipitation-treated.
TF	Solution heat-treated and precipitation-treated.
TD	Solution heat-treated, cold worked and naturally aged.

The 'yellow brasses' are the more readily available and commonly used, with zinc contents varying between 34 and 40%.

Alpha brass contains zinc retained within the basic copper structure. This exists in the range from 100% Cu to 64 Cu–36 Zn and has good cold working properties.

Arsenical brass is a 70 Cu–30 Zn α-brass with small additions of arsenic. It has good corrosion and forming properties.

Basic brass is a stamping quality used to establish a 'basic' price for all other copper alloys, hence its name.

Cartridge brass is a 70 Cu–30 Zn alloy with excellent deep drawing properties. It was originally used for shells and is now used for components requiring spinning or flanging.

Duplex brasses, 62–58 Cu and 38–42 Zn contain both α and β phases, they are superior for hot working.

A grade simply referred to as 63/37 is widely considered to be the industry's general purpose material; it is normally bought with no reference or stipulation.

Gunmetal is a cast alloy of composition Cu–10 Sn–2 Zn. Other gunmetals substitute lead for some of the tin up to a maximum of 7%, (see below under bronzes).

Table 4.5 Some important copper-based alloys.

	Relevant specifications	Composition (%)	Condition	0.1% Proof stress (N mm^{-2})	Tensile strength (N mm^{-2})	Elongation (%)	Hardness (VPN)	Characteristics and uses
					Typical mechanical properties			
Brasses	BS 2970/5:CZ106	30 Zn	Annealed Hard	77 510	325 695	70 5	65 185	*Cartridge brass*: deep-drawing brass, having maximum ductility of the copper zinc alloys
	BS 2870/5:CZ108	37 Zn	Annealed Hard	95 540	340 725	55 4	65 185	*Common brass*: a general purpose alloy suitable for limited forming operations by cold-work
	BS 2870/5:CZ123	40 Zn	Hot-rolled	110	370	40	75	Hot-rolled plate used for tube plates of condensers. Also as extruded rods and tubes. Limited capacity for cold-work.
	BS 2870/5:CZ114	Mn ⎫ Al ⎬ up to Fe ⎭ 7% total Sn ⎱ 37 Zn	Grade A Grade B	230 280	465 540	20 15	– –	*High-tensile brass*: wrought sections for pump rods, etc. Cast alloys: marine propellers, water turbine runners, rudders. Locomotive axle boxes.
Tin bronzes	BS 2870:PB101	3.75 Sn 0.10 P	Annealed Hard	110 620	340 740	65 5	60 210	*Low tin bronze*: good elastic properties combined with corrosion resistance. Springs and instrument parts.
	BS 1400:PB1 C	10 Sn 0.5 P	Sand-cast	125	280	15	90	*Cast phosphor bronze*: mainly bearings cast as sticks for machining of small bearing bushes
	BS 1400:G1 C	10 Sn 2 Zn	Sand-cast	125	295	16	85	*Admiralty gunmetal*: pumps, valves and miscellaneous castings, particularly for marine purposes because of good corrosion resistance. Also statuary because of good casting properties.

Table 4.5 (continued)

	Relevant specifications	Composition (%)	Condition	0.1% Proof stress (N mm⁻²)	Tensile strength (N mm⁻²)	Elongation (%)	Hardness (VPN)	Characteristics and uses
					Typical mechanical properties			
Aluminium bronzes	BS 2870/5:CA101	5 Al Ni ⎫ up to Mn ⎭ 4.0% total	Annealed Hard	125 590	385 775	70 4	80 220	Imitation jewellery, etc. Excellent resistance to corrosion and to oxidation on heating, hence used in engineering particularly in tube form.
	BS 1400:ABI B	9.5 Al 2.5 Fe Ni ⎫ up to Mn ⎭ 4.0% each	Cast	–	525	–	115	The best-known aluminium bronze for both sand- and die-casting. Corrosion-resistant castings.
Cupro-nickels	BS 2870/5:CN105	25 Ni 0.25 Mn	Annealed Hard	– –	355 600	45 5	80 170	Mainly for coinage, e.g. the current British 'silver' coinage
	BS 3073/6:NA13	68 Ni 1.25 Fe 1.25 Mn	Annealed Hard	215 570	540 725	45 20	120 220	*Monel Metal*: Combines good mechanical properties with excellent corrosion resistance. Mainly in chemical engineering plant.

Publisher's note: British Standards are continually being updated. Readers are advised to contact British Standards Institution from whom complete editions of the standards can be obtained

Table 4.6 Copper casting alloys and their properties.

Alloy	Name	Properties	Applications
LG2	Leaded gunmetal	Corrosion resistance including sea water, good machinability.	Water and steam fittings up to 275°C, moderate duty bearings, intricate pressure tight castings.
LG4	Leaded gunmetal	Better suited for thicker sections, good machinability.	Many marine uses including pump bodies and other sea-water handling components.
PB 1/2	Phosphor bronze	Good wear resistance and high mechanical strength.	Heavy duty gears and wormswheels. Heavily loaded spindle nuts, couplings and bearings.
PB4	Phophor bronze	Less expensive than PB1.	Medium gears, bearings with high loads, more tolerant of inaccurate fit than PB1.
LB2	Leaded bronze	Able to absorb abrasive particles which become embedded.	Bearings with moderate load, moderate to high sliding velocity, hot mill bearings.
LB4	Leaded bronze	Tolerant of indifferent lubrication, good embeddability.	Moderately loaded bearings.
HTB1	High tensile brass	Good corrosion resistance.	General castings, used on marine components including propellers.
HTB3	High tensile brass	Good resistance to wear at low speeds under high loads	Rolling mill slipper pads, screwdown nuts, etc.
AB1/2	Aluminium bronze	Outstanding resistance to sea water, AB2 has best resistance to acid attack.	Water fittings and general purpose castings.
SB1	Silicon brass	Low lead content	General purpose castings including valves and water fittings.

Publisher's note: the information in this table has been compiled from BS 1400 (Cu based alloys).

High tensile brass contains additional manganese and iron; sometimes tin, aluminium or silicon are also used.

Nickel-silver is an alloy of copper, nickel and zinc. Its composition is similar to brass with the zinc content replaced by nickel by up to 20%. This metal is silver in colour which accounts for its name.

4.4 BRONZE

Bronzes are alloys of copper and 1–10% tin. Other types, named accordingly, contain 5–10% aluminium or 0.4–1% phosphorous. Another is silicon bronze with 1–4% silicon. Bronzes vary in colour from red through orange-yellow to white. They are tough, ductile, strong and corrosion resistant. The addition of phosphorous gives greater strength, corrosion resistance and casting ability.

Aluminium bronzes possess excellent corrosion and shock resistance, so they are used for stressed products in harsh environments.

Gunmetal, as mentioned above is an alloy of composition Cu–10 Sn–2 Zn. It performs well in marine environments and a variation which substitutes up to 7% lead for some of the tin is a good bearing metal in shell or cradle assemblies.

Manganese bronze is really a high tensile brass incorrectly named, along with 'Architectural' bronze. The latter describes two types of brass best suited to decorative applications.

Table 4.7 lists the compositions, names and applications of bronzes.

Table 4.7 Bronzes and typical applications

Name	Composition (%)	Applications
Tin bronzes		
BS 2870	3.8 Sn 0.1 P 96 Cu	A low tin bronze, good elastic properties combined with corrosion resistance, springs and instrument parts.
BS 1400 (PB1/C)	10.0 Sn 0.5 P 89 Cu	Cast phosphor bronze, mainly bearings, cast as sticks for machining of small bearing bushes.
BS1400 (Gl/C) Note 1	10.0 Sn 2.0 Zn 88 Cu	'Admiralty gunmetal', pumps, valves and miscellaneous castings, particularly for marine purposes because of good corrosion resistance, good casting properties.
Aluminium Bronzes		
BS 2870/5	5.0 Al Ni } 4 Mn } 91 Cu	Imitation jewellery, excellent resistance to corrosion and to oxidation on heating, used extensively in engineering in tube form.
BS 1400 Note 2	9.5 Al 2.5 Fe 1.0 Ni 1.0 Mn	Best known aluminium bronze for both sand- and die-casting, corrosion resistant castings

[1] Some gunmetals have the expensive tin replaced by zinc; this not only reduces cost but makes deoxidation with phosphorus unnecessary.

[2] Difficulties in casting these alloys arise from the rapid oxidation of aluminium at casting temperature, this has restricted their popularity.

4.5 GOLD

Gold is a relatively soft metal, yellow coloured, corrosion resistant but tarnished by sulphur or by-products. Gold is non-toxic and chemically inert.

White gold, a jewellers' alloy, has a composition Au–17 Ni–17 Cu–7 Zn.

For use in the electronics industry, gold is alloyed with silicon and immediately quenched (to prevent crystallisation) forming an amorphous material. This is usually supplied as 10 μm thick wafers.

Gold is the most malleable of metals and can be worked into 'leaf' form, 0.002 mm thick, by hammering rather than rolling. One gram can cover one square metre or make fine wire 2 km in length.

Gold is primarily used now as a protective coating against corrosion, heat or radiation, its applications are within the electronic, jewellery and decorative work areas.

Gold is normally applied by plating but certain ceramics and glass can be painted using 'liquid bright gold' and heat cured to bond the two materials.

Gold has been used quite a lot by dentists for crowns or caps etc., but has now been overtaken by more modern materials like ceramics.

In medicine gold sodium thiomalate, an odourless yellowish powder soluble in water, is used as an antirheumatic.

4.6 MAGNESIUM

Magnesium is the lightest of the metals normally used in engineering, being 65% the density of aluminium and 25% the density of steel.

The main applications are lightweight structural components for the auto and aircraft industry, where easy machining is an added bonus.

In its pure state magnesium can be used as a sacrificial electrode to protect other metals.

Table 4.8 gives the properties of magnesium based alloys. Additional information on applications is in Table 4.9.

Magnesium ignites easily when pure and is a fire hazard even when alloyed. Great care should be taken to guard against fire or the placement of any construction in a potentially hazardous position.

Magnesium is available as cast or wrought products. Some Mg alloys are very well suited to die casting so that complex items can be produced at very high and economical rates.

Another advantage of magnesium is that the power requirements for manufacturing are lower. Machining items in magnesium uses less than one fifth the power required to machine comparable steel items.

Apart from light structural components magnesium has applications in sound resonating diaphragms and sound-damping and shielding equipment.

Table 4.8 Some magnesium-based alloys.

	BS specification	Composition (%) (balance Mg)	Condition	0.2% Proof stress (N mm^{-2})	Tensile strength (N mm^{-2})	Elongation (%)
					Typical mechanical properties	
Cast alloys	2970:MAG.3	10.0 Al 0.3 Mn 0.7 Zn	Chill-cast Fully heat-treated	100 130	170 215	2 2
	2970:MAG.5	4.0 Zn 0.7 Ar 1.2 Rare earths	As cast Heat-treated	95 130	170 215	5 4
	2970:MAG.8	0.7 Zr 3.0 Th 2.0 Zn	Heat-treated	100	210	8
Wrought alloys	3370:MAG.S101 3372:MAG.F101 3373:MAG.E101	1.5 Mn	Rolled	70	200	5
	3372:MAG.F121 3373:MAG.E121	6.0 Al 0.3 Mn 1.0 Zn	Forged Extruded	155 140	280 215	8 8
	3370:MAG.S151 3372:MAG.F151 3373:MAG.E151	3.0 Zn 0.7 Zr	Rolled Extruded	170 215	265 310	8 8
	3372:MAG.F161 3373:MAG.E161	5.5 Zn 0.6 Zr	Heat-treated	230	315	8

Publisher's note: British Standards are continually being updated. Readers are advised to contact British Standards Institution from whom complete editions of the standards can be obtained.

Table 4.9   Magnesium applications

Generally magnesium alloys have a strength-to-weight ratio more than ten times that of steel and are easily machined. The alloys have good sound-proofing qualities and damping properties, high stiffness and are resistant to alkalies. Used for

- housing for machinery
- hand tools
- office equipment
- ladders
- ramps
- marine hardware
- non-stressed lightweight structural parts

Castings
Because magnesium does not solder to the die it is possible to cast small-diameter cored holes with little or no taper and to employ complicated coring. The preferred section thicknesses for magnesium die castings range from 1.5 mm to 5 mm with a minimum thickness of 1.2 mm being recommended. Very intricate parts with controlled surface textures and extremely close tolerances can be produced

Magnesium–lithium alloy
Originally developed for aerospace and military use such as vehicle protection armour and ammunition containers.

Magnesium–nickel alloy
When added to nickel or its alloys this has a deoxidising effect.

Magnesium carbonate
Used for insulating cover for steam pipes and furnaces, for making oxychloride cement in boiler compounds and as a filler for rubber and paper. Also used as a heat insulator.

Magnesium sulphate
$MgSO_4.7H_2O$ is commonly known as Epsom salts. Used for leather tanning, as a mordant in dyeing and printing textiles, as a filler for cotton cloth, for sizing paper, in water-resistant and fireproof magnesia cements, and as a laxative.

4.7 NICKEL

Nickel is a silvery white metal that is hard but ductile. It can be polished to a high grade finish and will retain this finish for a long time. Nickel has excellent corrosion resistance but in its pure state has limited uses. It is more commonly used as an alloying element. Nickel is also magnetic, a property which gives rise to other applications.

Nickel can be alloyed with copper to form bronzes, with steel to form stainless steel and with other metals to form corrosion resistant alloys like 'Nimonic' or 'Monel'.

An application for elemental nickel is for the sintered electrode plates in Ni–Cd batteries.

Nickel is the principal constituent of corrosion resistant alloys, therefore when combined with other elements like chromium, which ensures a low rate of oxidation, the end result is a particularly good high temperature material ideal for products like the resistance wires used in heating elements.

Trade names like 'Nimonic' and 'Inconel' describe families of high temperature alloys, typically Ni–20 Cr, which have high creep strength at elevated temperatures and are used where stiffness is needed above 900°C such as in aeroengine parts. These alloys are also in demand in comparatively low-temperature applications in the dairy and distilling industries.

Food and chemical processing installations make extensive use of nickel alloys.

The 'Monel' alloy consists of nickel and copper with carbon, manganese, iron, sulphur, silicon and traces of aluminium, titanium and cobalt. It is used in electronics and where high corrosion resistance is required. Another alloy formed with nickel is 'Permalloy' a metal with high magnetic permeability at low field strengths.

Nickel can be used to plate substrates of cheap base metals as a protective and decorative coating. The most widely used compound is nickel sulphate but nickel chloride provides a harder fine grain plate.

Table 4.10 gives nickel data.

Table 4.10 Nickel applications

Nickel is seldom used in massive form on its own except for electroplating anodes. When alloyed and in wrought or cast form it is suitable for jet engine parts, springs, switches and other technical applications. Wrought nickel alloys with chromium and iron are used for electrical resistance applications, while alloys with copper, molybdenum, manganese and silicon are used for magnetic applications in relays, magnetic shields and communication equipment.

Monel metal
This range of copper–nickel alloys is intended for applications requiring high corrosion resistance such as valves, pump parts, propeller shafts, heat exchangers, springs and similar.

Hastalloy
A chemical resistance alloy range for use in the chemical processing industries.

Inconel and Incolloy
High temperature alloys with good corrosion and shock resistance.

Nimonic
High temperature alloys: working range from 750°C to 940°C.

Nickel bronze
A tough, fine-grained corrosion resistant metal in which the nickel replaces tin. Used for bearings needing additional resistance to compression and shock loading.

Nickel cast iron
High strength alloy cast iron containing nickel. Similar to silicon, it assists graphite formation.

Nickel copper
An alloy of nickel and copper employed for adding nickel to non-ferrous alloys.

Pure
Used for sintered plates in nickel–cadmium batteries. Produced by vaporizing nickel carbonyl and depositing the nickel as a powder

4.8 SILVER

Silver is a white metal element which is soft and very malleable. Silver tarnishes easily in air by the formation of silver sulphide but this does not prevent its use since the base material is not lost. Silver is made use of as a protective barrier, somewhat expensive but very effective.

Silver is the most electrically and thermally conductive of all metals. Although pure silver can be obtained, it is normally alloyed with copper to provide workable sterling silver at Ag–7.5 Cu. In commercial silver the copper content is 10%.

Modern applications of silver include electrical contacts, solders, chemical equipment, batteries and electroplating. Silver compounds are used in the manufacture of photographic film.

Silver solder is a confusing term since these alloys are neither 'solders' nor silver. They are alloys with a silver content of 9–80%, the balance being copper and zinc, which are used in brazing. Heat is applied by a blowtorch or oxyacetylene flame. Silver soldered joints are tight, strong and electrically conducting at a relatively low cost. The solder composition is varied depending on the application and properties required, and the colour varies with the composition between silvery white and dull yellow. For example Ag–20 Cu–15 Zn has a melting point of 700°C; Ag–45 Cu–35 Zn has a melting point of 760°C.

There are many other less well-known uses for silver such as in a laminated coating, with TiO_2, on the inside of light bulbs reducing power consumption by 50% and prolonging bulb life. Silver is also widely used as a catalyst, laboratory reagent and antiseptic in compounds such as silver chloride, silver fluoride and silver nitrate.

A medical application is to combine silver with a protein and use it for its specific antiseptic and bacteriostatic actions: Argyrol is one such product, which has low toxicity. Silver potassium cyanide is used as a bactericide and antiseptic (as well as in silver plating): this is a useful but deadly substance.

Silver has specialist uses in medicine in anti-depressants and as a low toxicity anti-bacterial agent (e.g. Argyrol).

4.9 TIN

Tin is a soft malleable metal suitable for foil manufacture; tin foil can be as thin as 0.005 mm, though tin foil has been significantly replaced by aluminium foil for domestic use. Tin is used in alloys to form brasses, bronzes, pewter and solders. The physical properties change radically when alloyed with even small amounts of other metals; lead will soften tin, arsenic and zinc will harden it. An addition of as little as 0.25% nickel can increase tensile strength by 200%, while 2% copper is needed to modify tensile strength by 150%.

Tin is alloyed with other metals to give solders with melting points in the range 370–420°C.

Tin plate is mild steel sheet coated on both sides with pure tin. This is used to make corrosion resistant, non-contaminating, food cans, though tinning is being superseded by other coatings and laquers now. Drawn copper wire for electrical uses is usually tinned to aid the adhesion of plastic insulation. Tin is highly reflective when polished and can be used for mirrors. It solders easily, of course, and is slightly harder than lead.

Most tin is used for coating or alloying, rather than on its own. 'Terne' is an alloy of lead and tin used for plating.

Tin is used in the electronic industry for capacitor liners; other industrial applications are bearing linings, cooking vessels, pewterware and tubing for the food industry.

White bearing metal is a soft cast alloy of Sn–8 Pb; normal die casting grades of white metal are Sn–13 Pb–5 Cu.

Tin organisations exist to promote the use of this material: see information in the Appendices to Chapter 29.

4.10 TITANIUM

Titanium is a comparatively light hard metal, although more dense than aluminium it is 45% less dense than steel but with the same tensile strength. Ti has a strength-to-weight ratio greater than any other structural metal: 30% greater than steel or aluminium. Titanium maintains its strength over a temperature range of 250–540°C. A problem is the very high cost of titanium: approximately double that of stainless steel. Titanium has very good corrosion resistance because of the formation of a protective oxide coating.

Stainless steel utilises titanium; in pearlite steels it acts as a deoxidiser and in very small amounts, 0.02–0.05%, it increases the yield point and gives welded parts which need not be normalised after assembly. In austenitic steels the titanium retards intergranular corrosion.

Applications include aerospace components, gas-turbine blades, valve bodies, chemical-processing equipment, and electrodes in chlorine batteries. Titanium is used for surgical implants, like joints and pins, and surgical instruments.

Titania, the oxide TiO_2, is white and very opaque. It is used as a filler in plastics, paints and synthetic fibres. Because of its inertness at comparatively low temperatures it is acceptable for a wide range of medical components.

By reacting TiO_2 and carbon black together and sintering the material compounded into a small chip, a very hard cutting tool is produced, the popular carbide tip. This is lighter and cheaper than tungsten carbide but unfortunately more brittle. Table 4.11 shows data and information regarding the use of titanium.

Table 4.11   Titanium applications

High-purity titanium has a relatively low tensile strength, 216 N mm^{-2}, and a high ductility, 50%, but the strength can be raised considerably by alloying.

The relative density of titanium is only 4.5 and suitable alloys based on it have a high specific strength. Also creep properties up to 500°C are very satisfactory with fatigue limits high. These alloys are therefore very suitable for applications in the compressors of jet engines, as well as turbo generators, gas turbines, condenser tubing and rotors. Structural forgings for Concorde were produced from titanium alloy IMI Ti 680 (strength 1300 N mm^{-2}).

In pearlite steels titanium acts as a deoxidiser. When present in amounts of 0.02 to 0.05% it increases the yield point of plain-carbon steels. Weldability is promoted without the necessity for normalising.

In austenitic stainless steels the element is utilised to retard intergranular corrosion.

Titanium carbide
Compounded and reacted at 1800°C to form a hard crystalline powder. Compacted with cobalt or nickel for use as cutting tools or heat resistant parts. Lighter in weight and cheaper than tungsten carbide but more brittle.

Titanium oxide
Titania is an important pigment used in paint and textiles, white in colour with off colours produced by adding ground rutile ore.

4.11   TUNGSTEN

Tungsten is a hard, dense, silvery white, brittle metal with a high electrical conductivity. It has the highest melting point of all metals and can be worked quite easily if pure. Once contaminated, for any reason, it becomes very brittle.

Tungsten is readily coated onto other materials by vapour deposition or flame spraying, to form a protective covering. It can be used as a heat barrier in solar energy devices, since even at high temperatures it remains corrosion resistant.

When alloyed with other metals like copper and nickel it can and is used as shielding against radiation because this alloy has a density of up to 45% greater than lead. Tungsten is also used in armour plating and armour piercing shells.

The best known compound of this element is tungsten carbide, W_2C, used in high-speed cutting tools (Table 4.12). W_2C is also used to make high-temperature elements in furnaces and vacuum-metallizing equipment. When supplied in wire format, it is used as filaments for light bulbs. Another application is the central electrode in a TIG welding torch.

Tungsten silicate, WSi_2, is a ceramic used as a coating for electrical resistance and refractory applications.

Table 4.12 Ceramics and borides for cutting tools

Ceramics	Bonding metal/alloy
Tungsten carbide W_2C	Cobalt
Titanium carbide TiC	Molybdenum, cobalt or tungsten
Molybdenum carbide Mo_2C	Cobalt
Silicon carbide SiC	Cobalt or chromium
Titanium boride TiB_2	Cobalt or nickel
Chromium boride Cr_3B_2	Nickel
Molybdenum boride Mo_2B	Nickel, nickel/chromium

4.12 ZINC

Zinc is a silvery white metal with a bluish cast used for galvanising; making brass bronze or nickel silver and in architectural flashing. It is probably best known by the general public for its use as the outer case in batteries, in other words, the negative electrode in a zinc–carbon cell.

The most widely used zinc die casting alloy is called Mazak, this is Zn–4 Al–3 Cu, which gives good rigidity and strength but can be brittle or even swell during use if contaminated with impurities. This is countered by ensuring that die casting alloys are made from zinc referred to as the 'four nines' which is 99.99% pure. The same applies to the use of powdered zinc in batteries, since dendritic growth is complicated by impurities and internal short circuits can occur.

Zinc is rarely used for structural purposes but it is applied as a coating to steel by dipping, spraying or plating. Zn is extensively used as sacrificial anodes on ships and constructions like bridges. For commercial applications it is normally alloyed with other elements like aluminium, copper, magnesium or iron. Zinc is not suitable for stressed components or assemblies since it will creep under continuous stress loading.

The application of a protective coating on steel components is nearly always referred to as galvanising, but there are actually four methods of applying the zinc. Table 4.13 shows the different methods, their advantages and disadvantages.

Being non-toxic, zinc is in demand as a white pigment in paint manufacturing.

Zinc production is used approximately 40% for galvanic coating, 30% for die-casting, 18% for brass manufacture, 5% in a rolled form and 7% for other applications.

The metal is available in plate, sheet, rod and wire forms, can be extruded, bent, rolled, stamped and spun. It is environmentally acceptable because of its low cost, energy saving and comparatively pollution-free processing.

Table 4.13 Zinc coating methods

Process	Features	Advantages	Disadvantages	Comments
Hot dip galvanising	Coating integral with steel, process pre-clean treatment essential, shot blasting promotes a more vigorous reaction, colour: light grey.	Versatile widespread use, only limitation is size of bath, provides protection where spray cannot.	Coating contains alloy layer, etching required prior to painting.	Bath temperature 450–465°C. 50 μm on thin steel up to 150 μm on thick steel.
Sheradising	Matt uniform coat, normally used on small components, thinner coat than hot dipping, diffused coating provides chemical bond, colour: dark grey.	An alloying coating, good adhesion, continuous and very uniform, close control, hardest of all zinc coatings, good key for paint.	Limited by barrel size.	Typical thickness 25 μm, process temperature 370°C, just below the melting point of zinc.
Spray coating	Frequently used as a base for organic finishes, usually applied to the finished components.	Good mechanical inter-locking provided part is firstly grit blasted.	Coatings are porous but will fill up with corrosion products.	Generally 100–150 μm thickness, thicker coatings are possible.
Zinc paint	Used alone or as zinc base primer under conventional paints, formulated with a high proportion of zinc dust pigment to provide conductivity.	Uniform, any pores fill with reaction products, suitable for anything that can be painted, sprayed or dipped.	Performance varies, tight controls required, sensitive to poor preparation.	Up to 35 μm in one coat.
Impact plating	After impact plating parts have to be sealed or chromated, plated film itself is a porous alloy film consisting of impacted platelets.	Innovative dry plating technology, high corrosion resistant coating treatment, cold process, no heating effects.	Needs post treatment to seal off porosity, variable coat, no metallurgical bond to base steel.	Film weight of 8 to 12 grams.

5
Polymers

To the person in the street 'plastic' means one material. Hand them an object made of acrylic and another made of low density polythene (LDPE) and the only comment might be that one is harder than the other. The materials designer, on the other hand, should perceive the type, group, generic family, strengths etc., the method of manufacture and the process that provides the finished article, as well as coatings or finish.

It is the job of the engineer to know and understand, or be able to find out, the differences between various plastic materials. You should know the tensile strength of LDPE compared with acrylic, be able to find out their comparative values of percentage elongation, look up the maximum working temperature of both materials, find the contact to give prices per tonne of each and so on.

These are only a few of the physical properties which can be measured, quantified and specified when selecting a plastic for a particular application.

What about their uses, assemblies or handling? Say, for example, that carbon dioxide gas has to be transferred from a dispensing machine to an instrument. PVC tubing is cheap, flexible and easily worked but not so easily handled as a raw material, so consider silicone. Good, but how do you fit/bond/hold the end fitting? Reconsider again, what about polyurethane? Suitable? Yes. Adhesive bond? Yes. Acceptable to the customer? Yes. So in this example we select PU.

The example above is a simple way of highlighting the questions to be answered by the designer when it comes to plastics and their selection. To aid designers and provide a quick reference text on plastics this chapter lists the generic groups, gives advantages and disadvantages and provides details of applications. It is easy to see what materials are already in use and use this knowledge to jump-start your selection; a selection which you must still justify, not copy from other applications – they could have got it wrong!

5.1 GENERAL PROPERTIES OF POLYMERS

There are about 600 types of plastic available with suppliers making many variations of their own; then there are mixtures of many kinds, giving about 4500 options to choose from.

I cannot cover all the variations available but it is helpful to consider a synopsis of the generic groups, then take each family in more detail to indicate the direction you need to follow.

It is important not to put too much emphasis on comparing sets of numerical values for polymer properties. Most effort should be put into finding out how these properties relate to the use of the material in practice. Elimination of unsuitable groups of polymers is the most productive way to start, gradually working towards the ideal choice.

There are some complicated classifications of plastics available, not to mention the effect on these base materials of fillers, additives, pigments and fibres. Additives not only improve the original properties of the polymers but may provide completely new compounds. These classifications are useful in some circumstances, but for our purposes we will start simply by considering the more useful and widely used groups: thermoplastic polymers, thermosetting polymers and thermoplastic elastomers. Table 5.1 shows the characteristics and features which classify a polymer into these groups, and lists examples. Polymers are often known by abbreviations: some of these are listed in Table 5.2.

It is useful to know how to identify these materials easily and quickly. Figure 5.1 shows a three stage method using water and a naked flame, sometimes messy but easy to use.

Over the years the use of plastics for medical devices has increased as has the tendency towards the use of disposable products. The use of different plastics is not equal and is primarily down to cost and physical properties with Figure 5.2 providing a rough indication of the materials commonly used and their comparative distribution.

Table 5.3 shows some medical applications of processed polymers, mostly for disposables but also for reusable product groups. Manufacturing methods can modify the basic properties of the raw material.

Although tables of material properties should not be the only criterion for polymer selection, it is, of course, important that they should be consulted and compared against the stipulated target values laid down in the product brief.

Table 5.4 shows various properties of the more common plastics; not all the polymers nor all the materials tests, but this indicates the vast amount of information available. If you ask then values specific to your application can be supplied by the manufacturers. Figures 5.3 to 5.5 show comparative values for isolated properties.

The values shown are only comparisons since additional data are needed in real situations, e.g. to determine maximum working temperature one needs

Table 5.1 Polymer classification

Category	Stiffness	Condition (once moulded)	Characteristics	Examples
Thermo-setting	Rigid	Fixed once moulded to shape and set, cannot be softened by reheating	Structure due to the formation of coulent bonds between chain molecules, once formed the shape is maintained, some cold-setting variations produced by mixing reagents at ambient temperatures	Silicone Epoxy Melamine Bakelite Urea formaldehyde Phenol formaldehyde Casein Polyurethane (thermosetting variety Polyester unsaturated alkyl resins
Thermo-plastic	Covers the range from rigid to flexible; varies with type, fillers and compound	Can be reheated and remoulded repeatedly	Becomes fluid on heating, may require some pressure assistance; when heat removed no longer remains fluid; fillers like talc, glass fibres, glass beads are added to increase density and strength	PVC PVA PTFE Polyethylene (HDPE, LDPE) Polyamides (nylon) Acetal Modified PTO Cellulose Nitrate Polycarbonate Polypropylene Polysulphone Polyurethane Polystyrene ABS PVF CTFE FEP
Thermo-plastic elastomer	Flexible	Softens on the application of heat	Have characteristics of both plastics and elastomers, can be processed on normal equipment	Nitrile rubber Isoprene rubber Butadiene rubber Acrylic rubber Urethane rubber Ethylene propylene rubber EVA Neoprene rubber Chlorinated polythylene

Table 5.2 Polymer abbreviations

ABS	acrylonitrile–butadiene–styrene copolymer	PAS	poly(aryl sulphone)
		PB	polybutadiene
ABS(HH)	high heat ABS	PBT	poly(butylene terephthalate)
ABS/PC	ABS–PC copolymer	PBTP	fir retardant PBT
Acetal (ST)	super tough acetal elastomer	PC	polycarbonate
ACS	acrylonitrile–chlorinated polyethylene–styrene copolymer	PCTFE	polychlorotrifluoroethylene
		PE	polyethylene
BR	butadiene rubber	PEEK	polyetheretherketone
CA	cellulose acetate	PEG	poly(ethylene glycol)
CAB	cellulose acetate butyrate	PEI	poly(ether imide)
CAP	cellulose acetate propionate	PEO	poly(ethylene oxide)
CEE	co-ether ester (TPE)	PES	poly(ether sulphone)
CMC	carboxymethyl cellulose	PET	poly(ethylene terephthalate)
CN	cellulose nitrate	PF	phenol-formaldehyde
CP	cellulose propionate	PFA	perfluoro alkoxy alkane
CPE	chlorinated PE	PI	polyimide
CPVC	chlorinated PVC	PIB	polyisobutylene
CR	polychloropene	PIR	polyisocyanurate foam
CTA	cellulose triacetate	PK	polyketone
CTFE	chlorotrifluoroethylene	PMMA	poly(methyl methacrylate)
DAP	diallyl phthalate	PMP	poly(methyl pentene)
E-PTFE	expanded PTFE (Gore-Tex)	POM	polyacetal (polyoxymethylene)
E/P	ethylene–propylene copolymer	PP	polypropylene
EC	ethyl cellulose	PP(COP)	PP copolymer
ECTFE	ethylene–chlorotrifluoroethylene copolymer	PP(homo)	PP homopolymer
		PP(MF)	modified fire retardant PP
EEA	etherester amide	PPG	polypropylene glycol
EMA	ethylene–methacrylate copolymer	PPO	poly(phenylene oxide)
EP	epoxy resin	PPOX	poly(propylene oxide)
EPDM	ethylene–propylene–diene copolymer	PPS	poly(phenylene sulphide)
		PPVC	plasticised PVC
EPM	ethylene–propylene copolymer	PS	polystyrene
EPR	elastomeric ethylene–propylene copolymer	PSU	polysulphone
		PTFCE	polytrifluorochloroethylene
EPT, EPTR	elastomeric ethylene–propylene–diene copolymer	PTFE	polytetrafluoroethylene
		PTMG	polytetramethylene glycol
ETFE	ethylene–tetrafluoroethylene copolymer	PTMT	poly(tetramethylene terephthalate)
EVA	ethylene–vinylacetate copolymer	PU	polyurethane
FEP	fluoro(ethylene–propylene) copolymer	PVA	poly(vinyl acetate)
		PVAL	poly(vinyl alcohol)
GF	glass fibre	PVB	poly(vinyl butyral)
HDPE	high-density polyethylene	PVC	poly(vinyl chloride)
HIPS	high-impact polystyrene	PVDC	poly(vinylidene chloride)
IIR	butyl rubber (elastomeric isobutylene–isoprene copolymer)	PVDF	poly(vinylidene fluoride)
		PVF	poly(vinyl fluoride)
IPN	interpenetrating polymer network	PVFM	poly(vinyl formal)
		PVOH	poly(vinyl alcohol)
IR	polyisoprene rubber	RTV	room temperature vulcanising silicone rubber
LCP	liquid crystal polymer		
LDPE	low-density polyethylene	SAN	styrene–acrylonitrile copolymer
LLDPE	linear low-density polyethylene	SB	styrene–butadiene copolymer
MF	melamine formaldehyde resin	SBR	styrene–butadiene rubber
NBR	elastomeric acrylonitrile–butadiene (nitrile rubber)	SBS	styrene–butadiene–styrene copolymer
NC	nitrocellulose (cellulose nitrate)	SMA	styrene–maleic anhydride copolymer
NR	natural rubber		
OL	olefinic based PE	SMC	polymer for large constructional panels
PA6, PA66	polyamides (nylon)		
PAA	poly(acrylic acid)	TPE	thermoplastic elastomer
PAEK	polyaryletherketone	TPU	thermoplastic PU
PAI	polyamide–imide copolymer	UF	urea-formaldehyde resin
PAN	polyacrylonitrile	UPVC	unplasticised PVC
PAPI	polyamide–polyimide copolymer	XLPE	cross-linked PE

Table 5.3 Manufacturing methods and applications

Processing technique	Typical products and components
Extrusion	
Tubing	Blood and i.v. tubing, catheters
Film	Blood and i.v. bags, packaging, ostomy bags
Sheet	Oxygen masks, rigid packaging, orthopaedic devices, containers
Injection moulding	Labware, containers, machine components, valve, syringe parts, needle hubs, administration set fittings, catheter fittings, forceps, scalpels, tubes: used for disposables
Thermo forming/ vacuum forming (on sheet)	Incubator covers, machine casings, lab equipment, disability aids, rigid packaging, trays
Blow moulding	Containers, drainage bottles, packaging
Rotational moulding	Blood containers, X-ray equipment, electromedical machine cabinets, disability aids, bins
Compression moulding (thermoset plastic)	Instrument components, lenses, hearing aids
Structural foam moulding	Equipment enclosures, consoles, orthopaedic devices, disability aids
Composite moulding (often hand lid)	High strength casings, X-ray couches, prostheses, implants
Casting	Various machine and equipment components

to know cross-section and bending moment; the cost table changes from week to week let alone over the years.

As mentioned, specific values can readily be obtained from the material suppliers, in fact once they have your name on their mailing list you will be inundated with information. Table 5.5 shows a list of engineering polymers, their trade names and the company which you can contact for data.

Table 5.6 shows applications of polymers in a wide range of industries.

Table 5.7 illustrates medical applications.

Table 5.8 gives properties of polymers for medical applications.

Table 5.9 shows their advantages and disadvantages.

Table 5.10 indicates possible joining methods.

Table 5.11 gives values for shrinkage on injection moulding, which is discussed in more detail later.

These tables are intended as a guide since there are about 55 individual test results which can be consulted, describing physical, electrical, thermal, mechanical and chemical properties.

At the end of this book there is a glossary of terms used in this section.

After this general discussion of polymer properties and applications follows more detailed consideration of different materials.

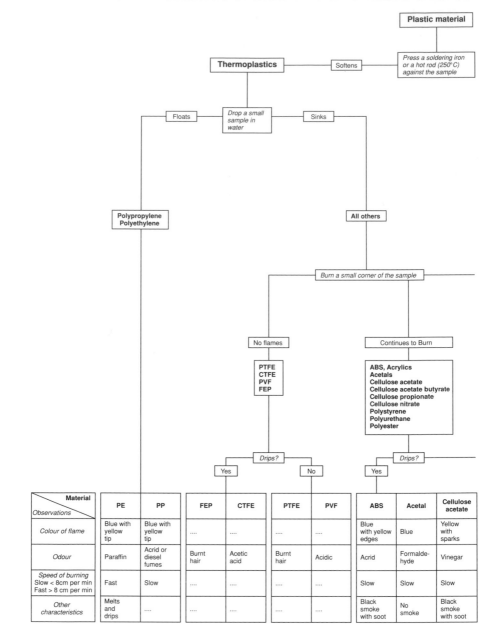

Figure 5.1 Identification of plastics by a three stage method. (Original source unknown.)

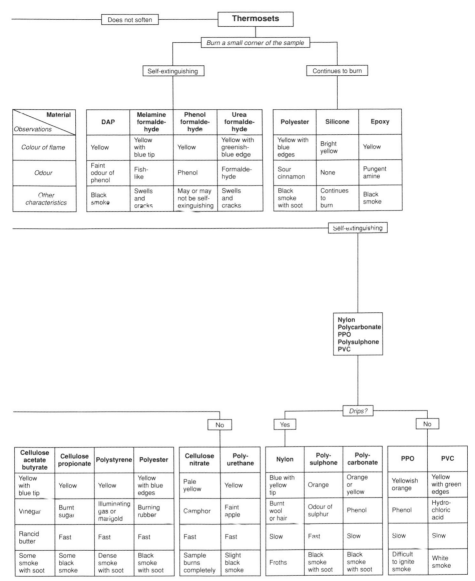

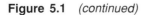

Figure 5.1 *(continued)*

Table 5.4   Properties of plastics. (Original source unknown.)

Properties		ASTM test method	ABS polymer	Acetal	Acrylic	Cellulose acetate
Mechanical						
Tensile strength at						
break (p.s.i.)		D638	4800–6300		7000–11 000	1900–9000
Elongation at						
break (%)		D638	5–70	25–75	2–10	6–70
Yield strength (p.s.i.)		D638	4000–5500	9500–12 000		
Compressive strength						
(rupture or yield) (p.s.i.)		D695	4500–8000	18 000 @ 10%	12 000–18 000	3000–8000
Flexural strength						
(rupture or yield) (p.s.i.)		D790	8000–11 000	14 000	13 000–19 000	2000–16 000
Tensile modulus						
(10^3 p.s.i.)		D638	230–330	520	380–450	
Compressive modulus						
(10^3 p.s.i.)		D695	140–300	670	370–460	
Flexural modulus						
(10^3 p.s.i.)	21°C	D790	250–350	380–430	420–460	1200–4000
	93°C	D790				
	120°C	D790				
	150°C	D790				
Izod impact (ft. lb/in						
notch, 3.2 mm thick						
specimen)		D256A	6.5–7.5	1.3–2.3	0.3–0.5	1.0–7.8
Hardness	Rockwell	D785	R85–105	M94	M85–105	R34–125
	Shore	D2240				
Thermal						
Coef. of linear						
thermal expansion						
(10 x 6in/in°C)		D696	95–110	100	50–90	80–180
Deflection						
temperature	(264 p.s.i.)	D668	205–215	255	165–210	111–195
flexural load, °F		annealed				
	(66 p.s.i.)		210–225 annealed	338	175–225	120–209
Thermal conductivity						
(10 × 4 cal –cm/						
sec–cm²–°C)		C177		5.5	4.0–6.0	4–8
Physical						
Specific gravity		D792	1.01–1.04	1.42	1.17–1.20	1.22–1.34
Water absorption						
(3/2 mm thick)						
(24 h saturation)		D570	0.20–0.45	0.25–0.40	0.1–0.4	1.7–6.5
Dielectric strength						
(3.2 mm thick)						
(V/mil)		D149	350–500	500	400–500	250–600

kPa = p.s.i. × 6.894; b = dry, as moulded; c = to equilibrium with 50% humidity.

Table 5.4 *(continued)*

Polyamide (nylon)	Poly-carbonate	Polyethylene (LDPE)	Polyethylene (HDPE)	Polypropylene (HIPS)	Poly-styrene	Poly(vinyl-chloride)	PTFE
12 000b; 11 000c	9500	600–2300	3100–5500	4500–6000	7500	6000–7500	2000–5000
60b; 300c 8000b; 6500c	110 9000	90–800 800–1200	20–130 3000–4000	100–600 4500–5400	2.5	40–80	200–400
15 000b (yld)	12 500		2700–3600	5500–8000		8000–13 000	1700
17 000b; 6100c	13 500			6000–8000		10 000–16 000	
	345	14–38	60–180	165–225	450	350–600	58–80
	350			150–300			60
420b; 185c	340	8–60	100–260	170–250		300–500	80
					50		
					35		
0.8–1.0b; 2.1c R120b; M83b	14 M70	No break D40–51	0.5–20 D60–70	0.4 1.0 R80–102	0.4 M75	0.4–20 D65–85	3 D50–55
80	68	100–220	110–130	81–100		50–100	
167b	270	90–105	110–130	120–140	200	140–170	
474b	280	100–121	140–190	225–250		135–180	250
5.8	4.7	8	11–12	2.8		3.5–5.0	6.0
1.13–1.15	1.2	0.910–0.925	0.941–0.965	0.900–0.910	1.05	1.30–1.58	2.14–2.20
1.0–1.3	0.15	<0.10	<0.01	0.01–0.03		0.04–0.4	<0.01
600b	380	450–1000	450–500	600		350–500	480

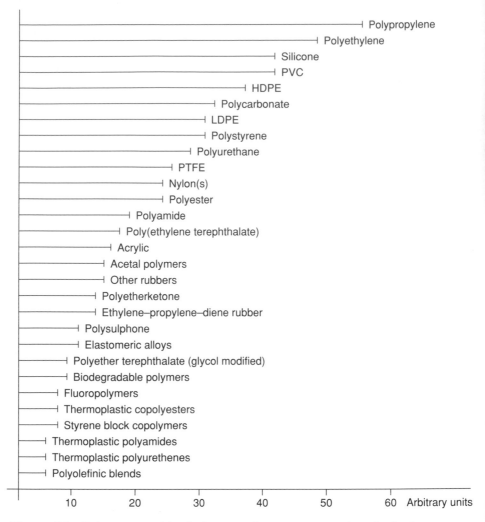

Figure 5.2 Polymers used in device manufacture: comparative distribution.

5.2 COMMONLY USED THERMOPLASTIC POLYMERS

Thermoplastic materials can be repeatedly softened by heating so they are easily formed. The molecular chains flow freely on heating but become entangled and fixed when cold.

5.2.1 *ACRYLONITRILE–BUTADIENE–STYRENE COPOLYMER (ABS)*

ABS is a popular and easily worked thermoplastic polymer. It is easy to join, bonding readily with the majority of solvents, exhibits low moulding

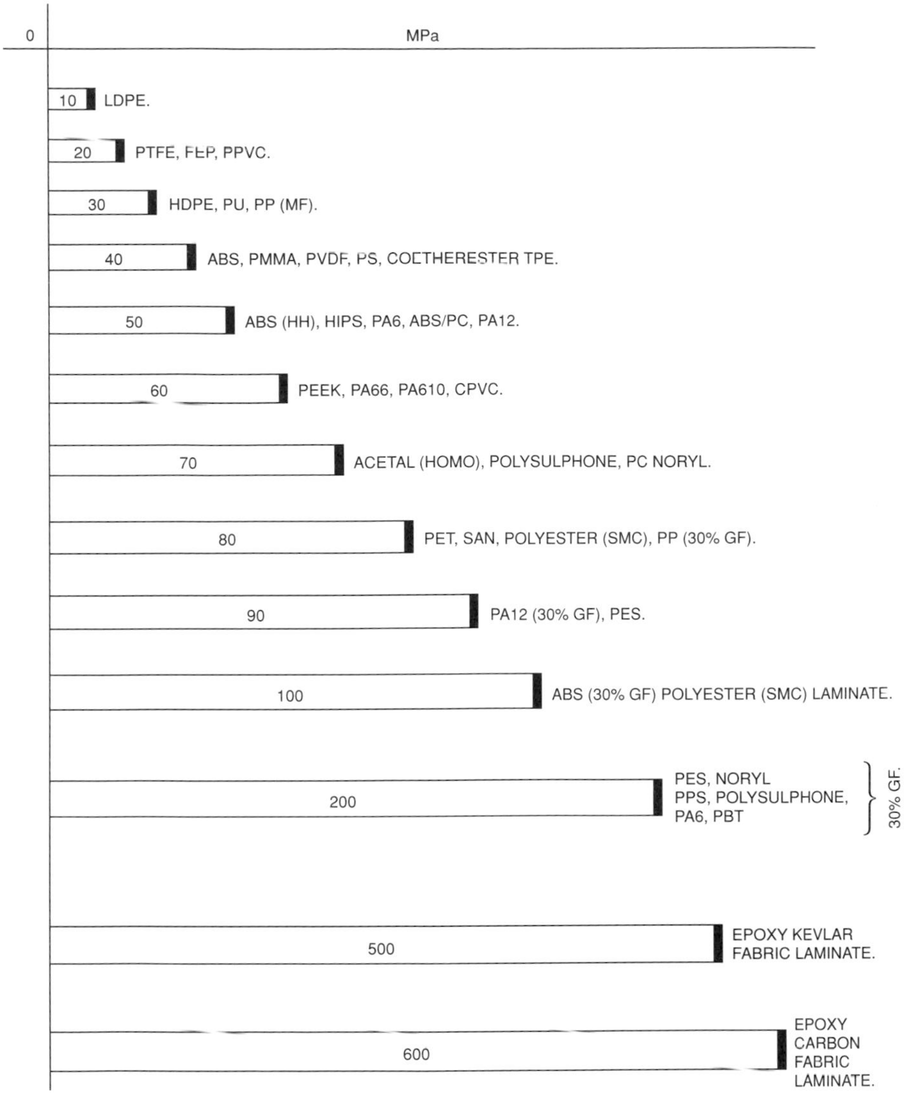

Figure 5.3 Tensile strengths of polymers.

shrinkage and is comparatively tough. ABS can be electroplated, provided correct preparation is carried out and flash coatings applied, so it is decorative. ABS can be used within a wide temperature range: –20 to +80°C.

ABS can be moulded, extruded, vacuum formed or machined and is a versatile material. When high strength is required ABS can be loaded using various fillers or additives; it can also be modified by mixing with other polymers like PC, PVC, PS, etc. ABS is available in impact and fire retardent grades.

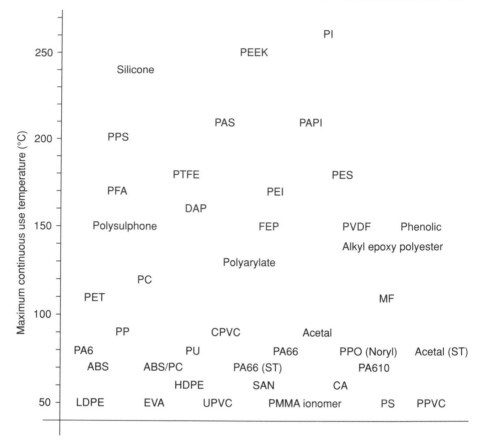

Figure 5.4 Maximum operating temperatures for polymers.

Care should be taken regarding pigments, as some will affect other properties or methods of assembly, e.g. ultrasonic welding is normally very easy with ABS but if incorrect pigments are used then welds can be significantly weakened.

Advantages of ABS are:

- varied combinations of physical properties,
- easily worked and processed,
- easily joined and fabricated,
- easily machined,
- low cost, and
- can be gamma treated.

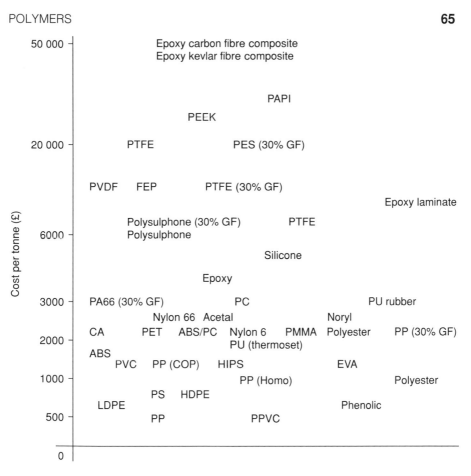

Figure 5.5 Material cost of polymers (based on 1992/3 data).

Disadvantages of ABS are:

- low resistance to solvents,
- low maximum working temperature, and
- low wear resistance.

ABS is used for containers, 'phone sets, tubes, auto trim and disposable forceps. Plated versions are used as plumbing fittings and taps, or decorative boxes. Also there are some restricted applications as reflective panels.

5.2.2 ACETALS (POLYOXYMETHYLENES, POM)

POM is a crystallised polymer of formaldehyde, being one of the most stable and strongest of the thermoplastics.

Table 5.5   Engineering polymers and trade names

Generic name	Trade name	Manufacturer/Registered trademark of
PTFE	Halon TFE	Ausimont
	Teflon TFE	DuPont
	Fluon	ICI
	Hostaflon TF	Hoechst Celanese
E-PTFE	Gore-Tex	W.L. Gore
FEP	Neoflon FEP	Daikin
	Teflon FEP	DuPont
PFA	Neoflon PFA	Daikin
	Teflon PFA	DuPont
PVDF	Kynar	Elf Atochem
	Forflon	Elf Atochem
PSU	Udel	Amoco
PET	Valox	GE Plastics
PC	Lexan	GE Plastics
PEEK	Victrex PEEK	Victrex Ltd.,
PAEK	Ultrapel PAEK	BASF
PK	Kadel PK	Amoco
PAS	Radel	Amoco
PES	Ultrason E	BASF
PPS	Ryton	Phillips
	Supec	GE Plastics
	Fortron	Hoechst Cleanese
LCP (Liquid crystal polymer)	Vecra	Hoechst Celanese
	Xydar	Amoco
PA (Nylon)	Zytel	DuPont
	Rilsan	Elf Atochem
	Kevlar	DuPont
PE	Dacron	DuPont

It can be added to, filled, reinforced and stabilised against UV degradation. POM is resistant to organic solvents (except phenols), with a maximum working temperature of 110°C and a low friction value.

Advantages of POM are:

- excellent fatigue and creep properties,
- good wear resistance, and
- good resistance to solvents.

Disadvantages of POM are:

- low resistance to acid and alkalis,
- poor resistance to UV degradation, and
- high percentage mould shrinkage.

POM is used for gears, reciprocating parts, springs, kettle bodies, audio and video cassette components and disposable lighter bodies. It is sometimes compared with polyamides (nylon) because of a better creep resistance.

Table 5.6 Polymer applications

Acrylics	Automatic parts, dials and handles, lenses, brush-backs, hospital equipment, display material signs, light fittings, inspection panel covers, machine guards, skylights, some telephones, sanitary ware
Acrylonitrile–butadiene–styrene (ABS)	Telephone handsets, housings for consumer durables, food containers, luggage, refrigerator liners, safety helmets, radio cabinets, tote boxes, car fascia panels, instrument clusters
Cellulosic plastics	
Cellulose acetate (CA)	Toys, beads, electrical parts, steering wheels, packaging sheeting, toothbrushes, cosmetics, windows in window cartons
Cellulose acetate butyrate (CAB)	Moulded or extruded parts for metallisation (reflectors etc.), outdoor signs, automobile tail-light covers, tool handles, toothbrushes, piping
Cellulose propionate (CP)	Automotive parts, telephone housings, toys, radio/TV parts, toothbrushes, sunglass frames
Epoxides	Chemically resistant paints, adhesives, electrical insulation, chemical and wear resistant jointless flooring, road coatings, laminates, powder coatings, repair kits, filament wound pipes, tanks and pressure vessels
Ethylene vinyl acetate (EVA)	Flexible extrusions tubing and hose, sachets, sheathing, cable coverings. Closures, gaskets, handle grips, shoe soles, disposable gloves, box liners, packaging film, inflatable toys
Fluorinated polymers	
Fluorinated ethylene propylene (FEP)	Coil formers, valve holders, wire insulation, electronic components, encapsulations and fluidised bed coatings
Polytetrafluoroethylene (PTFE)	Gaskets, packings, valves, sintered metal bearings, rigid and flexible pipes, membranes, wire insulations, non-stick coatings for kitchen utensils, heat sealing equipment, covers
Polytrifluorochloroethylene (PCTFE)	Extruded sheet, profile and film, gaskets, pump sealants, dispersion coatings, liquid level indicators
Ionomers	Shoe heel tips, hammer and mallet heats, bottles, skin packaging, coating, shoe soles, shoe stiffeners, meat packaging, flexible packaging
Melamine formaldehyde (MF)	
Unfilled	Usually occurs in laminate form as surfacing for tables etc.
α-Cellulose filled	Noted for durability, hardness and good electrical properties, suitable for appliance housings, writing equipment, handles, lighting fixtures, instruction panels
Nylons	
PA 6	Moulded mechanical parts, gear wheels, bushings, automobile and refrigerator door closures, mixer valves, switch housings, cable clamps, pipes, tubing, filaments, stockings, clothing, zips
PA 66	As for Type 6
PA 11	Electro/mechanical components such as cams, housings, guides, terminal blocks, transformers and bobbins, reinforced hose, components in copiers, calculators
PA 12	Injection moulded parts for automotive, electric and electronic and precision machine industries. Semi-rigid or flexible tubing for fuel lines, air brakes, pressurised air lines. Cable and wire sheathing, chill roll and blown film. Powder coatings

Table 5.6   *(continued)*

Phenol formal- dehyde (PF)	
Unfilled	Adhesives, laminates, pulp mouldings, particle board
Woodflour/cotton/ flock filled	Bottle tops, electrical parts, fuse boxes, heat-resistant close- tolerance mouldings, toilet seats
Polyacetals (POM)	Load-bearing mechanical parts, small pressure vessels, aerosol containers, gears, automobile, engineering products
Polycarbonates (PC)	Camera components, electrical apparatus, sterilisable ware, lamp covers, safety helmets, sterilisable transparent feeding bottles for babies
Polyesters (PET)	
Resin	Unreinforced resin for buttons, surface coatings. Filled resin for imitation marble, flooring, pipe joints, mortars and body stoppers
Dough moulding compound	Protective housings, connectors, cowls, offering non-corrosion, durability, good electrical performance and high strength
Sheet moulding compound	Outlets in the electrical, building, motor engineering and furniture industries that compete on a cost basis
Polyethylenes	
Low Density (LDPE)	Housewares (bottles, bowls, buckets, containers), spouts for detergent cans, shoe parts, toys, packaging film, garment bags, sheet, piping for domestic, industrial and agricultural use, cable and wire insulation and sheathing, paper, cellulose and foil coating, carpet backing, monofilament, cold water storage tanks
High Density (HDPE)	As for low density polyethylene. Materials have greater rigidity, specially suitable for large carrying cases, housings, closures, appliance parts
Polyphenylene oxide	Valve bases, switches, housings, meter cases
Polypropylene (PP)	Domestic, hospital and laboratory ware, textile, automotive, electrical and industrial usages. Containers and closures, crates, toys, blown containers. Film fibre for baler twine, ropes, sacks and carpet backing. Fibre for carpet face yarns.
Polystyrenes (PS)	
Conventional	Packaging (disposable and others), dishes and utensils, refrigerator parts, emblems, signs, displays, toys, novelties, combs, brush-backs, lighting fixtures, rigid containers, house- wares
Toughened (HIPS)	Wheels, helmets, valve parts, refrigerator parts, electric fan blades, toys, housewares, containers, battery cases, refrigerator linings and trays
Styrene acrylonitrile	Cups, tumblers, trays, toothbrush handles, refrigerator components, lenses, cosmetic items, hi-fi covers and cases, packaging
Urea formaldehyde (UF)	
Cellulose filled	As for filled MF but unsuitable for dinner ware. UF resins are used for similar applications to those shown under unfilled PF

Table 5.6 *(continued)*

Vinyl polymers	
Rigid polyvinyl chloride (PVC)	Extrusion of piping, profiles and sheet in applications requiring chemical inertness and scuff-resistance combined with light weight. Plastisols for toys, leathercloth, etc. Plastic guttering, high clarity bottles, formed packaging trays, moulded containers
Rigid vinyl chloride/acetate	Similar applications to those for PVC but widely used in the manufacture of calendered sheet used for toys, novelties, wall coverings, displays, templates
Rubber modified PVC	Same as for PVC

Table 5.7 Medical applications of polymers

Material	Applications
Polyethylene (HDPE, LDPE)	Containers, cups, spike protectors
Polypropylene (PP)	Containers, syringes, slide clamps, mini-dripper
PVC	
Flexible	Tubing, sheet, bags, flexible containers, catheters
Rigid	Rod, moulded parts, connectors, Luers
Polyester (PET)	Containers, moulded parts, oxygenator
Polystyrene (PS)	Labware, syringes, containers and Petri diskes, moulded parts, Luer connections
ABS	Moulded parts, cannulae, tubes, i.v. spikes, Luers
Polycarbonate (PC)	High wear parts, filler joints, Luer fits
Acrylic (Perspex, Diakon)	Moulded parts, i.v. spike, Luer connectors
Cellulosic	Burettes, tubes
Fluoroplastics	Flexible thin walled tubing
Thermoplastic elastomers	Film, bags, plugs, flexible tubes
Polyurethane (PU)	Film, tubing (flexible and rigid), containers
Polyamide (Nylon)	Packaging film, catheters, moulded parts
Silicone rubber	Padding, tubing, catheters, flexible seals, film

5.2.3 ACRYLICS

Acrylic is very resistant to UV degradation, and can be modified to create alloys which will increase its impact strength and toughness. Acrylic is sometimes extruded into thin film and bonded or laminated to clear ABS sheet to provide alternative windows which are tough, unbreakable, clear and UV resistant. Easily machined and fabricated, acrylic bonds well and will polish (after machining) back to clear. The good optical properties mean acrylic can be used for manufacture of lenses or fibres for light transfer.

Table 5.8 Properties of polymers for medical applications. Reproduced with permission from *Medical Device and Diagnostic Industry*, Guide to Medical Plastics, April 1994. Copyright © 1994 Canon Communication LLC

Polymer material	Specific gravity	Sterilisation		Visual clarity	Tensile strength at yield (MPa)	Elongation to break (%)	Stiff or ductile	Relative ease of processing	Leading medical uses
		Steam (at 121°C)	Radiation (25 kGy)						
PVC									
Flexible	1.21	Yes	Yes	Clear	17.2	350	Ductile	With extreme care, can burn	Film, bags, tubing, moulded parts
Rigid	1.45	Distorts	Yellows	Clear	44.8	0.5–150	Stiff	Easy	Containers, film, moulded parts, caps
Polyethylenes (all types)	0.88–0.96	Marginal to poor	Yes	Cloudy to clear	27.5	500–1000	Ductile to stiff	Easy	Labware
Polystyrenes	1.05	Distorts	Yes	High clarity	41.4	2–5	Very stiff	Easy	Containers, syringes
Poly-propylenes	0.9	Yes (stabilized)	Yes	Cloudy to clear	34.5	500–700	Ductile	Easy	Containers, moulded parts
Thermoplastic Polyesters	1.35	Distorts	Yes	Clear	54	50–300	Stiff	With care	Moulded parts, packaging, films
Copolyesters and copoly-ester blends	1.2–1.31	Distorts	Yes	Clear	45–56	110–300	Ductile	With care	
Thermoplastic Elastomers									
Elastomeric alloys	0.9–1.2	Yes	Yes	Opaque 3–11		300–600	Ductile	Easy	Moulded parts, film, tubing, stoppers, bags
Styrene block copolymers	0.9–1.2	Marginal	Yes	Trans-lucent and opaque	5.2–18.6	550–1200	Ductile	Easy	
Polycarbonates	1.20	Yes	Yes	Clear	62	110	Ductile	With care	Moulded parts
ABS	1.06	Distorts	Yes	Opaque and clear	48	2–30	Ductile	Easy	Moulded parts

Table 5.8 *(continued)*

Polymer material	Specific gravity	Sterilisation		Visual clarity	Tensile strength at yield (MPa)	Elongation to Break (%)	Stiff or ductile	Relative ease of processing	Leading medical uses
		Steam (at 121°C)	Radiation (25 kGy)						
Acrylics (standard and impact grades)	1.19	Distorts	Standard grades yellow	High clarity	69	5–60	Stiff	Easy	Moulded parts
Polyurethanes Aliphatic	1.15	Distorts	Yes	Clear	41–48	200–1000	Ductile	Easy	Film, tubing, components
Aromatic	1.15	No	Yes	Clear	41–48	200–1000	Ductile	Easy	
Nylons	1.04–1.14	Yes	Yes	Clear and cloudy	62–83	59–100	Ductile	With care	Packaging film, catheters
SAN	1.08	Distorts	Yes	High clarity	76	3	Very stiff	Easy	Moulded parts
Cellulosics	1.19–1.23	Distorts	Yes	Clear	6.9–48	10–50	Ductile	Easy	Burettes, tubes

Table 5.9 Advantages and disadvantages of polymers for medical applications. Reproduced with permission from *Medical Device and Diagnostic Industry*, Guide to Medical Plastics, April 1994. Copyright © 1994 Canon Communication LLC

Polymer	Advantages	Disadvantages
PVC	Low cost. Rigid and flexible grades. Seals by any method: solvent, heat, RF, sonic. Sterilises by any method. Good clarity.	Extractable plasticizers, heavy metals, and heat stabilizers. Moulding and extrusion require special expertise. Rigid PVC grades are sensitive to thermal degradation and can discolour or burn during processing.
Polyethylenes (HDPE, LDPE)	Low cost. Easy processing. Very ductile. Very low extraction. Easy to heat seal. Many grades and types available.	Some grades can be cloudy. Hard to join by solvent or adhesives. Distorts at steam sterilisation temperature.
Polystyrenes (PS)	Low cost. High clarity. East moulding. Many grades available.	Stiff and brittle unless impact modified. Distorts in steam sterilisation.
Polypropylenes (PP)	Low cost. Easy processing. Very ductile. Very low extraction. Easy to heat seal.	Hard to join by solvent or adhesives. Marginal distortion in steam sterilisation. Degraded by radiation sterilisation unless stabilised form is used. Poor low-temperature impact strength.
Thermoplastic polyesters	Moderate cost. High clarity. Very low extractables. Compatible with lipids and alcohols.	Drying essential. Specialised processing required. Long processing cycle. Distorts in steam sterilisation.
Copolyesters and copolyester blends	Low to medium cost. Excellent chemical resistance. Ductile. Sterilisable by gamma radiation and EtO.	Drying essential. Distorts in steam sterilisation. Good mould cooling required.
Thermoplastic elastomers	Low extractables. Biocompatibility. East and cost of processing. Flexibility and sealing characteristics.	Steam sterilisation marginal. High cost.
Polycarbonates (PC)	Excellent combination of physical properties. Very strong, very ductile, very clear. Sterilisable by any method. Moderate cost.	Extremely brittle when not properly dried. Hydrolytic instability. Requires high heat to mould. Crazes on exposure to common solvents. Limited exposure to autoclave cycles.
ABS	Excellent blend of physical properties. Many grades available. Moderate cos. Clear grades available. Solvent bonds well. Seals by any method except RF.	Distorts in steam sterilisation. Typically opaque.

Table 5.9 (continued)

Polymer	Advantages	Disadvantages
Acrylics	Exceptional clarity. Excellent processability and dimensional stability. Bonds well. Moderate cost. Available in standard and impact-resistant grades.	Standard grades brittle. Distorts in steam sterilisation.
Polyurethanes (PU)	Excellent flex fatigue life. Good physicals, clarity. Bonds well. Sterilisable by radiation and EtO. Excellent resistance to lipids and a variety of solvents.	High cost. Aromatic polyether type is known to release ppb trace amounts of a cytotoxic and carcinogenic diamine-methylene dianiline (MDA) after prolonged autoclaving. Aliphatic-based polyether is free of MDA, but distorts. Must be dried.
Nylons (PA)	Good clarify. Heat resistant. Strong. Ductile. Steam sterilisable.	High extractables, although non-toxic. High cost. Special solvents required for bonding. Requires controlled drying.
SAN	Excellent clarity. Low cost. Easily moulded	Distorts in steam sterilisation. Brittle. Contains trace acrylonitrile toxic monomer.
Cellulosics	Excellent clarity. Tough and flexible. Moderate cost. Solvent bonds well.	Distorts in steam sterilisation. Uses plasticiser. May extract.

Table 5.10   Bonding and joining polymers

Material	Solvent bondable to self	RF bondable to self	Heat bondable to self	Ultrasonically bondable to self
ABS	✓		✓	✓
Acetal			✓	✓
Acrylic	✓		✓	✓
Cellulosic, butyrate	✓		✓	
Eva	✓	✓	✓	
Nylon			✓	✓
Noryl	✓		✓	✓
Polycarbonate	✓		✓	✓
Polyester		✓		
Polyethylene				
HDPE			✓	✓
LDPE			✓	✓
Polypropylene			✓	
Polystyrene	✓		✓	✓
Polyurethane			✓	✓
PVC				
Flexible	✓	✓	✓	
Rigid	✓	✓	✓	✓
Polysulphone	✓		✓	✓

Table 5.11   Average shrinkage on moulding

Polymer	Mould shrinkage (%)
ABS	0.6
Acetal	2.0
Acrylic	0.4–0.8
Acrylic rubber	0.6
Cellulosic proprionate	0.4
Butyrate	0.5
Nylon (PA)	1.2
Noryl	0.6
Polycarbonate (PC)	0.6
Polyester (PET)	2.0
HDPE	2.5
LDPE	3.0
Poly(phenylenesulphide) (PPS)	0.4
Polypropylene (PP)	2.0
Polystyrene (PS)	0.6
PVC	
Rigid	0.5
Flexible	1.0–5.0 varies with plasticiser

Advantages of acrylic are:

- good weathering and UV resistance,
- excellent light transfer,
- good wear resistance,
- stable once formed,
- easily fabricated, and
- can be gamma treated (but will discolour, returns to original but can take up to 90 days).

Disadvantages of acrylic are:

- low resistance to solvents (something of an advantage in fabrication),
- low temperature resistance, and
- poor mechanical properties.

Acrylic is used for lenses, panels, toughened windows, light diffusers and fibre optics.

5.2.4 POLY(METHYL METHACRYLATE) (PMMA)

PMMA is a hard transparent polymer, which is tough, resistant to impact and used as an alternative to glass. It is very easily fabricated and used to build models or visual presentations. A common trade name for PMMA is Perspex; another is Lucite.

Advantages of PMMA are:

- good UV resistance,
- dimensionally stable,
- easily fabricated,
- good decorative appearance, and
- good electrical track and arc resistance.

Disadvantages of PMMA are:

- easily attacked by solvents,
- physical properties poor when stressed, and
- low maximum working temperature, 50°C.

PMMA is used for covers, baths, lenses and out-door signs. Implantable grade PMMA is used in intraocular lenses and orthopaedic cement.

5.2.5 CELLULOSIC POLYMERS (CP, CAP, CAB, CA)

These are ideal materials for decorative finishes, providing an excellent gloss. Celluloses have low friction and are tough but not suitable for impact components. Celluloses are good coating materials and were originally used as Cellophane for food packaging. Grades can be modified to provide alternative options (as in the abbreviations shown above): cellulose propionate, cellulose acetate propionate, cellulose acetate and cellulose acetate butyrate.

Advantages of celluloses are:

- tough (at low temperatures),
- good light transmission, and
- good visual appearance.

Disadvantages of celluloses are:

- attacked by solvents,
- low heat tolerance, and
- flammable.

Cellulose nitrate is used for table tennis balls, cellulose acetate is used in the film and photography industry. Cellulose acetate butyrate is used for goggles, toothbrush handles, and mainly blister packs.

5.2.6   FLUOROCARBON POLYMERS

These have high resistance to most chemicals, low friction and good electrical properties. It is best to view the individual materials in their own right: FEP, PTFE, PVDF, PVF, PFA, ETFE and PCTFE.

Fluorocarbon polymers have excellent high temperature tolerance; the maximum working temperature for the group is 150–180°C.

Wear resistance is excellent and useful, and the coefficient of friction is very low. The applications are specialised but widespread.

Advantages of fluorocarbon polymers are:

- resistant to UV,
- good chemical resistance,
- excellent wear resistance,
- high temperature tolerance, and
- fire resistance.

Disadvantages of fluorocarbon polymers are:

- poor physical strength,
- processing problems, and
- expensive.

These polymers are used as bearing surfaces and protective coatings.

5.2.6.1   Fluorinated Ethylene–Propylene or Fluoro (ethylene–propylene) Copolymer (FEP)

FEP is similar to PTFE in its properties but is easier to manipulate and form. It can be moulded by normal methods and is sometimes referred to as a melt-processable version of PTFE. FEP has a lower temperature tolerance than PTFE but at 200°C is still considered to be very useful. The impact strength is very high.

Advantages of FEP are:

- moulding grades available,
- good impact strength,
- low coefficient of friction, and
- excellent chemical resistance.

Disadvantages of FEP are:

- expensive, and
- the least stiff of the fluorocarbon polymers.

FEP is used as a protective film or coating against corrosion, for electrical terminals and for coating within the food and chemical industries.

5.2.6.2 Polytetrafluoroethylene (PTFE)

PTFE is resistant to the majority of chemicals, has a low coefficient of friction and is very good as a bearing material. PTFE can be used continuously at a high temperature of up to 250°C. However, PTFE is difficult to work with and has a bad reputation for bonding or attachment to other materials. Since it does not melt fully when heated certain difficulties are associated with processing, welding and manufacture.

PTFE can be loaded with various fillers to enhance physical properties like stiffness. Sintering allows the manufacture of bulkier components and coatings can be applied by spraying.

Advantages of PTFE are:

- non-flammable,
- excellent chemical resistance,
- excellent electrical resistance,
- excellent heat tolerance,
- good high temperature tolerance, and
- acts as a bearing surface.

Disadvantages of PTFE are:

- difficult to bond or join with other materials, and
- low tolerance to gamma sterilisation (will crack and become very brittle in a short time).

PTFE is used to coat cooking items and for dry bearings, as an internal lining for tanks or container vessels, in high temperature electrical applications such as relay parts or wire insulation. It is also used as a coating to aid insertion of instruments, or to prevent adhesion of blood products. Expanded

PTFE membranes are used in filters and the pore size can be controlled to suit various applications. Expanded PTFE (Gore-Tex) is also used for prosthetic purposes such as surgical patches and vascular grafts.

5.2.6.3   Poly(vinylidene fluoride) (PVDF)

PVDF has similar properties to PTFE but is better suited for gamma sterilisation, although inferior in chemical resistance. It has good general chemical and abrasion resistance, and this ability can be increased by the addition of glass or carbon fibres.

Advantages of PVDF are:

- can be moulded,
- better wear resistance than PTFE,
- strongest of the fluorocarbon polymers, and
- can be gamma treated.

Disadvantages of PVDF are:

- lower chemical tolerance than PTFE, and
- poorer electrical properties than PTFE.

PVDF is used for heat shrink tubing, wire insulation, pipe fittings and for limited nuclear industry components.

5.2.6.4   Poly(vinyl fluoride) (PVF)

PVF is a tough fluorocarbon but with limited applications. Newer materials have mostly superseded PVF. Normally it has good chemical resistance. One application still using this material in quantities is in the lamination of printed circuit boards.

5.2.6.5   Polyfluoralkoxy Alkane (PFA)

This is a high temperature continuous use material, used as an alternative to FEP. Although it can withstand temperatures to 250°C and has similar characteristics it is expensive in comparison to its more common family member, FEP.

5.2.6.6   Ethylene–Tetrafluoroethylene Copolymer (ETFE)

This is an example of development for specific applications. Du Pont produced this material as an alternative to PTFE and FEP, which has improved hardness. It is a tough, malleable fluorocarbon with surface hardness similar to nylon. The improved physical properties are, however, coupled with a reduction in chemical resistance and temperature tolerance.

5.2.7 POLYAMIDES (PA, NYLON)

Polyamides are strong, abrasion resistant, flexible, multi-use materials. They are resistant to some solvents but absorb others like alcohol and water. Nylons can be filled or reinforced with many substances, e.g. talc, glass fibre, carbon black and metal filaments.

Nylons are very free flowing during moulding and fill cavities well, even down to small shaped flanges or diameters. Care should be taken with the quality of mould tools, especially split lines and insert fits.

The polyamides are a large family group. Nylon 6, 6.6, 6.9, 6.10, 6.11 and 6.12 are aromatic and transparent with 6 and 6.6, being the more widely used for general engineering. A significant different is in the percentage water absorption for each group. For example, under saturation conditions nylon 6 has the highest value at 12%, whereas nylon 6.12 absorbs less than 2%. This influences the choice of nylon for electrical applications.

Transparent nylon has properties competitive with acrylics and polycarbonates but is more expensive; it also has a slightly lower light transmission value. Nylon is a good tough strong material which should be considered as an alternative when assessing SAN, PMMA or PS for applications, even though its resistance to UV is lower. A trade name for an aramid fibre is Kevlar®, DuPont.

Advantages of nylons in general are:

- excellent moulding properties,
- good physical properties,
- improved stiffness when filled,
- comparatively low cost, and
- can be gamma treated

Disadvantages of nylons are:

- low resistance to acids,
- poor electrical insulation,
- low heat resistance,
- maximum working temperature 80°C,
- high percentage moisture absorption, and
- may exhibit a brownish colour shift after gamma sterilisation.

Nylons are used for a wide range of engineering applications from support pads to gears, including handles, covers and cheap toy components. In medical applications, nylon is used for surgical sutures and blood transfer tubing.

5.2.8 POLYAMIDE–IMIDE (PAI, PAPI)

These are tougher and stronger than the nylons. They have chemical resistance and can be moulded easily. Some post processing may be required to ensure that the full mechanical properties are utilised. The range of working temperature is a useful 0–250°C.

PAI and PAPI can be applied in liquid form and baked to remove the carrier or solvent, leaving a coating which is chemically resistant and has low friction. They are good electrical insulators, although coatings should be carefully checked for pin holes. PAI and PAPI have good solvent, UV, microwave and radiation resistance but may work out expensive when the processing costs are considered. These polymers are used for engine components, printed circuit boards and electrical connections.

5.2.9 POLYARYLATES

Polyarylates are tough, offer good electrical insulation, are dimensionally stable and have good weathering properties. Polyarylates can be moulded but high temperatures are required. They are transparent with excellent UV and heat resistance and provide an alternative to polysulphone or polycarbonate.

Polyarylates are used as electrical connector covers, housings, lamp mirrors and bottles.

5.2.10 POLYSULPHONE (PSU)

Polysulphone is regarded as a good engineering plastic with a comparatively high continuous running temperature tolerance of 180°C. In the medical device industry, its chemical resistance and the availability of high quality certified material makes it an excellent choice.

PSU is a solid hard material with a good abrasion resistance. It is highly resistant to acids and alkalis but susceptible to organic solvents. It can be reinforced by glass fibre or mineral fillers, and is also available as a plating grade, or even alloyed with ABS. PSU is a tough resilient material with excellent dielectric strength and resistance to chemical attack.

Advantages of PSU are:

- continuous running temperature of up to 180°C,
- transparent,
- autoclaveable, and
- can be gamma treated.

Disadvantages of PSU are:

- stress cracking if exposed to organic solvents,
- expensive, and
- some difficulties in processing if temperatures not correctly managed.

PSU is used for medical sterilisation trays, suction bottles, respirators and drug administration access ports. It is also used for filter bowls and microwave cookware. Other applications are in general electrical, electronic and engineering components requiring high performance at elevated temperatures.

5.2.10.1 Poly(aryl sulphone) (PAS)

This is similar to PSU but with better chemical resistance. It is a stiff, strong material with good physical and mechanical properties, heat tolerance is very good, up to 200°C for continuous use. It is used for electrical connector bodies, parts of relays and switches.

5.2.10.2 Poly(ether sulphone) (PES)

This polymer is stable up to 180°C. It is tough, rigid and has good mechanical properties. It is in between PSU and PAS in terms of physical, chemical and mechanical properties. It can be reinforced, if necessary, by the addition of glass or carbon fibres. PES is used in printed circuit boards, sockets, connector blocks or housings. The applications are similar to those of PSU.

5.2.11 *POLYBUTADIENE (PB)*

This thermoplastic polymer is a linear polyolefin, tough and good against abrasion, exhibiting moisture retention and electrical insulation. It can be used alone or in laminated sheets, forming a lining for containers. PB is flexible and conforms well. It is used for underfloor heating pipes, abrasive slurry pipes or as a lining for either.

5.2.12 *POLY(BUTYLENE TEREPHTHALATE) (PBT)*

PBT is a thermoplastic polyester. It is used mainly with fillers for applications requiring rigidity and toughness. It competes with nylon and acetal for strength and uses like handles, plugs or gears. It is also used for integrated circuit carriers, brushes and electrical connectors.

Advantages of PBT in general are:

- stiff, hard and strong,
- tough and resilient,
- high temperature tolerance with exceptional short term peak resistance, and
- good coefficient of friction.

Disadvantages of PBT are:

- high percentage moulding shrinkage,
- difficult to process, and
- high heat loss.

5.2.13   POLYCARBONATE (PC)

This is a tough, clear, hard material but is easily scratched. Because of its excellent optical properties it is used for lenses, light barriers and decorative models. PC has good electrical properties and is capable of being effective (mechanically and electrically) in the range –40 to 130°C. Although attacked by solvents this is an advantage for fabrication and permits easy assembly or repositioning, so polycarbonate is good for the construction of prototypes or presentational models.

PC is easily machined and the scratches created are quickly polished out. Many grades are available including glass-fibre reinforced PC and PC–ABS alloys. PTFE lubricated PC is also available. A common trade name for polycarbonate is Lexan.

Advantages of PC are:

- excellent impact resistance,
- easy to fabricate,
- high light transmission,
- good heat resistance, and
- can be gamma treated.

Disadvantages of PC are:

- attacked by solvents,
- susceptible to stress cracking,
- easily marked (low abrasion resistance),
- expensive, and
- processing difficulties.

It is used for electrical housing, models, capacitors and reflectors. Transparent types are used for lenses, glasses and riot shields.

5.2.14   POLY(ETHYLENE TEREPHTHALATE) (AMORPHOUS PET)

This is a clear thermoplastic with good light transmission qualities, ideal for heat forming from sheets to manufacture packing trays or carriers. More importantly it can be gamma treated. It is blow moulded to form bottles and cosmetic containers. When supplied in thin film format it is used for capacitor insulation, photographic and X-ray film. Because of its electrical insulating properties it is sometimes more suitable for electrical fittings than other polymers.

Advantages of PET are:

- high stiffness and strength,
- excellent barrier characteristics, and
- transparent.

Disadvantages of PET are:

- high percentage moulding shrinkage.

5.2.16 POLYETHYLENE (PE)

Polyethylenes (polythenes) are tough, have very little moisture absorption, good chemical resistance and good electrical insulation. PE forms a useful bearing surface with a low coefficient of friction.

The properties of polyethylenes depend on the length and degree of branching of the polyolefin chains. Some designations are:

- LDPE, low density polyethylene,
- LLDPE, linear low density polyethylene,
- HDPE, high density polyethylene,
- XLPE, cross-linked polyethylene,
- UHMWPE, ultra-high molecular weight polyethylene.

Polyethylenes are used in such diverse applications as bottles and cable insulation to toys. As the molecular weight and strength increases then so do the specific applications. Some uses are blow or rotary moulded petrol tanks, blown shrink film, extruded pipes for gas or water and the ubiquitous polythene bag. Chlorinated polyethylene (CPE) can be alloyed with PVC to form a tough protective film.

Advantages of polyethylenes are:

- cheap,
- can be easily processed and even blown to very thin film,
- general chemical resistance is good,
- good electrical properties, and
- can be gamma treated.

Disadvantages of polyethylenes are:

- comparatively low strength,
- poor UV resistance,
- high percentage moulding shrinkage, and
- flammable.

PE foam has good chemical and barrier properties and can be thermoformed. It is more expensive than polystyrene foam but more resilient and is used for packaging of items sensitive to impact, acoustic cladding and water tank insulation.

Polyethylenes are used for packaging medical devices and for disposables. UHMWPE is used for the acetabular component of artificial hip joints.

5.2.17 POLYIMIDE (PI)

This thermoplastic polymer has excellent physical characteristics, especially abrasion resistance, and a high operating temperature at 250°C with outstanding resistance to radiation. It is used as the adhesive and bonding agent for diamond wheels, in bearings, and as an insulating coating. The high running temperature plus bearing properties suit it for use in compressor parts. The insulating properties favour printed circuit board manufacture and capacitor separators.

PI can be gamma treated. It can be moulded (with care) but is very expensive, though for some applications the gains in physical properties can make it a cost effective choice.

Advantages of PI are:

- non-flammable,
- low creep even at elevated temperatures,
- good insulation properties,
- high temperature tolerance, and
- can be gamma treated.

Disadvantages of PI are:

- expensive,
- low impact strength,
- attacked by alkalis and hydrolysis, and
- care needed in processing.

5.2.18 POLYKETONES

Polyketones are high temperature materials suitable for a number of electrical applications. The derivative polyetheretherketone, PEEK, is used when support is needed for items like electrical sockets or electronic connections.

Polyketones are resistant to radiation and most solvents but polyetherketone, PEK, is better suited for higher temperature applications.

Polyketones are gamma treatable and are used in the medical, space and nuclear environments. The maximum temperature for long-term use is 240°C. There are good abrasion and wear properties and comparatively high strength, but these polymers can be expensive and sometimes difficult to process.

5.2.19 POLY(METHYL PENTENE) (PMP)

This thermoplastic has good temperature resistance but is brittle. The transparent grade has good clarity and its chemical and dimensional stability are equalled only by polypropylene, PP. Because of its good tolerance to temperature variations it can be autoclaved repeatedly. It is expensive and has a high percentage moulding shrinkage but the medical applications at the moment are numerous, e.g. optical glasses, petri dishes and containers requiring frequent sterilisation.

5.2.20 POLY(PHENYLENE SULPHIDE) (PPS)

PPS has good chemical and solvent resistance with a medium to high temperature tolerance up to 190°C. It can be gamma treated as well as autoclaved, and will maintain dimensional stability with both methods of sterilisation. It is used as a replacement for phenolic electrical housings, as coatings for the chemical industry and for internal components for pumps.

5.2.21 POLYPROPYLENE (PP)

Polypropylene is a popular material, easily processed and handled. It has good resistance to the majority of chemicals but is susceptible to heat and abrasion. Excellent impact properties make polypropylene ideal for containers, protective housings and fluid containers. PP can be quite difficult to fabricate or join with other polymers, but there are a wide range of grades to minimize problems and various methods of joining both chemical and mechanical. PP can have a very good hinge effect and many containers make use of this feature to provide a cap which is an integral part of the product. This feature aids manufacture, requiring only one moulding and no assembly time.

Advantages of PP are:

- cheap,
- easy to process,
- excellent chemical resistance,
- good overall physical strengths,
- low moisture absorption,
- stable to 90°C for continuous use, and
- some gamma treatable grades are available.

Disadvantages of PP are:

- poor UV resistance,
- high percentage moulding shrinkage,
- gas permeable,
- high creep, and
- difficult to bond.

PP is used extensively for pipes, containers, handles and buckets, in battery containers and for critical medical components. When modified with rubber it is used for auto bumpers; if talc-filled, stiffness increases and the temperature tolerance increases. Work is in progress to evolve new grades and uses for this (and other) polymers. Development work is being carried out by Shell Chemicals on a new polypropylene to be used in the petrochemical industry as an insulating barrier. This insulation would protect the pipes used to transport the crude oil from the North Sea against corrosion and be able to withstand the thermal stress from hot oil at 110°C on one side and sea water at 5°C on the other.

5.2.22 POLYSTYRENE (PS)

There are various grades of polystyrene. The impact resistant material is toughened with polybutadiene elastomer. PS can be formed in many ways: extruded, moulded, blown film, sheet, formed or rotary moulded. Polystyrene is the most stable and radiation resistant polymer in the thermoplastic family. It has good general mechanical properties, which can be modified to provide an even wider choice. It is readily attacked by solvents which can be an asset when fabricating a prototype or finished product (e.g. Airfix kits + PS cement).

Advantages of PS are:

- cheap,
- stiff and strong,
- good electrical characteristics,
- easily processed,
- low percentage mould shrinkage,
- good transparency,
- easily fabricated and machined, and
- can be gamma treated.

Disadvantages of PS are

- brittle,
- low UV tolerance,
- flammable,
- low heat resistance,
- attacked by many solvents, and
- low stress resistance.

Polystyrene has a multitude of uses from blow moulded boxes and bottles, to cassette containers, cheap toys and disposable forceps. When compounded for structural foam applications include large machine housings, packaging or even furniture. It is well known in food trays and egg boxes.

5.2.23 STYRENE–ACRYLONITRILE (SAN)

SAN is a thermoplastic copolymer of styrene (75%) and acrylonitrile (25%). It is an amorphous polymer with superior chemical and heat resistance to polystyrene. The impact characteristics of SAN are excellent; it is strong, tough, rigid and transparent, with good optical properties.

Advantages of SAN are:

- comparatively cheap
- rigid, strong, tough
- slight blue tint in transparent grades,
- good acid and alkali resistance,
- very little trouble processing, and
- can be gamma treated.

Disadvantages of SAN are:

- light transmission inferior to PMMA,
- higher water absorption than styrene, and
- low heat resistance, 55°C.

SAN is used for domestic products such as toothbrush handles, work surfaces or covers. It is also used for external battery cases, dials, optical contact lenses, medical waste and disposable fluid containers.

5.2.24 POLY(VINYL CHLORIDE) (PVC)

PVC is a very widely used but controversial plastic. It is discussed at length in Chapter 6. The comments here are for the sake of completeness of this polymer survey.

5.2.24.1 Plasticised Poly(vinyl chloride) (PPVC)

PPVC is an excellent plastic for injection moulding. Care needs to be taken to avoid chloride corrosion of tooling and mould parts. PPVC can also be used for extrusion or dipping. Plasticisers added to PVC improve plasticity, for more rigid grades PVC can be cross-linked.

Uses of PPVC vary from a critical electrical high-voltage insulating covering for cables to a simple garden hose. Medical applications vary from external tubing requiring food grade to catheters and implants needing full material clearance and certification.

The cross-linked grades are used for heat-shrink tubing and adhesive tape.

PVC can be gamma treated but unmodified grades will discolour to varying degrees from a slight brown tint to smoky black. There are gamma-stable grades available if the finished colour is of importance.

Advantages of PPVC are:

- easy to process by most methods,
- cheap,
- tough, with excellent elongation properties,
- flexible or rigid grades available,
- excellent UV tolerance, and
- can be gamma treated.

Disadvantages of PPVC are:

- can corrode tooling and process equipment,
- low heat tolerance,
- low creep resistance, and
- problems with disposal.

5.2.24.2 Unplasticised Poly(vinyl chloride) (UPVC)

UPVC is well known as the material of replacement window frames. Various alloyed and modified grades are available: UPVC can be alloyed with ABS, SMA, or acrylic, UV stabilised, filled or high impact grades exist.

A copolymer of PVC and PP is used for blow moulding and thermoforming. A copolymer of PVC and VC increases the protection against water vapour and is used for stretch film applications.

Advantages of UPVC are:

- cheap,
- good chemical resistance,
- good UV resistance,
- stiff, tough, strong, and
- can be gamma treated.

Disadvantages of UPVC are:

- processing must be monitored and is sometimes difficult
- low solvent resistance, and
- low heat tolerance, 50°C.

UPVC is used for gutters, modified UPVC is used for window frames, copolymers are used for film and bottle manufacture.

5.3 COMMONLY USED THERMOSETTING POLYMERS

Thermosetting polymers are materials which solidify after forming and cannot be softened again. The molecular structure changes on heating so that the long chain molecules are irreversibly cross-linked.

5.3.1 POLYURETHANE (PU)

PU is an excellent material with a wide range of applications and variable methods of manufacture. Available as an elastomer, a foam (rigid or flexible), a sealant, an adhesive or as a moulding grade. It is made by reacting polyethers, polyesters and polycaprolactone.

Advantages of PU are:

- low thermal transfer,
- quick, easy process,

- good adhesion strength,
- cheap tooling for rotary injection moulding, and
- can be gamma treated.

Disadvantages of PU are:

- low heat tolerance,
- toxic isocyanates, and
- poor tolerance to UV.

Rigid PU is used for packaging, large housings, simulated wood effect allows for fabricated furniture or work tops and buoyancy floats. Flexible PU is used for tubing, pipes, rollers, car bumpers and for coating fabrics.

5.3.2 SILICONES

Silicone polymers exist as liquids, semi-solids, soft or hard solids, depending on the molecular weight and degree of polymerisation. Although they can be soft, silicones are thermosetting polymers supplied as one- or two-part compounds which require heat treatment to cure after processing. They can be formed by moulding, extrusion or casting.

Silicones have very good resistance to chemical and solvent attack. They have excellent heat endurance characteristics. For electrical insulation, thermosetting silicones offer some of the best options open to the designer. The temperature tolerance is good at 260°C.

Silicones can be reinforced or filled with a variety of cheap materials. They are obtainable in coloured soft (from 15 Shore 'A') or hard grades.

Regarded as inert once cured, silicone tubing is used extensively in the medical world to carry gases and solutions, for wound drainage etc. Silicones are implanted for various prosthetic purposes including finger joints, female sterilisation and mammary implants. Adverse publicity about breast implants has caused concern that is not yet resolved.

5.3.3 POLYIMIDE (PI)

Polyimide is one of the most temperature resistant plastics with a continuous working limit of 260°C and the ability to withstand 300°C for short periods. PI also functions well at very low temperatures.

PI is dimensionally stable with good tensile and impact strength values and little creep. Electrical arc resistance is good. PI is gamma treatable and transparent to microwaves, it is also expensive.

PI is used for valve seats and piston rings in the auto industry, and for applications in nuclear engineering.

5.3.4   UNSATURATED POLYESTER

This thermoset can have a range of properties by modifying the base resin to produce finished goods that can be hard and brittle or soft and flexible. It has good chemical resistance, good physical properties and an outstanding strength-to-weight ratio. Unsaturated polyester is tougher than melamine, phenolic or urethane and cheaper than epoxy. It has poor solvent resistance compared with the other thermosets, and relatively poor heat tolerance with a maximum working temperature of 130°C. It is used for electrical parts or auto components, and as linings for tanks and concrete containers.

5.3.5   PHENOLIC RESIN, PHENOL FORMALDEHYDE (PF)

Phenolic thermosetting resin in a good electrical insulator, but may show signs of stress if incorrectly used. The physical properties are moderate but with good heat resistance.

Advantages of PF:

- low cost,
- heat tolerance up to 185°C with fillers (150°C without), and
- easy to machine.

Disadvantages of PF are:

- limited colour choice, and
- brittle.

Laminates with PF are better known under the trade name Tufnol, and are used for various components. Phenolic resins have to a large extent been superseded by modern engineering plastics, e.g. PPS replaces phenolic electrical housings because it is less brittle, has greater temperature tolerance, is easier to form and is just as good an electrical insulator. Phenolic resins are still used in chipboard and plywood, and as a chemically resistant coating for metals.

5.3.6   MELAMINE RESIN

Melamine is a hard thermoset used quite a lot in the electrical industry. It is electrically stable even under conditions of high humidity. Melamine has good chemical resistance but can be attacked fairly easily by strong acids and alkalis. The maximum continuous use temperature is 100°C. Impact strength is poor. At lower temperatures it can withstand considerable mistreatment. The uses are diverse, from high voltage components to coloured decorative laminates (Formica) and tableware.

5.3.7 EPOXY RESIN

Epoxy resin is formed by mixing two components, resin and hardener: the ratio determines the final physical properties. The resin is usually rigid, hard and brittle, but by suitable choice of mixing ratio a much tougher material with high impact strength can be produced. Epoxy resin is used to bind fibres in composite materials: glass fibre, carbon fibre and metal fibres have been used. Particulate fillers are used to add bulk and reduce cost, or for specific enhancements. Examples are glass beads, talc, chalk and silica.

Epoxy is used to encapsulate parts, and to coat base materials to provide protection against chemical, physical or abrasive attack. It can act as a sacrificial bearing or wear coating. Epoxy is sometimes used as an adhesive (and gap filler) when difficult materials need to be bonded (see Chapters 8 on adhesives and 9 on corrosion protection).

Advantages of epoxy are:

- excellent electrical and chemical resistance,
- inert once mixed and cured,
- high temperature tolerance 170°C, and
- can be gamma treated.

Disadvantages of epoxy are:

- expensive,
- toxic as individual component parts,
- heat generation while curing,
- time required for mixed compound to cure,
- for some compounds the actual ratio of mixing is critical to obtain maximal physical properties.

5.4 THERMOPLASTIC ELASTOMERS (TPE)

Thermoplastic elastomers are polymers which have the properties of both rubbers and thermoplastics. They can be conventionally injection moulded to provide cheap well defined shapes, but have high elasticity like rubber. The polymer chains are cross-linked in an amorphous structure when cold. Tensile stress aligns the molecules giving elasticity, and heat breaks the cross-links allowing the material to flow.

5.4.1 THERMOPLASTIC URETHANE (TPU)

TPU is probably the most widely used thermoplastic elastomer. It has the highest abrasion resistance of all TPEs, good strength and tear resistance but a comparatively low maximum continuous operating temperature of 70°C. There are three types of thermoplastic urethanes: polyester-urethane, polyether-urethane and caproester-urethane. All are linear polymeric materials. Uses vary from critical O ring seals and diaphragms to show soles and V belts. This material is extruded to form windscreen wiper blades. The hardness can be varied by modification, between 70 Shore'A' and 65 Shore 'D'.

5.4.2   STYRENE–BUTADIENE–STYRENE COPOLYMER (SBS TPE)

This material has excellent flexibility even down to –40°C but the maximum continuous working temperature is only 45°C. It has low resistance to UV degradation and solvents, and exhibits creep. SBS is used as an adhesive and gap filler, for wire insulation and in footwear.

5.4.3   ETHERESTER AMIDE (EEA TPE)

EEA has poor resistance to solvents but good impart strength at low temperatures. It is used as an insulating covering for cables and for shoe soles.

5.4.4   OLEFINIC ELASTOMER (OL TPE)

This elastomer is used extensively in the auto industry for grills, panels, mud flaps, bumpers etc. It is well suited to this type of application since it remains flexible down to –35°C, although under load it will creep. It is also used as an impact modifier for PP.

5.4.5   CO-ETHER ESTER (CEE TPE)

CEE has a very useful range of working temperature: –50 to 80°C. A modified version maintains properties up to 135°C. It is one of the most costly of the TPEs and has good adhesive qualities. CEE is used for transmission belts, specialist tubing, liquid transfer pipes, and fuel tanks. Sometimes it is used as an impact modifier for PVC.

6
Poly(vinyl chloride) (PVC)

PVC is probably the most maligned and misunderstood material used in medical device manufacture and other industries. As mentioned in Chapter 5, PVC has had a bad press of late, particularly from the environmentalists, but contrary opinions are rarely heard as the manufacturers prefer to keep a low profile. In this chapter I hope to present the facts, so that you are better informed when evaluating whether to use PVC or an alternative.

6.1 PVC PRODUCTION

PVC, poly(vinyl chloride), is produced from vinyl chloride monomer (see Figure 6.1). The monomer is made by reactive combustion of ethylene and chlorine. Chlorine is produced from sodium chloride (salt) and ethylene is derived from oil. Vinyl chloride is flammable and highly reactive, so it is stored in liquid form under pressure. PVC is made by polymerisation of the monomer, which is achieved by dispersing it as droplets in water containing certain catalysts. Polymerisation occurs and most of the monomer is converted to polymer. The polymer is a white powder which is filtered from the water, care being taken to ensure than no unconverted monomer is allowed to contaminate the product.

 PVC was first produced industrially in about 1910, with commercial applications like vinyl records developing from 1930. It was not until the 1970s that it was found that long-term exposure to vinyl chloride monomer

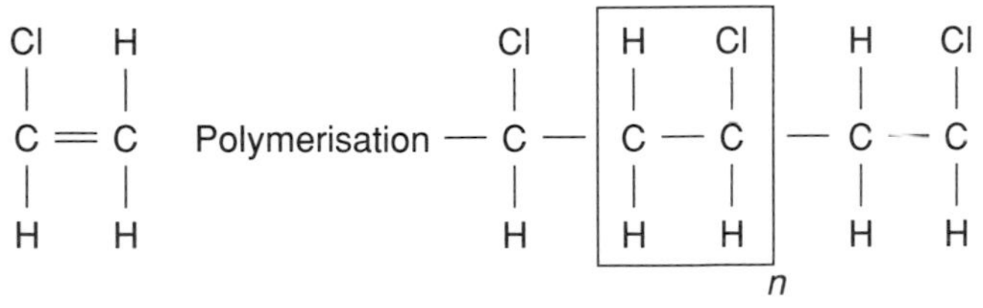

Figure 6.1 Structure of poly(vinyl chloride).

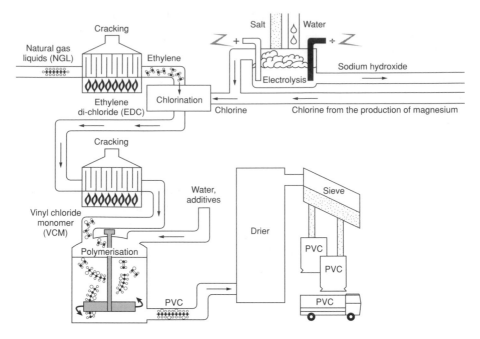

Figure 6.2 Diagram of PVC manufacture. © 1992 Norsk Hydro Polymers a.s. of Norway: first published in *PVC and the Environment* by Hydro Media and reproduced with permission.

could result in forms of cancer. This discovery resulted in major changes to the manufacturing facilities and methods of handling the raw materials and products. Significant changes were necessary to ensure the complete elimination of unreacted monomer from the polymer. There was concern about the further processing of PVC and its use in food and medical applications. A comprehensive directive from the EEC, 80/766/EEC was compiled to ensure safe manufacture and use of PVC.

The manufacturing process for PVC is shown in Figure 6.2.

There is more detailed discussion of types of PVC, their pros and cons, and applications, in Chapter 5.

6.2 ADVANTAGES OF PVC AND APPLICATIONS

PVC is one of the cheapest polymers to produce because the ethylene and chlorine used are produced from the abundant raw materials oil and salt. The price of PVC is fairly stable on the world market.

PVC is lightweight, cost effective, tough, easily processed, non-reactive and can be manipulated by a large number of industrial processes. The range of applications includes children's footballs, inflatable structures, drainage pipes and medical transfusion tubes. PVC is a versatile material with very many uses in building, industrial, domestic and medical applications.

PVC is easily maintained, can be coloured, made opaque or transparent.

Modified PVC can withstand normal gamma sterilisation doses without any detrimental changes.

PVC can be used for waterproofing textiles.

Less energy is needed to produce raw PVC than any other plastic. PVC manufacture also consumes less energy than the production of many other materials. Figures 6.3 and 6.4 illustrate the energy advantages of PVC. Owing to the good mechanical properties and low density, items made of PVC are lighter than comparable items made of other materials. For example, to give the same capacity as a 45 g PVC bottle, a 500–700 g glass bottle would be needed. Similarly an extruded PVC pipe requires only 15% the amount of energy needed to produce a cast iron pipe of the same dimensions, and the plastic pipe would last longer. Also the energy cost of transporting lightweight PVC items is considerably less than that for similar items in other materials.

Conventional packaging can be reduced in volume and weight by the use of PVC sheet or vacuum formed containers. Similarly in the automotive industry the use of PVC parts can reduce the weight of a vehicle and hence the energy cost and fuel consumption. Another reason to use PVC in vehicles is the resistance of the plastic to degradation from fuel or oil.

PVC has significant electrical insulation attributes, is weather resistant, resistant to UV degradation and resistant to fire. These qualities all contribute to safety features.

6.3 DISADVANTAGES AND PROBLEMS WITH PVC

Chlorine is a dangerous substance which must be stored very safety. About one third of the chlorine produced is used for PVC manufacture, the rest is used for other purposes, and some of the available chlorine is wasted because there is no use for it, it is a by-product of other processes.

Vinyl chloride is carcinogenic and is a cause of two types of liver cancer. Exposure to vinyl chloride has to be strictly limited. It is also highly flammable so safety precautions are required.

PVC is very inert and so it is not biodegradable. Disposal by land fill is not recommended so carefully controlled incineration is required. Without strict control of the incineration temperature there can be toxic emissions.

PVC should be incinerated at or above 500°C, although it will burn from 400°C. Combustion of PVC produces carbon dioxide and carbon monoxide, which are relatively safe. Combustion also produces HCl gas, which should be removed from the flue by scrubbers. HCl is an obnoxious irritant which damages lungs and eyes.

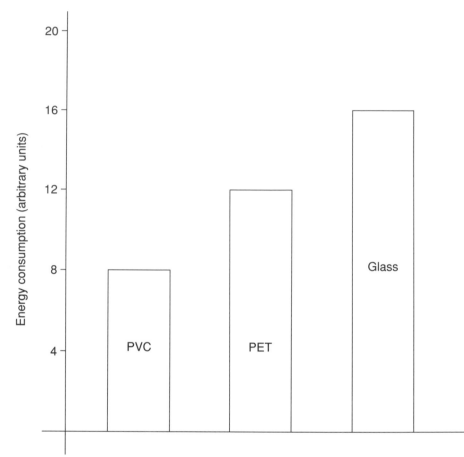

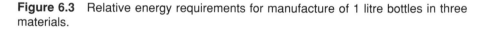

Figure 6.3   Relative energy requirements for manufacture of 1 litre bottles in three materials.

Flue scrubbing devices are normally employed in domestic refuse incinerators, these make safe the gaseous products leaving a residual ash. Ignition temperatures are shown in Figure 6.5. An example of an incinerator layout is shown in Figure 6.6. If released, the HCl would contribute to acid rain, another reason for using flue scrubbers.

Some modern systems utilise a method called the '3R Process' developed by Professor Vogg. This uses the hydrogen chloride produced to react with heavy metal residuals in the fly ash of incinerators, with the actual solids left being easier to dispose of.

There are still arguments about the formation of dioxins during refuse incineration but studies leave doubt about contribution of PVC to this problem.

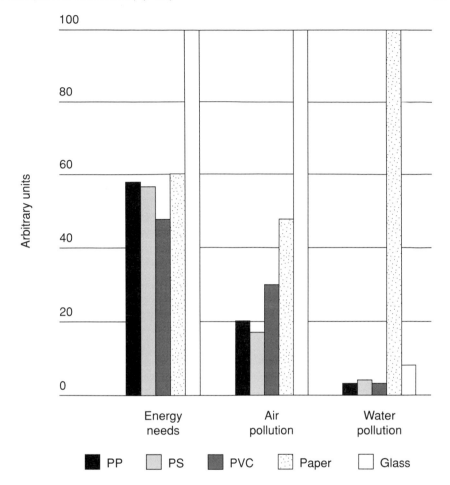

Figure 6.4 Relative energy requirements and pollutant production for food containers. These results are from the production and use of 250 ml containers in lots of 1000 in Germany. © 1988 Norsk Hydro Polymers a.s. of Norway.

Some stabilisers used in PVC contain heavy metals: their use is inappropriate for food or medical applications.

Plasticisers are used to increase the flexibility of the final PVC formed. They can migrate from the PVC into liquids that are in contact. This migration is most marked into oily or alcoholic-based substances but many other liquids are also affected. The selection and 'locking in' of plasticisers for PVC used for food or medical purposes is critical. For reference look up EEC regulations 81/432/EEC and 82/711/EEC.

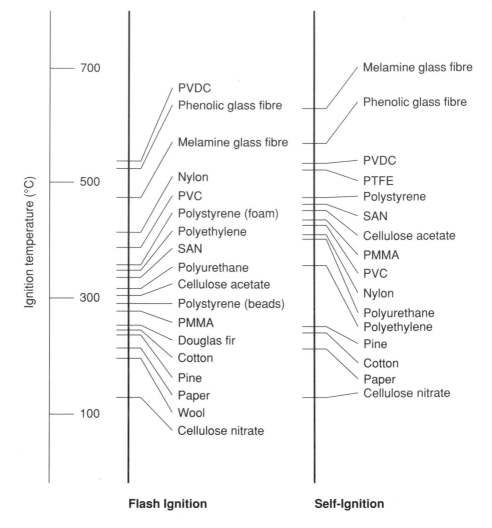

Figure 6.5 Ignition temperatures of various materials.

In some medical applications certain blood products can migrate into PVC containers or tubes. Selection of materials can modify this problem.

The ethylene necessary for PVC manufacture comes from oil which is a fossil fuel and a finite resource. As stocks decrease, in time, ethylene can be expected to become more expensive.

The environmental implications of PVC manufacture and use give rise to controversy which is not yet resolved. There is further discussion in Chapter 28. Figure 6.7 shows the 'chlorine circle' for the manufacture, use, recycling, incineration and cleaning of PVC.

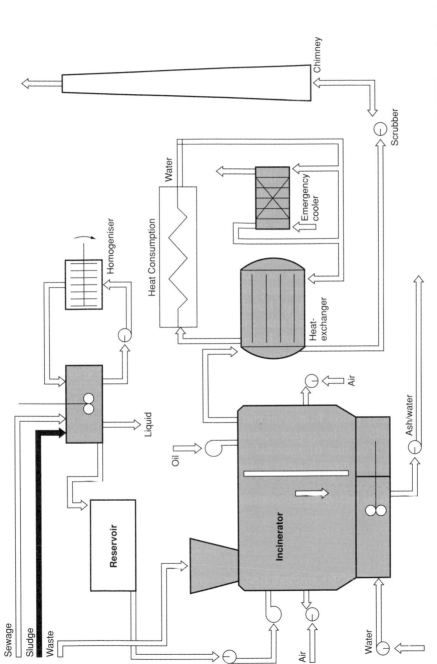

Figure 6.6 Incinerator for PVC waste. © 1992 Norsk Hydro Polymers a.s. of Norway: first published in *PVC and the Environment* by Hydro Media and reproduced with permission.

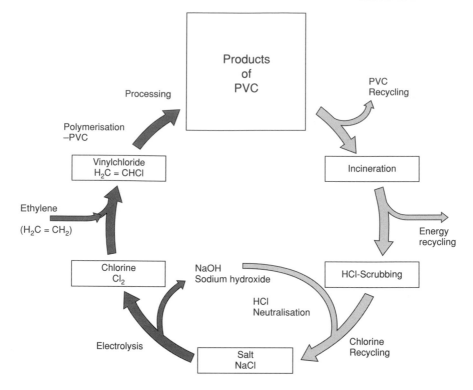

Figure 6.7   The chlorine circle for PVC recycling. © 1992 Norsk Hydro Polymers a.s. of Norway: first published in *PVC and the Environment* by Hydro Media and reproduced with permission.

In 1995 Germany lifted restrictions on PVC for use in building work. This was in response to detailed market research commissioned by the Federal Office of the Environment.

6.4 MIGRATION IN PVC

As mentioned above under disadvantages, there can be a problem with ingredients of some PVC formulations migrating into liquid phases with which the PVC is in contact. Some additives in PVC are toxic, and as PVC is used for food and medical purposes there are concerns.

This problem is particular to PVC because the additives used to enhance its physical properties are not chemically bonded to the base material. Under particular circumstances they may leach out.

Although it is recognised that this migration occurs, especially into food packaging, the tiny quantities of substances which migrate are generally considered to be so small as to be harmless. Even so there are strict national and international regulations about the types of polymers used and the additives incorporated for specific applications.

For a number of years there has been concern about the plasticisers used in PVC to increase its flexibility, for use in food, medical and domestic items. The concern is based on the belief that these plasticisers may cause cancer. This belief arises from research carried out on rats and mice in which the animals were fed massive doses of raw plasticisers over a long period of time. Now there is doubt about the relevance of the results of these experiments to low dose exposure in humans. The EC Scientific Committee on Food could not reach agreement about the toxicity or carcinogenicity of PVC plasticisers, but imposed maximum levels for contamination. These levels apply to food packaging and daily intakes by physical contamination as well as medical contact with tissues and especially blood. Short-term use limits the amount of plasticiser which leaches into the blood and is now permitted.

It has been estimated that we consume, on average, 2 g per year of plasticisers and the EC Scientific Committee on Food considers that there is no health hazard from the permitted plasticisers at this level of consumption. Table 6.1 lists the permitted additives.

Migration is a two way process. As well as ensuring that no toxic substances leach out of the PVC to food, tissue or blood there is testing continually being carried out to monitor, quantify and prevent absorption of body fluids or food components into the PVC.

Research has been conducted to verify the acceptability of vegetable and mineral oils, blood products, fatty foods and so on, in contact with PVC.

As an example of the testing techniques used, sheets of PVC are suspended in solutions of selected media and left for 8 weeks at 37°C with tests on every 7th day. Flexibility is monitored and compared with originally measured cold flex deflection. This indicates the plasticiser content. Table 6.2 shows the different effects of water and vegetable oil based media.

6.5 MEDICAL APPLICATIONS OF PVC

In this section I will concentrate on the medical market applications of PVC since the other industrial and domestic uses (like window frames, pipes and insulation) are well known and are discussed in Chapter 5. Some of the advantages of PVC are specific to blood or tissue contact, and some cannot be duplicated by any other material.

Advantages of PVC relevant to medical devices are as follows.

- PVC can be modified from its natural rigid state by the addition of plasticisers to give a range of flexible or semi-rigid plastics.
- PVC can be injection moulded, extruded, compression moulded, blow moulded, rotary moulded or dipped to provide a wide range of forms.

Table 6.1   Additives used in the manufacture of PVC

Additive	Approximate content (%)
Antistatic agents	0.2–2
Biostabilisers	0.5–1
Blowing agents	0.5–1
Colourants	0.1–2
Fillers	5–50
Flame retardants	2–5
Impact modifiers	2–10
Lubricants	0.5–1
Plasticisers	10–50
Process enhancers	< 1
Viscosity modifiers	0.5–2

Table 6.2   Percentage decrease in flexion of PVC after 8 weeks exposure to various media

Medium	Standard medical material	Extraction-resistant material
Simulated stomach contents[a]	No apparent changes	No apparent changes
Simulated gastric juice[b]	No apparent changes	No apparent changes
Milk	No apparent changes	No apparent changes
Vegetable oil (blended)	89	40
Prosparolarachis oil	41	20

[a]10% soya + 20% cream + 70% custard powder, adjusted to pH 1 and diluted with water to a ratio 3 : 7.
[b]2 g NaCl + 3.3 g pepsin in 7 ml conc HCl and mixed with 1 l water and checked to a pH 1.2.

- PVC is easily bonded by a large number of solvents.
- PVC is cheap.
- Depending on additives the material can be made crystal clear, fully opaque or translucent.
- PVC is an electrical insulator with a dielectric strength of MVm^{-1}.
- PVC can have barium sulphate added to make it radiopaque. Stripes of radiopaque material are incorporated in catheters.
- PVC can be sterilised by ETO or gamma treatment.
- Any colour of PVC can be created to aid identification or aid sales.

The principle medical applications of PVC are:

- blood and blood product storage bags,
- drainage catheters,
- blood tubing for transfusion sets,
- transfer cannulae,

- drip chambers,
- enema packs,
- intravenous solution giving sets,
- needle hubs, Luer fittings, Y tubing joints,
- urology collection bags and catheters.

For many years the PVC manufacturers have worked on developing materials from which leaching of plasticiser is either very low or nil. The resulting plastics now on the market are used extensively for lay-flat or calendered film which is used to make bags for storing intravenous solutions and blood. These low-loss PVCs are also used for wound drainage, gastric tubing and intravenous solution kits.

Sub-assemblies built up by device manufacturers may require pressurised joint components moulded from rigid PVC. Such products are simple to produce but excellent in quality, examples are Luers, taps, enema nozzles and drip-chamber compartments.

The clarity of PVC sheet is important for applications such as oxygen tents used in intensive care units. To make these tents PVC sheets are fabricated by welding. Special shapes or requirements can be achieved on site. The tents are safe, can be sterilised, have a soft textile 'feel' and there is no limit to size. The clarify makes observation of the patient easy, and if the patient is conscious they have all-round vision and suffer less trauma than being in a translucent or opaque enclosure.

PVC is sometimes used to sheathe catheters made of other materials that might be less patient-friendly. The PVC can be extruded over the finished catheter or applied as a coating to components. The PVC protects both the device and the patient from any harmful effects of the insertion, by physically supporting the catheter and reducing friction. Examples are angiographic catheters used to explore and expand restricted arteries, and flexible fibre optics where the glass bundle fibres could be broken.

Nasogastic feeding tubes are used in the treatment of infants and others who cannot feed orally. The tube must be small enough to cause no discomfort, must transport food or medication and should not interact with any of the body fluids with which it comes into contact. Conventional PVC and other flexible polymers become brittle after long-term use as feeding tubes, so they have to be replaced regularly which is inconvenient and potentially traumatic for the patient.

Hydro Polymers in collaboration with others pioneered the development and manufacture of a material which could meet the demanding criteria specified above.

PVC enema kits are inexpensive and allow the option of patients administering their own treatment at home.

Continuous ambulatory peritoneal dialysis (CAPD) is a method of dialysis in which the treatment solution is slowly perfused into the abdominal cavity.

The patient is fitted with a PVC bag which obviates the need for a hospital place. Compared to the capital-intensive bedside dialysis machines, this makes dialysis available to far more people.

A less obvious medical application is the use of PVC for floor coverings. Shaped and welded it can form a smooth surface which aids cleaning and the removal of potential infection within hospitals. PVC flooring can be loaded with conducting particles to form an anti-static surface which reduces the risk of explosion present when using oxygen, anaesthetic gases and electrical equipment.

With each new operation, treatment, transfusion etc. there must be assurances of no cross-infection. PVC allows the use of inexpensive disposable products to the benefit of the patient.

New formulations and applications for PVC are being developed. Their manufacturers are now well aware of the need to assuage toxicity and environmental safety concerns, so I feel the use of PVC will actually increase not decrease over the next twenty year.

Dioxin emissions from incinerators can now be reduced to 0.1 ng m^{-3}, chlorine use is still talked about but PVC is not now the main problem. Recycling methods have improved to the extent that used PVC articles can be cleaned, stripped and granulated for reuse without any major problems. In Holland a project is underway to evaluate the recycling of blood bags. Toxicity may be the last remaining problem, and there have been no major changes over the last twenty years except for the recent introductions of new plasticiser, TOTM, (tri-2-ethyl-hexyl-tri-mellitate). Its toxicity and metabolic pathway is still under investigation.

Owing to its versatility, ability to be formed by a variety of methods, continued (and predicted) low cost and a growing acceptance clinically, the medical device industry is more likely to seek new applications for PVC rather than promote a reduction in use.

6.6   ACKNOWLEDGEMENTS

I wish to thank Norsk Hydro Polymers for background information and some of the illustrations.

7
Other Materials

Medical devices are mostly made with the well-known metallic and polymeric materials described in previous chapters. There are, however, other materials that are not so easily classified but which may come into their own when their particular properties are required.

As they are less widely used, non-metallic non-polymeric materials may be overlooked in your material selection process, so some of them are described here to prompt your thoughts. This survey is not comprehensive, but should give you an idea of possibilities.

I have not covered here the modern generation of specially developed biomaterials which have very specific uses and may be custom-made for one application. The trend is towards composite materials which can mimic the properties of biological material (e.g. a polymer–ceramic composite to substitute for bone); after all natural materials are very often composites. Information about such developments can be found in research journals and conference proceedings.

7.1 BAKELITE

Bakelite is a trade name for paper, cotton or glass fibre laminates bonded with thermosetting resin (Union Carbide Corp.). Because of this Bakelite has excellent strength and stiffness at elevated temperatures. It is also an excellent electrical insulator and is ideal for board fittings for electronic equipment. Bakelite is chemically resistant, has good mechanical strength and a low coefficient of expansion.

The paper laminates are split into five groups all bonded together with phenolic resin, the cotton laminates are split into seven groups of which five are combined with phenolic resins, the remaining two by epoxy. The coarseness of the cotton weave determines the final physical strength and in turn the appropriate applications. The largest category is the glass fibre laminates with nine groups all with specific uses and material bases ranging from melamine to epoxy.

7.2   BARIUM

Barium is a white soft metal used in compounds with other materials as a pigment or an additive for specialised industrial lubricants. In medicine there are two main applications. Barium sulphate is radiopaque and is given to patients in a 'barium meal' as a means of imaging the digestive tract. Barium sulphate is also added to polymers and thermoplastic elastomers to make them visible by X-ray. The barium sulphate is inert and creates no problems in the body. It is acceptable for all forms of sterilisation whether ETO, gamma or autoclave.

7.3   CADMIUM

Cadmium is a plating material used to protect base metals from corrosion, as a yellow pigment in paint and as one of the electrodes in Ni–Cd rechargeable cells. Because Cd is highly toxic there are dangers to those processing it and difficulties of long-term disposal so it is increasingly being replaced by other materials.

7.4   CARBON

The industrial uses of carbon are mostly for graphite. 'Carbon black' is used in pigments in inks, paint and rubber and as a filler in battery plates (electrodes). Activated carbon is an absorbent used in filters, waste treatment systems and for removal of toxins from fluids. Extruded graphite rods are used as the sacrificial electrodes in high-voltage electrical applications, while ground graphite rods are the current transfer central electrodes in most domestic zinc–carbon and zinc–chloride batteries.

Carbon and graphite components are produced by three methods: machining, moulding or extrusion (the last two requiring oven baking to cure after the initial processing). Low volumes are best made by machining because the costs of moulding or extrusion tools and their processing equipment are very high and are normally only affordable for long-run, high-quantity production. Graphite is favoured for machining because of its strength and its ability to be manufactured to tolerances approaching those of metal working.

Probably the best known medical application is as spun carbon fibres either in long strands or in fine woven cloth. Carbon fibres have an exceptional strength-to-weight ratio, are resistant to chemicals and have special electrical properties. Carbon fibre braids are used to repair or replace ligaments – in time the carbon fibres break down and the material is dispersed in the body, after acting as a scaffold for new tissue.

Carbon-fibre reinforced composites have been used for bone prostheses and repair.

Carbon-fibre reinforces composites are used in aerospace, automotive and sporting applications.

Pyrolitic carbon is a special form which has a glassy surface that carries an electric charge. It is antithrombogenic and has been used in cardiovascular applications.

7.5 CERAMICS

Ceramic is a general term for four groups of inorganic materials which are formed by the application of pressure and heat to their base ingredients. These materials have an extremely diverse range of uses from builders bricks to sanitary bowls. The four groups are as follows.

- Bonded ceramics: in which oxide crystals are held together by glassy matrix.
- Amorphous ceramics: otherwise known as glasses. Man-made versions are used for lenses, bottles and windows.
- Cements: a group which may contain either crystalline or amorphous phases.
- Crystalline ceramics are single phase materials.

The compressive strengths of the ceramics are exceptional, but they are very stuff and brittle. If designing with ceramics, it is necessary to keep them in compression and to eliminate stress concentrations. Ceramics are exceptionally hard and this feature is used in abrasives, cutting tools and for wear resistance. For example, synthetic polyester fibres include a titania filler, TiO_2 (see section 4.10) which causes rapid wear of yarn guides in fibre processing plants. Substituting ceramic yarn guides reduces the wear problem. Table 7.1 lists some hardnesses.

Ceramics are strong in compression but weak in torsion and bending. They are very brittle and undergo significant shrinkage during forming by sintering, which has to be allowed for in tool and die making.

Bulk uses of ceramics are well known, as in refractory bricks, water pipes electrical insulators, construction materials etc. There are many other smaller scale applications. Table 7.2 shows examples of ceramic glasses and their uses.

The most commonly known engineering ceramic is probably silicon carbide which is used in grinding wheels. Other compounds include carbides, borides and nitrides.

Ceramics can be used instead of metals for high-temperature bearings. They have a lower coefficient of thermal expansion and low coefficient of friction which means lower running temperatures and less consumption

Table 7.1   Knoop hardness of common ceramics

Material	Knoop hardness
Diamond	7000
Boron nitride	7000
Boron carbide	2900
Silicon carbide	2600
Alumina	2000
Hardened and tempered steel (for comparison)	700

Table 7.2   Uses of ceramic glasses

Glass	Applications
Borosilicate 70% SiO_2	Heat resistant cooking items, glass seals on pressurised battery cells, laboratory 'glassware'.
'Soda' glass 72% SiO_2	Bottles, plateglass, windows.
Lead glasses	
50% SiO_2	Lamps, valves and electronics
40% SiO_2	Optical fittings and lenses

of lubricant. The low density (60% less than steel) means lower centrifugal stresses. The example considered was a ceramic ball hot isostatically pressed from silicon nitride.

One classification of ceramics is as follows.

• Whiteware: china, tiles porcelain and electrical insulation.
• Refractories: fireclay, furnace linings, bricks and mortar.
• Porcelain enamels: protective coating for metal substrates.
• Structural clay: bricks, tiles and pipes.
• Glass: moulded transparent components.

Ceramic parts are produced in various ways. Manufacture can be by wet or dry bag pressing, mechanical pressing, extrusion or slip casting.Once compacted the material is sintered to bring out the full physical, mechanical, chemical and temperature resistant properties.

Advantages of ceramics include:

• high mechanical strength,
• resistance to abrasion and wear,
• low friction,
• dimensionally stable,
• excellent chemical resistance, and
• hard surface finish.

Table 7.3 Comparative surface hardness, nominal scale

Material	Hardness
Diamond (gemstone)	10
Sapphire (gemstone)	9
Alumina (aluminium oxide)	9
Topaz (quartz gemstone)	8
Quartz (crystallised silicon dioxide)	7
Tool steel (high carbon, H & T)	6.5
Silica (silicon dioxide)	5.5
Glass (silica + soda ash + lime)	5.5
Carbon steel (plain, not heat treated)	5
Limestone (natural rock)	3.5
Copper (pure)	3
Gypsum (plaster board)	2
Talc (magnesium silicate)	1

Disadvantages include:

- cost per component,
- high tool cost,
- brittle, and
- low resistance to shock.

There are even machinable grades available now: just buy a block and make your own components! Table 7.3 shows some comparative surface hardnesses.

7.6 DIAMOND

Diamond is a hard crystalline form of carbon. If pure it is colourless: various 'tints' occur due to contamination. Diamond is formed under great pressure and heat, so diamond is very temperature resistant and is used in high precision hot running optics. Industrial diamond is used in abrasives for grinding and lapping and as point cutters for drilling.

Diamonds are the hardest of all naturally occurring materials and Table 7.4 shows the Moh's hardness scale with diamond at the top. This is a scale in which each mineral in the list can scratch the one below it, any other material can be classified by which mineral will scratch it. Diamonds are used in testing machines to provide quantative hardness values: the Moh's scale is a comparative ranking. Rockwell and Vickers' machines each utilise a diamond pyramid to quantify values; the Brinell test uses a hardened steel ball.

Approximately 6 tonnes of natural diamonds are made available each year by the mine owners, but industrial use is mainly of the synthetically manufactured types. These extremely useful grades are made by compressing

Table 7.4 Moh's scratch test for surface hardness

Mineral	Moh's scale
Diamond	10
Corundum	9
Topaz	8
Quartz	7
Orthoclase feldspar	6
Apatite	5
Fluorite	4
Calcite	3
Gypsum	2
Talc	1

graphite at 800 000–1 800 000 psi at temperatures of 1500–2400°C, with a catalyst of chromium, nickel or another metal, which forms a thin film between the base graphite and the slowly forming diamond crystal. Much higher temperatures and pressures would be necessary, putting up the cost and process difficulties, if no catalyst were used.

These synthetic crystals can be used as contacts in high-running temperature thermistors, as glass cutters, mounted on oil drilling tips, crushed to form powder and added to lapping or polishing paste. Crushed diamond is compounded with rubber to form grinding wheels (bonded compounds of epoxy or other adhesives are used): the diamond powder size determines the wheel grade, final use, and which materials can be machined in this way. There are newer, more exotic, applications of these industrial synthetic diamonds since the manufacturing process has been able to grow single crystals to a particular size or configuration. One of these uses is in microsurgery where a single diamond crystal is mounted onto a scalpel holder, back lit by fibre optics in the handle, and used as a cutting tool by ophthalmic (eye) surgeons.

7.7 LATEX (NATURAL RUBBER)

Latex is a sticky white liquid tapped from special trees. Natural latex from tropical trees was the only source of rubber until 1945, then artificial rubbers became available. Synthetic latex is manufactured by emulsion polymerisation techniques from styrene–butadiene copolymer, acrylate resins, polyvinyl acetate and other similar compounds. Small latex particles are formed, 0.05–0.15 μm in diameter, which are superior to the natural type and can be used as binders, in paints or coatings.

Raw natural rubber cannot be used directly as an engineering material since it is in a thermoplastic state and any deformation when stretched is permanent, because the long chain molecules only have van der Waals forces

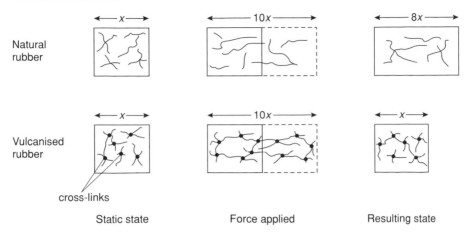

Figure 7.1 Structures of natural rubber and vulcanised rubber before and after deformation.

between them. When the raw material is vulcanised the van der Waals forces are replaced by cross-links and the material becomes elastic. This is illustrated in Figure 7.1.

Vulcanising was first started commercially by Goodyear in 1839. He used sulphur to make the cross-links between polyisoprene molecules. In modern treatment a vulcanising agent and other compounds are added to the raw material to provide alternative physical properties, e.g. carbon filler increases both strength and abrasion resistance.

The stiffness of the finished rubber depends on the extent of cross-linking which is determined by the amount of vulcanising agent used. A number of polymer chains will remain unlinked, and they are susceptible to oxidation. This reduces the elasticity and the rubber becomes brittle or 'perishes'. To overcome this problem antioxidants are added to the original mixture.

Styrene rubber, a synthetic rubber, is a copolymer of butadiene and styrene and was developed in the USA in the early 1940s. It has very similar physical properties to natural rubber but could be easily and cheaply manufactured from less costly and more readily available base materials. It does not rely on a limited natural resource. Styrene rubber is used for car tyres, hose pipes and electrical insulation.

Other synthetic rubbers are neoprene, butyl rubber and nitrile rubber. Table 7.5 shows the rubber types and the monomer(s) involved. Neoprene is an expensive rubber because the vulcanising is carried out with metallic oxides such as MgO or ZnO. Butyl rubber has the advantage of being the most chemically resistant of the rubbers and is impermeable to oxygen and other gases. Nitrile rubber is a high temperature material but expensive. Table 7.6 shows applications against each rubber type. Rubber parts can be

Table 7.5 Rubber types

Rubber	Monomer
Natural	Isoprene
Neoprene	Chloroprene
Styrene rubber	75% butadiene and 25% styrene
Butyl rubber	87% isobutylene and 2% isoprene
Nitrile rubber	Butadiene and acrylonitrile

Table 7.6 Rubber applications

Material	Uses
Natural rubber	Diaphragms, ballons, thin wall dipped profiles, condoms
Neoprene	Gaskets, sheathing, hoses, V belts, padding and sound insulation, O rings
Styrene rubber	Car tyres, footwear, hose pipes, conveyors, electrical insulation
Butyl rubber	Air bags, inner tubes, diaphragms, hoses, tank linings
Nitrile rubber	Gaskets, cable insulation, seals, O rings

produced by a large number of methods, most commonly by extrusion and injection moulding but also by compression transfer moulding, blanking (from extruded sheet), die cutting and dipping.

7.8 FUSED QUARTZ (SODIUM DIOXIDE)

Quartz is a melted compound of natural minerals or sand. When artificially manufactured it is called fused silica. This material has very good thermal and chemical resistance with excellent compressive strength and because of its low thermal expansion it is suitable for applications such as optical flats or precision mirrors.

Silica has high transparency and is used on good quality windows or from protective viewing ports in hazardous conditions. It is totally unaffected by all acids except hydrofluoric acid and is only mildly attacked by caustic alkalis. The high melting point of 1700°C gives rise to some electronic component support applications.

7.9 SHAPE-MEMORY METAL

Shape-memory metal is a nickel–titanium alloy which can be deformed and then return to its original shape on the application of heat. It is now used instead of some of the more traditional electromechanical assemblies, in particular bimetallic strips.

Discovered by scientists in the Naval Research Laboratory in 1962, shape-memory was an effect observed in certain nickel–titanium alloys. It was found that below particular temperatures these alloys could be deformed into new shapes (up to 8% deformation) and then could be returned to the original shape if the temperature was raised above the fixing level. This could be made to occur a number of times with no adverse effect on the metal.

In the early 1970s a company called Raychem developed two groups of alloys with shape-memory effect: one used β–brass and was named 'Bettalloy' the other used Ni–Ti and was called 'Tinel'. The company emphasis is now on Tinel. Tinel alloys combine excellent shape-memory properties, good mechanical and physical characteristics and are cost effective in manufacture. They are strong, resistant to corrosion and stress fatigue, and are dimensionally stable in temperature extremes.

Tinel alloys have been used to create a range of products as diverse as a high-pressure pipe coupling, mechanical fasteners, super-elastic wire, and thermally and electrically operated actuator springs. The shape-memory phenomenon results from a crystalline phase change known as the martensitic transformation. When the metal is cooled below a certain temperature the highly twinned martensitic phase that forms is clearly visible in a microscopic view of the surface. Under examination it contrasts sharply with the higher temperature austenitic phase. Tinel alloy is very soft, similar to solder, during the 'cold' martensitic phase and can be deformed by up to 8% in tension, compression or shear. When heated the martensitic state becomes unstable and the alloy returns to its strong austenitic state and recovers its original form.

The composition of the alloy determines the temperature range involved and can be modified to suit the working environment. The transformation can be reversed, but it should be noted that the temperature at which it occurs is different during heating than in cooling. The cycle can be repeated indefinitely.

To illustrate the operation of this effect and its application to actual products here are a few examples.

1. 'Cryofit' couplings are tubular components machined 2–3% smaller than the diameter of the tubing to be joined. When cooled to the martensitic state the soft metal is expanded to be a slide fit to the tubes and it is placed over the join of two tubes. When allowed to heat up to ambient temperature the coupling constricts to grip and seal; the clamping stresses can reach 100 000 p.s.i., providing a uniform clamp which is repeatable over and over again. Figure 7.2 illustrates the Cryofit coupling.
2. Cryocon connections are gas tight, highly effective electrical connections requiring no external housing or fitment, ideal where size or weight (and access) is limited. They offer excellent protection in corrosive conditions.

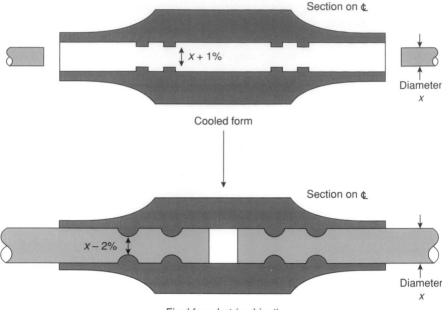

Cooled form

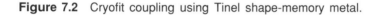

Final form hot (ambient)

Figure 7.2 Cryofit coupling using Tinel shape-memory metal.

3. The 'Split-fit' is initially a ring but can be cooled and deformed into the shape of an ellipse. Figure 7.3 shows the two stages. Once fitted and allowed to heat up the ring regains its shape and closes the split tangs of the connector.
4. Finally, an example of a thermal activator (heated either by direct temperature change or electrically) contained within a tailored housing. On one side a standard steel spring pushes against a dedicated Tinel spring as shown in Figure 7.4. At low temperature the shape-memory spring is soft and allows a bias to the steel spring, as the temperature rises the Tinel spring becomes stiffer and stronger pushing against the steel spring and allowing the piston controlling the fluid or whatever to move across. Daimler–Benz make use of this method to control oil pressure in their automatic shift systems.

7.10 TUFNOL

Tufnol is an engineering composite supplied in many forms.

- Cotton laminate.
- Paper–phenolic laminate.

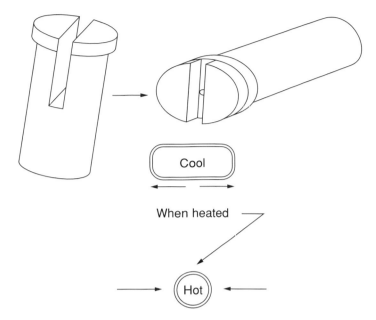

Figure 7.3 Split-fit connector using Tinel shape-memory metal.

- Paper–epoxy laminate.
- Epoxy–cotton laminate.
- Asbestos–phenolic laminate.
- Polyester–glass mat laminate.
- Glass-fibre laminate.

These forms are designed to offer a very wide range of physical properties from heat tolerance bands of 90°C to 300°C or compressive strengths up to 420 MPa. The laminates are made by laying-up resin-impregnated sheets of either paper or cotton or whatever the base material; once stacked together they are pressed and heated. This cures the resin and forms a solid sheet. By using different reinforcing sheets the Tufnol material can be modified to meet mechanical, electrical and chemical property requests from customers.

The phenolic paper grade is used as an electrical insulator and is very stable in humid and high voltage conditions. Although low on the strength and toughness scales compared with other grades, this is the cheapest and most suitable non-metallic alternative.

The cotton-phenolic grade is the most common with excellent wear resistance, good strength and good toughness characteristics. It is split into subgroups by varying the coarseness of the cotton weave. The wider, stronger types are used for components requiring more in-built strength and on physically larger jobs. When good surface finish, close dimensional tolerances

Tinel spring

Steel spring

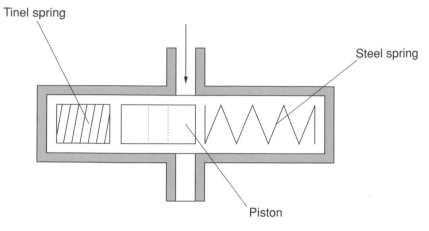

Piston

Closed (cold)

Sections on ℄

Tinel spring extended

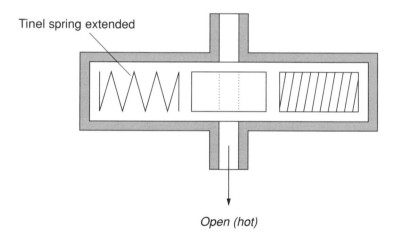

Open (hot)

Figure 7.4 Thermally activated valve using Tinel shape-memory spring.

or high strength in thin sections is needed then a finer grade weave is appropriate.

The asbestos laminates are better suited to high-temperature applications than the paper or cotton grades, but this high temperature tolerance is at the detriment of the electrical properties, and there are now stringent health and safety requirements for working with asbestos.

The epoxy–paper and epoxy–cotton laminates have excellent electrical properties, good dimensional stability and wear resistance. They are easy to machine and maintain a good surface finish.

Glass fibre grades have high strength and dimensional stability. The high fibre content dictates the applications since it is not wear resistant, nor is it so easy to machine as the other grades.

Care should be taken with any grade when machining a component from solid. The laminated grain structure provides both strength and weakness, depending upon the direction of each layer. It is essential that the correct section is chosen to ensure that the laminates give strength in the optimal direction for the use. This also applies even when no load bearing is destined for the part but some complex machining is necessary.

7.11 BIODEGRADABLES

When biodegradable materials are mentioned everyone will have their own interpretation of the word. For the manufacture of medical devices we need biodegradable materials which are:

- able to be sterilised by ETO, gamma or steam,
- easy to make into usable products,
- degradable in its selected environment, internal or external, without additional substances having to be applied,
- sufficiently stiff and strong enough,
- not too expensive,
- safe for the patient, and
- safe for the environment.

It is becoming increasingly important to promote these types of materials because of the awareness now being shown by the medical and environmental lobbies. The first degradable applications and probably the most well-known were degradable surgical sutures. These were introduced in 1967 by Schmitt and Polistina in the USA when they patented an application using polyglycolic acid (PGA). This was very closely followed by Dexon, another USA product, which was called an absorbable suture. The next new player to enter this market was Ethicon with a product called Vicryl, a 92:8 glycolic acid–lactic acid copolymer. Ethicon has been quite prolific, in the early days between the mid-1970s and the late 1980s developing many new and exciting variations. The acceptance of these materials by the scientific bodies and the general public has allowed the evolution of many innovative applications. Table 7.7 shows some examples.

Controlled drug release is a new field which is developing rapidly, because of the limited control conventional methods of application give for drug introduction. Modern ways of producing drugs allows their mixing, placement or application to be modified quite easily, it's the carrier which presents the bigger challenge. Table 7.8 shows methods of drug transfer and application.

Table 7.7   Classification of some biocompatible devices

Biocompatible groups	Applications
Permanent fixtures	Hernia support, fracture plates and pins
Biodegradables	
Temporary fixtures	Ligament repair and support
Absorbed devices	Drug delivery ssytems, sutures
External devices	Protective films

Table 7.8   Methods of drug delivery

Drug in solution	Spike/bag
	Needle and syringe
	Oral
Drug absorption	Patches
	Implanted capsules
	Impregnated bandage
	Nasal spray
	Topical creams

Bayer Plastics have developed a biodegradable polymer designed and formulated for the packaging industry. It is fully acceptable to the environmentalist lobby, and there is proof that the polymer will interact with the other materials it is buried with and instigate a bacteriogical deterioration to take place.

As an example of a biodegradable medical product, think of a simple spring clip, moulded in biodegradable plastic. This could be applied to a blood vessel or similar, and clipped shut to clamp the vessel. Over the next year or so it would be absorbed into the body but the damaged vessel or tube would remain closed. This might be to close blood vessels when removing the gall bladder, or maybe for clamping fallopian tubes. The idea is yours to evolve free of charge. Figure 7.5 illustrates this concept.

The two examples above which describe the disposable packing and the speculative product concept, depend on soluble biodegradable plastics. The next material is different. A company called Zeneca has launched a degradable polymer group under the trade name of Biopol. Biopol polymers are produced from natural plant based resources by a chemical manufacturing process which uses sunlight as the primary energy source. The polymers are stable, moisture resistant (under normal storage and use), can be processed by conventional methods and have the properties normally associated with more traditional plastics. The material can be disposed of in the standard way or will degrade, ideally when compounded with household waste. Alternatively it can be recycled and used again, then eventually incinerated with no toxic residue.

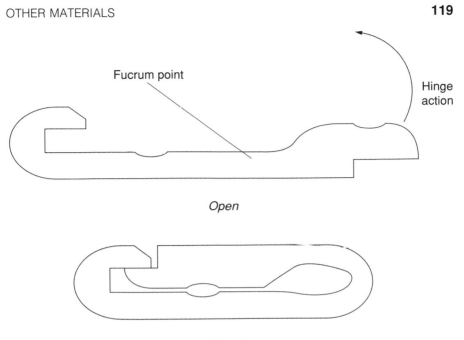

Fucrum point

Hinge action

Open

Closed

Figure 7.5 Biodegradable vessel clamp idea.

Biopol materials are thermoplastic polyesters composed of hydroxy-butyrate (HB) and hydroxyvalerate (HV) units incorporated randomly throughout the polymer chain. The final chemical structure of PHB/V copolymers is shown in Figure 7.6. The Biopol cycle is shown in Figure 7.7 It is produced by fermentation of a sugar feedstock by naturally occurring micro-organisms. The physical properties vary depending upon the HV content, so the flexibility and tensile strength can be modified to give a range which resembles the physical properties of polyethylene and polypropylene. Table 7.9 shows a comparison of values with the two polymers mentioned.

Here are some actual product examples of Biopol biodegradables in use, the potential is unlimited.

- Linien and Sanara bottles: shampoo and skincare product containers. These are stable enough to hold their form even in the high moisture environment of a bathroom.
- Cup, knife and fork: paper cups coated in Biopol resin. Knife and fork resistant to grease, moisture and heat.
- Garden: compost bags, plant pots, fertiliser bags. Use and return to the compost pile.
- Fishing nets: if lost they will sink to the sea floor and then degrade with minimal effect on marine life.

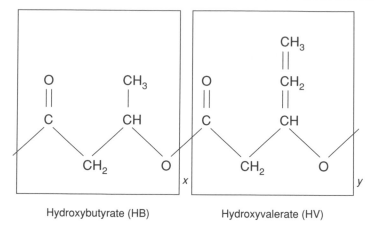

Hydroxybutyrate (HB)   Hydroxyvalerate (HV)

Figure 7.6   Structure of hydroxybutyrate–hydroxyvalerate copolymer.

Table 7.9   Comparative polymer properties. Reproduced by permission of Monsanto Company

Property	Biopol	LDPE	PP
Melting point (°C)	136–162	105–110	160–168
Melt flow index (g/10 min)	5.8	1.1–22	0.3–4.0
Young's Modulus (kPa × 10^3)	400–1000	100–200	1400–1800
Tensile strength (kPa × 10^2)	200–310	80–100	250–350
Elongation at break (%)	8–42	150–600	400–900

- Food packaging: at present under evaluation by the FDA and the European Commission. No leaching of toxins to product or food.

It is likely that more biodegradable materials will be developed and soon become available. A full definition of biodegradability could be as follows: the susceptibility of a substance to decomposition by micro-organisms, specifically the rate at which compounds may be chemically broken down by bacteria or natural environmental factors. Easily biodegraded species include ethanol, benzoic acid, benzaldehyde, ethyl acetate. Less easily degraded species include ethylene glycol, isopropanol, diethylene glycol and triethanddiamine. Resistant to biodegradation are methanol, monoethanolamine, methylethylketone, and acetone. But there are additives that will accelerate biodegradation in polyethylene, polystyrene and other 'common' polymers.

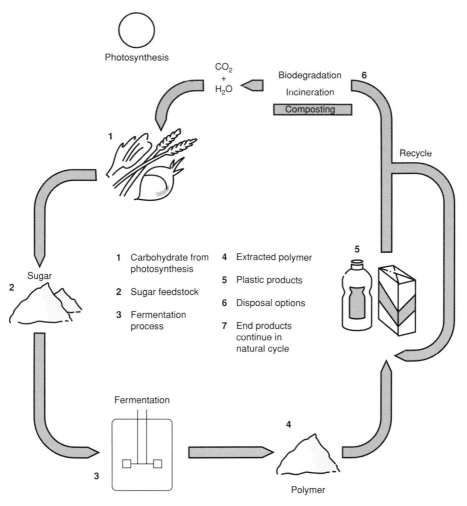

Figure 7.7 The Biopol cycle. Reproduced by permission of Monsanto Company

7.12 ACKNOWLEDGEMENTS

Information for the biodegradables section was kindly provided by Zeneca Bio Products, Cleveland, UK; the Biopol business is now owned by Monsanto Company, St Louis, MO, USA.

8
Adhesives

Long gone are the days of just one pot of glue was used for all jobs and never trusted unless there was mechanical fixation as well. Now there are adhesives to bond metals, plastics, fibres, glass and anything else you can envisage.

Dissimilar materials, different types of surface finish, hostile environments, hot or cold: all circumstances are provided for with modern adhesives. In special cases the manufacturers will devise a custom adhesive just for you. Years ago adhesives were poor and, deservedly, they were not taken seriously in engineering. Now high quality adhesives have a very different reputation, and some bonded joints are stronger than those made by traditional methods, see Table 8.1.

Adhesives should be carefully selected from the huge range available so that their particular properties suit a specific application. Information and assistance is available from manufacturers and suppliers to aid the selection process. Help available from suppliers may include:

- knowledge of prior applications,
- test results for bonding, shear and tensile stress,
- physical testing of an assembly,
- samples for your own assessment,
- information on new types, grades, methods of applying either on the market now or about to be launched, and
- advice on joint design.

From my experience, once they become aware of any new uses you may have then the support is overwhelming.

You need to be aware of the area of use, what heat there will be, any light bright or otherwise, will the bond be wet at any time, types of materials to be bonded, loading, safety considerations and many other factors. Once you have assessed these requirements you will be able to narrow down the options for adhesive bonding. Then call an adhesives company and obtain samples. Build the joint or a simulation and then destroy it. Check that the failure load is in excess of that in the design brief and all is well.

Adhesives are usually defined as materials that are used to create a bond between other materials. As solvents can create a bond between other

Table 8.1   Advantages and disadvantages of adhesive joints

Advantages	Disadvantages
• Able to join dissimilar materials. • Normally cheaper method than mechanical methods. • Generally hidden. • Dual properties of sealing and bonding. • Easy application, can also be restricted to one side only. • Production application can more easily be automated. • Lower internal stresses after curing. • Minimum joint distortion. • Majority of adhesives will sterilise by ETO and gamma without problems. • Excellent strength-to-weight ratio. • Lower capital cost investment.	• Base materials may be toxic. • Susceptible to bad process control and effect on joint (surface preparation). • Continuous use normally limited to below 130°C. • Joint normally permanent. • Joint design critical. • Existing surfaces textures affect the finished bond strength. • Cleaning and surface preparation critical. • Joint size proportional to finish strength. • Generally no warning prior to joint failure. • Still regarded by a large number of people within the manufacturing industry as a 'black art'.

materials I will include them. Adhesives may be supplied in the form of a paste, powder, film, cement, resin or liquid. They are all characterised by the materials on which they react, the degree of tack, the strength of the bond, the speed of cure and durability.

8.1   TYPES OF ADHESIVES

8.1.1   ANIMAL GLUE

Animal glue contains proteins obtained from boiled down animal waste products. The glue is soluble, applied as a highly viscous liquid and forms a strong bond with materials like paper, wood or leather. There is resistance to moisture, and the bond is cured by drying. The cost is very low, but there are problems due to the smell of finished goods and during processing.

8.1.2   STARCH GLUE

Starch glue is based on cornstarch with a high affinity for paper and is used for little else. The bond is sensitive to moisture and the glue is applied as water dispersions with a low temperature cure.

8.1.3   ANAEROBIC ADHESIVE

This adhesive is usually an acrylic-based liquid, although it is sometimes supplied as a paste. It cures by the exclusion of oxygen when component parts are assembled which allows polymerisation to take place at a slow rate unless catalysts are added (normally by the manufacturer). Although anaerobic adhesive can be used as a gap filler, there are limitations to the gap size which can be filled successfully. The usual thrixotropic type can seal gaps up to 0.4 mm thick, but normal clearances should not exceed 0.1 mm. These adhesives are used extensively for threadlocking and retaining parts when dimensional errors would result in scrap. They are best suited for high volume mechanical assemblies and areas where pins, circlips etc., would hinder assembly times.

8.1.4   STRUCTURAL ANAEROBIC ADHESIVE

This adhesive differs from the former by being based on resin systems which cure to provide a flexible adhesive. It can be used to fill gaps of up to 1.5 mm and within a temperature range of –60 to 230°C. Other advantages of this anaerobic system are that it can be cured without heat or mixing, the compound can easily be stored, there are no pot-life restrictions, and it is easy to clean products and equipment because of the relatively slow cure time. Another important advantage is that of low toxicity levels, and no ingredient which could cause skin reaction. Because of this structural anaerobic adhesives have become quite popular.

8.1.5   HOT MELT ADHESIVE

This is a thermoplastic which is normally solid at room temperature. The plastic melts on heating, is applied to a surface and as it cools the adhesion takes place. Compression of the two surfaces for a few seconds will aid the process as the material gels. The low surface tension of the liquid plastic makes it suitable for a wide range of materials. The adhesive includes a tackifying resin, viscosity modifier and the all important base polymer. Blending allows a range of properties to suit different applications. The base polymer varies but is normally EVA, EEA, nylon or polyester. The first two are used for carton sealing and book binding with the polyester generally classed as the engineering version due to its physical strength. Limitations include the short bond time which causes a need for rapid assembly and a narrow band of application temperatures, (too high or too low and the bond is weakened significantly). The liquid polymer has bad adhesion to smooth surfaces, so it is necessary to roughen surfaces to provide a key or to use porous materials.

8.1.6 CYANOACRYLATE GLUE

Initially known as 'superglue' when first introduced in about 1960, this group of adhesives has evolved to dominate the market. This is mainly due to the ability to bond dissimilar materials and act on virtually everything, with some notable exceptions. Cyanoacrylate works by the base alkali being activated by small amounts of moisture, but because of the adhesives' molecular structure, acids strongly inhibit curing and delays can be up to three minutes or more if the surfaces are contaminated. Flat hard surfaces cure more rapidly than porous or rough surfaces. With certain modifications cyanoacrylate fluids can be supplied in gel form and these can achieve successful gap fills; claims of 0.5 mm have been made but this is a very specialist application with a vast list of restrictions. Joints and their finished bonds will be affected by too low a moisture content on the contact surfaces, too large a gap and contamination by acids or acidic materials. For the best results metals are better than plastics, which are better than elastomers. With the normal ethyl or methyl cyanoacrylate materials sometimes there is a white stain left once the joint is cured, this is caused by the adhesive vapours (vented while curing) condensing too quickly. This problem is easily overcome by using a slower curing butylester grade. To enhance the bonding and increase the number of materials which can be used, surface treatment which cleans and degreases is encouraged. Recent developments and requirements within the medical device manufacturing industry have caused the major adhesive companies involved to carry out validation tests with the result that there is now available a large number of validated, cynoacrylates on the market, accredited for human implantation. One problem with 'superglue' is skin contact, so take care!

8.1.7 REACTIVE ACRYLIC ADHESIVE

This is an acrylic based adhesive which came about from two other types already described: anaerobic and cyanoacrylates. A two-part compound which needs a surface application, it cures fairly quickly with about 80% final strength after only 10 minutes. The cure time, as with others, is dependent on the materials to be joined and the gap size. Figure 8.1 shows the strength against time curves for various gap sizes.

8.1.8 PRESSURE SENSITIVE ADHESIVES

These are normally applied to a carrier material which supports and allows easy application. First introduced in the 1940s, the basic requirements of the pressure sensitive adhesives were to maintain a permanent tackiness in ambient conditions and not to need activation by water, solvent or heat. There are three forms in which pressure sensitive adhesives tapes are

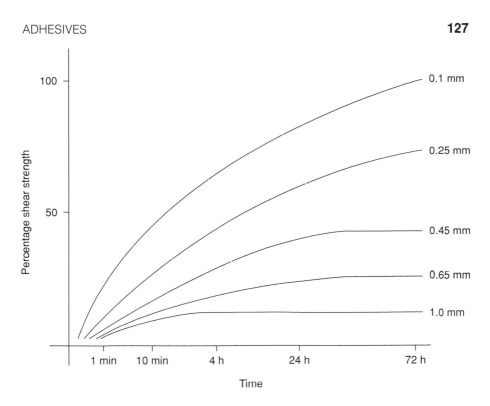

Figure 8.1 Adhesive cure strength and gap size.

supplied. The first is single coat like masking tape and sometimes backed by textiles, paper or metal; it can vary. This is used for domestic and industrial applications, packing etc. The second type is transfer coat. When the adhesive is pressed to a surface and the carrier removed, it leaves a thin film of the adhesive. If built up one on another it can be quite effective as a gap filler. The third type is double sided tape, which contains the carrier as normal but the adhesive has been applied to both sides. This requires a release paper on one side to allow handling and rolling of any quantity or length. Figure 8.2 shows the three types in cross section.

Pressure sensitive tapes are used worldwide with very little thought from the customer. They are cheap, simple and any size can be fabricated to suit the application. The carrier can be changed to provide additional features and properties. A disadvantage of this type of adhesive is that the final strength of the bond relies heavily on the carrier material and construction. Another disadvantage is that manufacturers are reluctant to make variations unless in large quantities.

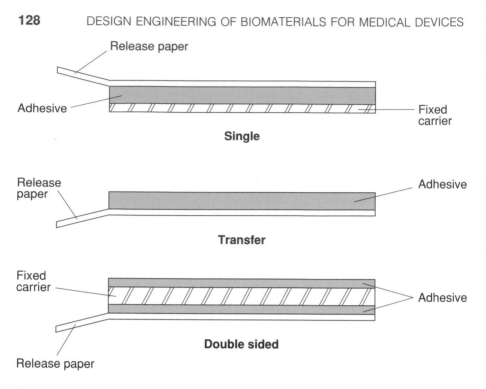

Figure 8.2   Three types of pressure sensitive tapes.

8.1.9   EPOXY ADHESIVES

Epoxy adhesive is normally associated with a two part system requiring exact measuring and mixing, but it can also be supplied in one part form which requires only heat to promote curing. The compound, once mixed or activated, solidifies by polymerisation when the ingredients combine. Heat aids the curing process and even accelerates it if applied externally, although there is significant self-heating during the initial chemical reaction. This self-heating can be detrimental to materials in contact if they have not been appropriately selected. A very simple rule to apply is the faster the set then the hotter the adhesive will become: check the individual components' tolerance to heat. The two part system comprises resin and hardener with the ratio determining not only the cure time but also the finished physical properties. One-part epoxy includes a catalyst which is activated by external heating. Epoxy adhesives are thermosetting and will soften slightly if heat is applied after curing but not enough to allow post manipulation. Resistant to the majority of commonly used chemicals, oils and solvents, most noticeable is its inertness once cured, a feature more and more being recognised by medical device manufacturers who use it widely for encapsulation rather than as an adhesive. The finished compound can be modified by different formulations to give a flexible or rigid, tough or brittle, clear or opaque, hard or soft material bonding to virtually all types of surfaces or substrates. The working temperature range is −150 to 200°C. Surface adhesion will be very poor if the workpiece is contaminated by any form of protein-based preserving oil. Another problem is the need to control the mixing ratio when using two part compounds because of the effect this has on the finished joint material. Working time with most epoxies is quite good, but support fixtures may be needed for the initial contact until the finished article can be self-supporting. Epoxy resins have a very low shrinkage rage so they can be applied to pre-stressed assemblies and create no additional stress within.

8.1.10   TOUGHENED ADHESIVE

This started life 25 years ago when epoxies were enhanced by the addition of rubber or liquid polymer compounds (the cured epoxy was found to have rubber particles about 1 μm diameter dispersed equally throughout). The resulting adhesive was tougher and had an improved peel strength. It was found that the particles prevented crack propagation, see Figure 8.3. There are three variations of the technique: toughened anaerobic, acrylic, or epoxy.

8.1.10.1   Toughened Anaerobic Adhesive

With enhanced peel strength and shock loading, this improved anaerobic adhesive is used for all types of lap joints.

8.1.10.2   Toughened Acrylic Adhesives

Supplied in all forms: liquid, thick resins and semi-solid thixotropic compounds. Some require an additional hardener to activate, others a mild surface primer. These are a versatile tool for assembly, but cannot be used on rubber-based materials or polymers like polyethylene or polyolefins with low coefficients of friction.

8.1.10.3   Toughened Epoxy Adhesives

Toughening is a suitable process for both types of epoxy, single and two part, but caution should be exercised when selecting the final application. Some of these adhesives produce a lot of heat on curing, which can damage the article.

8.1.11   SOLVENTS

Solvents are not usually considered true adhesives since the solvents them-selves evaporate away and do not form part of the finished joint. But as a

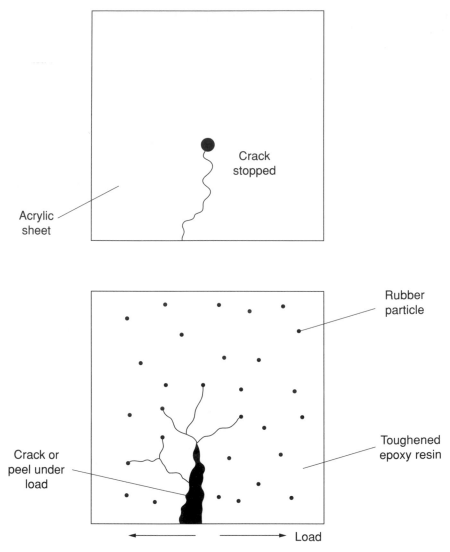

Figure 8.3 Crack-stopping by particulate toughening in epoxy resins.

carrier or a mechanism to seal two surfaces together the solvent is, in effect, an adhesive.

Directly applied solvents can seal and bond joints if there is dimensional accuracy in the components. This method is not applicable for gap filling.

When solids are dissolved in a solvent and then applied to a joint some gap filling is possible. Concentrations should be about 30%; if the solid content is more, high viscosity will result in poor wettability and impair the resulting bond. As with direct solvent application, the removal of the excess fluid either by evaporation or absorption is a limiting factor which may result in the need for a long open time. This approach is not recommended for structural or load bearing assemblies.

Both methods can create safety problems. COSHH and other Health and Safety regulations must be complied with. To achieve safe vapour concentrations ventilation is required. There are some toxicity problems that are poorly understood.

8.1.12 UV CURE ADHESIVES

UV adhesives are a one-part system in which a liquid is cured by exposure to ultraviolet light. (There are some which are cured by visible light.) The liquids have a wide range of viscosities of 100–10 000 MPa.s. They are used not only as adhesives but also to encapsulate or 'pot'. These systems are becoming very popular because of the speed at which the compound sets once exposed to the high intensity light. Not all the material used may cure because a direct line of sight is required to ensure that the polymerisation process occurs. Sometimes a secondary cure is necessary; this can be achieved by heat, moisture, oxygen, an activator or anaerobicaly. After curing, although the base material has hardened, you may find a residual surface tackiness. This can be eliminated or reduced by the application of heat or external fluids, but in many cases require new lamps or a different wavelength. UV systems are particularly favoured during production because of the ease of assembly, and time available to correct wavelength. UV systems are particularly favoured during production because of the ease of assembly, and time available to correct alignment before a high intensity 'zap'. At least one external component or surface must be transparent. UV cure adhesives offer a high strength bond with all the advantages of epoxy plus flexibility of application and, when used as an adhesive, a very good gap filling capacity. Storage of the base materials should be between 10 and 30°C to prevent crystals forming and, of course, protection from exposure to daylight is required.

Critical safety measure are needed to ensure that there can be no exposure of the operators' eyes or skin.

8.1.13 SILICONE ADHESIVES

These are supplied in both one and two part systems, curing by evaporation of solvents or as a result of chemical reaction. Silicone adhesives are compatible with a great many surfaces but are costly and must be protected from moisture before use. They have good shear, tensile, impact and peel strength, and excellent resistance to chemicals and solvents with good adhesion to nearly everything. The bond is flexible, and has high temperature resistance.

Table 8.2   Adhesive types

Adhesive Type	Advantages	Disadvantages
Start	Water applied. Little environmental problem.	Limited to use on paper.
Anaerobic	Easy production use. Seals most mechanical assemblies.	Will not seal gaps over 0.3 mm successfully. Cost.
Structured	No mixing needed. Cures at ambient temperature. Low toxicity.	No structural indication of potential failure.
Hot melt	Easily applied. Rapid bond strength. Flexible joint.	Low creep strength. Application temperature critical.
Cyanoacrylate	Rapid cure. Covers the majority of materials.	Expensive (relative?). Low tolerance to surface contamination.
Tape	Cheap. Easily used. Varied types.	Low creep loading. Bad temperature tolerance.
Epoxy	Inert. Tough. Adheres to most materials.	Two-part mix ratio critical. Low tolerance to surface contamination. Brittle. Base materials may be toxic.
Solvent	Easy to alloy. Hidden joint. Applies to most polymers.	Health and Safety problems. Toxic.

Table 8.3   Examples of applications of adhesives

Adhesive	Applications
Anaerobic	Thread locking, gasket seals, joint sealing, bearing mounting.
Cyanoacrylate	Flexible belt, 'O' ring manufacture, Printed circuit board assemblies, latex balloons to catheters, 'Instant' adhesive superglue.
Hot melt	Low temperature/load applications, book binding, packing cases and boxes, laminated sheet.
Epoxy	Needle hubs, potted encapsulation, metal to plastic assemblies, hostile environments, high pressure loads.
Solvent	Luer locks, i.v. sets, filter bodies, drainage bottles, tubing sets.
Tape	Wrapping, sticky tape, double sided tapes, transfer labels.
Pressure sensitive tape	Self adhesive labels, foam backed padded tapes.
UV adhesive	Needle hubs, stainless steel hubs to glass syringe, bond for soft PVC to rigid PVC in anaesthesia masks.

Either of the two types, air curing or chemical reaction, can be loaded with different fillers to vary the physical properties of the end result.

Adhesive types are summarised in Table 8.2 and applications in Table 8.3.

8.2 SURFACE PREPARATION

Many of the surfaces which require bonding will only provide a good joint if they have been properly prepared. This preparation could be a simple rub down with a cloth to remove minor particles, a degrease in solvents or a complete multi-part strip down. Many of the adhesives described in this chapter will not be successful if there is any form of surface contamination. Surface treatments present problems for bonding techniques, e.g. plating, painting or any form of coating. Certain material groups have their own particular restrictions like moulded plastics which may contain plasticisers or have been treated with a mould release agent. Some polymers have a low surface energy because of oxide films formed during storage. Most surface treatment does not just clean the areas to be bonded but also prepares the component for wetting by the adhesive. The following methods are those most commonly used.

8.2.1 PRIMER

A primer stabilises and strengthens the surface to accept the adhesive bond.

8.2.2 CHEMICALLY MODIFY

This is an alternative to abrasion, in which a chemical is used to modify the surface, either by chemically changing the surface layer or by mechanically building a key for the adhesive to lock to. An example is acid etching, in which an oxide film with roughened contours is created.

8.2.3 PHYSICAL ABRASION

This roughens the surface as well as removing contamination and weak areas. Grit blasting is a one method and another uses emery cloth. Speed is important and the treated surface should be used within a specified time.

8.2.4 FLAME

Flame treatment is used to change the surface of materials like acetal, PTFE, polythene and polypropylene, by exposing the area to be bonded to the oxidising part of a gas flame. Oxygen atoms are added to the surface structure which increases the effectiveness of the adhesive bond. There are obviously safety hazards.

8.2.5 SOLVENT

Solvent cleaning is used to remove oils, grease and general contaminants and release agents from polymers. Detergents are an alternative to toxic

Table 8.4   Surface preparation for adhesive bonding

Material	Suggested preparation
Polymer	
ABS	Degrease with methyl alcohol or isopropyl alcohol.
Styrene	
LDPE	For extra adhesion abrade with medium grade emery cloth
HDPE	or tape.
PU	Solvent – best form of adhesive.
PVC	Cyanocrylate second choice.
Metal	
Aluminium	Degrease with solvent, either immerse or vapour type.
Copper	
Carbon	Roughen the surface with emery tape or chemically etch for
Nickel/chrome	greater bond strength.
Steel	Cyanoacrylate first choice then epoxy.
Tin	
Zinc	
Others	
Brick	Degrease with solvent by wiping.
Ceramic	Scrub the surface with wire brush and sand blast if still
Glass	contaminated.
Concrete	Epoxy to encapsulate, or toughened anaerobic.

solvents, coupled with scrubbing (abrasion) this can be a cost effective and environmentally acceptable method. Care should be taken with some of the solvents when polymers are involved.

8.2.6   CORONA DISCHARGE

This technique is used primarily for polymers which have a low surface energy and create problems with the adhesive bonding. It increases the surface energy by incorporating oxygen into the surface.

Surface preparation suggestions are shown in Table 8.4.

8.3   ADHESIVE SELECTION

As discussed above, modern adhesives should be selected for specific applications taking many relevant factors into account. While there is much helpful advice available from suppliers, it would be wise to consult more than one opinion or company before you make a final decision.

The other important decision that you have to couple with adhesive selection is joint design. The joint must be designed for adhesive bonding, preferably for a specific adhesive, and not just be borrowed from a failed mechanical fixing method.

Many of the factors to be considered are shown in Figure 8.4.

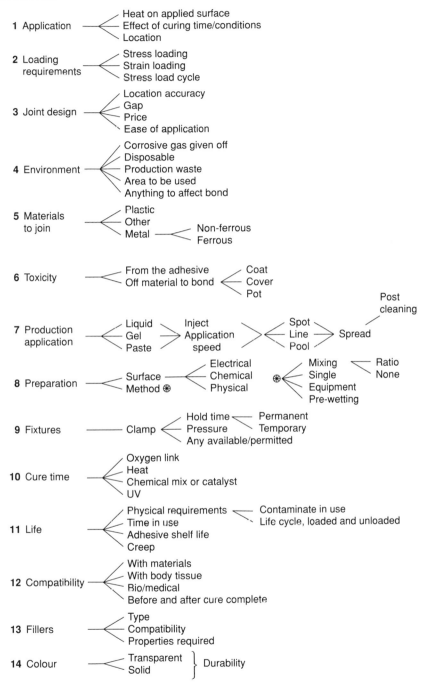

Figure 8.4 Selection criteria for adhesives.

8.3.1 MATERIALS INVOLVED

Metals, polymers, textiles: all have their own individual needs. Some must have surface preparation, some need physical restraints or supports, some should be considered as detrimental and changed.

8.3.2 LOADS

Consider the loads and stresses on the joint. Is it necessary to form a hermetic seal against gas or liquid? What about cosmetic implications?

8.3.3 SERVICE LIFE

How long must the joint endure? Must it survive the product or is a failure acceptable after a specified time? Storage time and service time?

8.3.4 JOINT DESIGN

Should a mechanical form be manufactured to accommodate the joint or should it be left as two mating surfaces? If a formal joint design is required then what form?

8.3.5 ENVIRONMENT

Many problems occur because of environmental effects. Consider both the effects of the environment on the adhesive joint, and any potentially toxic effects of the device or any treatment that it has had, on its host.

8.3.6 PRODUCTION ENGINEERING REQUIREMENTS

You must consider production needs, application methods, cure times and handling restrictions. Wettability and how the adhesive spreads is important. Is gap filling sufficient and what about pre-assembly requirements?

8.3.7 PRE-TREATMENT

If pre-treatment is required there are many factors to think about. What treatment, cost, time, does it need to be repeated, who can handle the solvents, etc?

8.3.8 BONDED APPLICATION

It may be necessary to convince sceptics of the validity of a bonded joint. In spite of various disadvantages listed here, you must make sure that the appropriateness of your proposed technique to the final application is the overriding consideration.

8.4   DESIGN OF ADHESIVE JOINTS

There are many opinions regarding the design of joints to suit adhesives, views which have been changed, questioned and vilified over the last ten years because of the advances and developments in the supply of adhesives.

There are still some basic principles which must be maintained to ensure a successful joint. Adhesives perform better in shear, tension and compression, so avoid peel or cleavage if possible. Figure 8.5 illustrates examples of adhesive joints.

Joints gain greater strength from increased width than length. If a lap joint is in shear the maximum stress is at the beam end. The bond can be improved by increasing the width rather than the length.

Materials to be joined should have the same coefficient of thermal expansion, or excessive shear stresses are produced. Also the adhesive should be modified or have fillers added if adverse temperature ranges are expected. Try to keep the actual bond line as thin as possible; this gives less chance of voids, slow or no cure and costs are lower because less adhesive is used. Select materials which require little or no-preparation, but if surface contamination is unavoidable, redesign the part to aid cleaning. Surface finish is important to the bond formed, so choose the right method of component manufacture. Try to evaluate the joint design by modelling and load testing. It is much better to scale test pieces and induced stresses in the lab, than to manufacture components and then test.

Figure 8.6 illustrates good and bad adhesive joint designs.

Examples of some of the more novel applications provide an insight into the use of adhesives, as well as helping potential choice of a group or type to use. But they also prove the great successes adhesives have managed in a comparatively short time.

8.5   DEVELOPMENTS WITH ADHESIVES IN MEDICAL DEVICES

8.5.1   LATEX BALLOONS

Latex balloons can be adhesive bonded to polyurethane tubes for use in high pressure catheters. Compatible with blood, there is no leaching or toxic contamination so any overspill of adhesive during assembly can be tolerated.

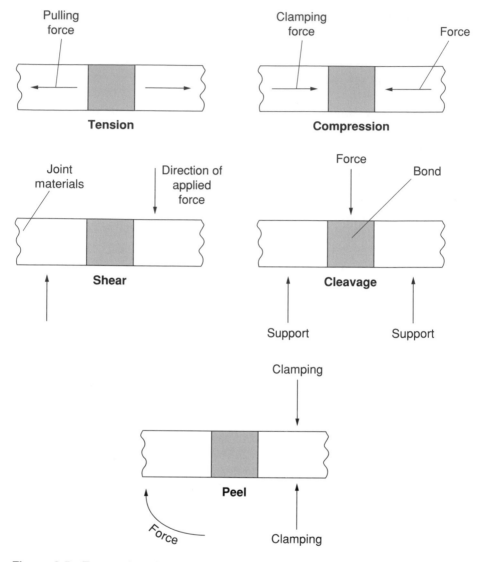

Figure 8.5 Types of strain at adhesive joints.

8.5.2 *TIP FORMING*

Tip forming is made possible by using the surface tension of one or two drops of adhesive to hold its smooth shape at the end of a stent or small diameter catheter; once solidified it produces a domed tip.

8.5.3 BONE REPAIR

In bone repair a viscous liquid, supplied in two parts, is mixed in an acid solution and then injected into the prepared site. Once injected it sets within 12 minutes and reaches final strength after only one hour. This system is designed to aid the healing of fractured hips, knees or wrists. A major advance is that over a long time the natural bone grows to replace the adhesive. This system is being trialled at the moment in four countries: France, Sweden, Netherlands and America.

8.5.4 WOUND CLOSURE

Instead of sutures, wounds can be closed with a tissue adhesive; a non-pigmented sterilised N-butyl cyanoacrylate. This bonds within seconds, holding the wound closed and sealed, with a little initial assistance from skin hooks which are then removed. It is claimed that scarring and trauma are reduced, and that because of the speed of closure there is less risk of infection. Made by Loctite and marketed under the name of Indermil, this adhesive also has a complete dedicated dispensing system.

8.5.5 UV CURING SILICONES

These glues are used to seal external tubing in ileostomy, urostomy and colostomy units. They are also used as the bonding agent in fabricated products such as endotracheal tube sets or urine drainage systems. Of course UV curing is not restricted to silicone, and alternatives are available to bond stainless steel needles to polymer hubs, dissimilar materials in anaesthesia masks, complete fascias to drainage containers and for sealing fibre optic catheter tips.

8.5.6 FIRBINOGEN TISSUE SEALANT

This is an adhesive to control blood leakage during surgery. Normally it is a two-part system consisting of donor fibrinogen and thrombin. It is used in general surgery, burns care and even during heart repair operations. The basic concept is to reduce the leakage caused within the chest cavity by the comparatively large number of small wounds which weep during and after surgery. This adhesive is made by Immuno A.G. of Vienna and marketed under the names Tisseal® and Tissvsol®. Another variation of this type of adhesive is a two part sealant which is mixed in the dispensing nozzle and used to 'plug' the hole left after a liver biopsy.

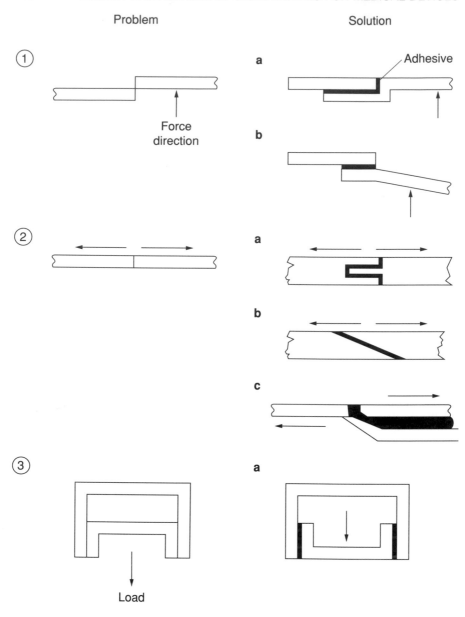

Figure 8.6 Designs for adhesive joints.

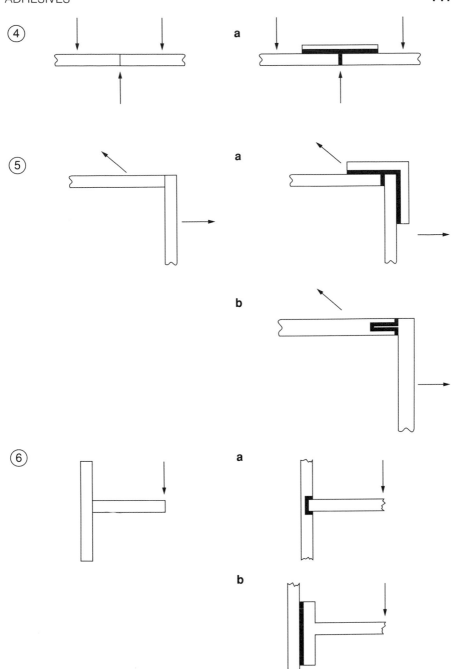

Figure 8.6 (*continued*)

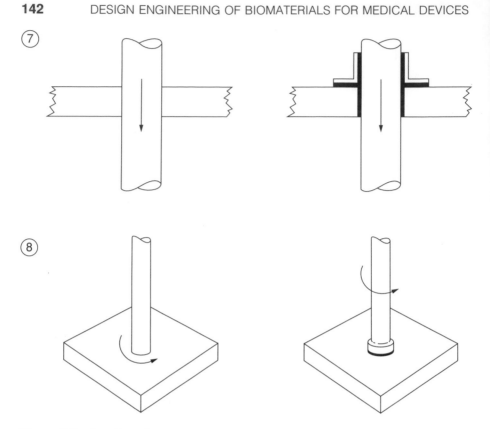

Figure 8.6   (*continued*)

Some people suggest that we have now reached the limit for using adhesives in medical applications, but I believe that there are many more applications which would benefit from the use of adhesives, and that with biomaterial and biochemical developments some invasive surgical procedures could become obsolete, replaced by simple day care visits and a 'pot of glue'.

9
Corrosion and Degradation

Inside the human body is warm and salty: a very corrosive environment. The body does not like to be tampered with and it invokes defence mechanisms when intruded. These factors make the body a hostile place for implanted materials.

Products that are not implanted are also vulnerable to corrosion from atmospheric conditions, during manufacture and storage, or in special settings such as during sterilisation.

Corrosion is by definition the degradation of metals and their alloys by electrochemical reaction with the surroundings. These surroundings may vary from strong acids or alkalis to a moisture laden atmosphere. These reactions are not always detrimental: for aluminium, copper and stainless steel a tenacious oxide covering is formed which effectively prevents any further growth of the oxide or other degradation, and serves to protect the base metal. For this reason aluminium and stainless steel are increasingly used for architectural purposes, and for instruments and articles visible to the public. Copper has been used for centuries to protect roofs; apart from the cosmetic appeal of the green colouring, the metal is easy to manipulate and helps to seal the roof's structure.

This protection on aluminium, stainless steel and copper means that it is not necessary to apply a secondary protective coating after manufacture, which can be a significant cost saving.

In the design of medical devices it is necessary to consider potential corrosion and degradation. There are two methods of prevention: either select a resistant material or protect the material from the harmful agents. Figure 9.1 illustrates a representation of the problem and some suggested solutions. Figure 9.2 shows some causes of corrosion.

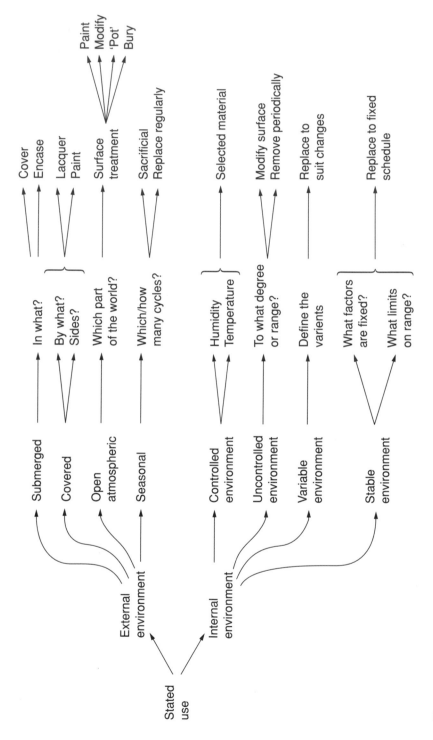

Figure 9.1 Choices of corrosion protection.

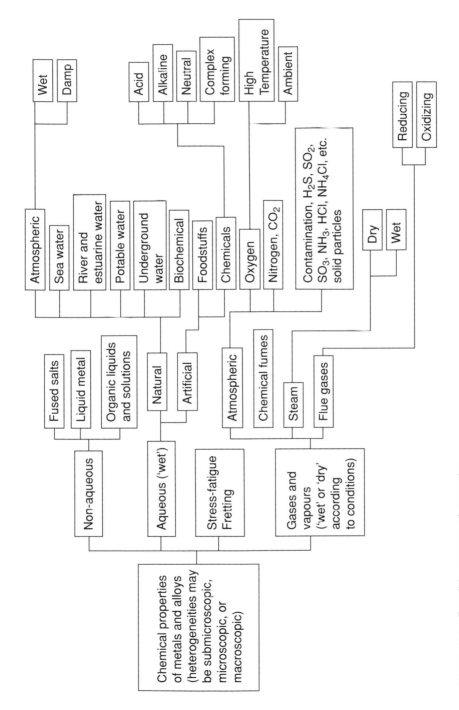

Figure 9.2 Possible causes of corrosion.

9.1 PROTECTION OR PREVENTION OF CORROSION

9.1.1 MATERIAL SELECTION

A correctly chosen material could solve corrosion problems in one go. Examples are needles made from stainless steel or instrument handles from aluminium. Alternatively, a polypropylene case may withstand 10 years in sea water. But be critical of these resistant materials, selection of copper for some environments can present a toxicity problem that will poison plant life.

9.1.2 SURFACE TREATMENTS

There are a number of methods which treat the surface of a metal and provide protection. These vary from simple heat treatment to complex ion implantation. Examples which best show this potential are blades, milling cutters and drills.

9.1.3 SURFACE MODIFICATION

This means changing or adding to the surface another coating which will survive the particular environment. The three most common methods are anodising aluminium, galvanising steel and plating metals or plastics.

9.1.4 SURFACE COATING

This includes painting and the application of epoxies and adhesive compounds. It is important that the coating adheres well to the base, and several layers or undercoats may be necessary.

So before you start to manufacture consider these points closely then select your material.

- Application: the actual end use.
- Location: environment, contamination, contained or not?
- Physical requirements: strength, size of item, finished weight, complexity of shape.
- Environment: wet or dry, hot or cold, extra problems.
- Users: skilled, unskilled, or automatic. What type of handling?

Listed below are various methods of treating metals and plastics that are commonly used in engineering and can be used for medical equipment where applicable.

9.2 SURFACE TREATMENTS AND COATINGS

9.2.1 ANODISING

Anodising is a general term given to the process of applying a hard coherent oxide coating to aluminium and some alloys by electrolytic methods. It is primarily for protection against corrosion but is sometimes applied for decoration or identification. The coating thickness and hardness can be varied to suit the application and with additional treatments dyes can be fixed to provide a permanent surface colour. The surface finish of the original workpiece is reproduced with a slight roughening, as there is no levelling effect. Any defects will be emphasised rather then hidden, so surfaces must be clean, well prepared and blemish free before treatment. Because the oxide coating is derived from the base metal itself, the corrosion resistance is dependant upon that same metal. The protection can be enhanced further by sealing the naturally occurring pores in the coating. There are a number of methods for sealing after anodising but normally immersion in boiling water is used to hydrate the oxide and form bulky by-products which plug the open pores. The ultimate is dichromate sealing (particularly good for marine and sea water splash conditions) which leaves within the coating a strong oxidising agent, this in turn helps to preserve the substrate from future attack. Surfaces can be painted after anodising, but owing to the inertness of the anodising, paint adhesion can be poor, so if the colouring is satisfactory why not leave it?

Anodising is normally grown to 50 μm thick for corrosion protection, this gives the best results and combination of properties at an economical cost. Remember that because of fixtures used to hold the components during the anodising process, there will always be small untreated areas and their location must be considered in the design.

Apart from corrosion protection, anodising is widely used to provide wear resistance, electrical insulation, decorative surface and temperature resistance (the melting point of the oxide is about 2000°C).

9.2.2 PLATING

The electroplating process normally applies a metallic coating to another metal substrate. There are plastics available now which can also be plated. The actual procedures vary depending upon the metal to be deposited and the substrate to be coated but in general it can simply be described as 'the transfer of metal from the anode (donor metal) to the cathode (substrate) in an electrolyte solution using electrical energy'. Plating provides a protective, and decorative, coat to the base material and imparts some of the properties of the donor metal. Materials that would not be suitable without protection can be plated and used with virtually no restriction. The added

Table 9.1 Metal plating combinations

Plating material	Steel	Zinc	PP	S/Steel	Al	PS	Copper	ABS	Brass
Cadmium	1								
Zinc	1								
Nickel	1, 2			5			1, 5		1, 5
Copper	4					4		3, 4	
Tin	1, 2, 3, 4						4		4
Chrome	2	2							
Silver	5						5		5
Gold	5						5		5
Copper/ nickel	1	1	5			5		5	
Cu/Ni/Cr	1	1	2	2, 5	1, 5	2, 5	1, 5	2, 5	2, 5

Key 1, Protection; 2, improved properties; 3, process protection; 4 base for further coatings or subsequent processing; 5, cosmetic appearance.

material can improve wear resistance, appearance, electrical conductivity or contact, better light reflection or even provide a more suitable surface for bonding additional materials. A multilayered approach, for example, is in the manufacture of printed circuit boards by electroplating copper to a phenolic sheet and then overplating with tin.

Coating thicknesses vary greatly but on average are between 0.003 and 0.05 mm for commercial applications.

The majority of metals can be plated but only a limited number of plastics are similarly treated, the more common ones being ABS, polysulphone, polypropylene and poly(phenylene oxide). There is loss of flexibility once the plastics are plated but this is outweighed by the lighter and more impact resistant assembly. Table 9.1 shows the more common combinations of base materials and their coatings, but should be viewed as an example of the frequency of use and not as recommended application partnerships.

9.2.3 ELECTROLESS NICKEL PLATE

Unlike conventional electroplating the electroless system operates chemically and, as its name implies, without electrical current. Coatings are deposited uniformly over the surface, overcoming one of the major drawbacks of the electroplating process. The resulting coat thickness is precise and even, easily monitored and controlled. This is a very viable, well used commercial process. Corrosion resistance is equal to that of stainless steel but is significantly cheaper because of the low cost of the substrates used. The hardness

Table 9.2 Suitability of materials for electroless plating

Best	Nickel, cobalt
Good	Aluminium, low-alloy or carbon steels, stainless steel
Fair	Require pre-treatment first: copper, glass, ceramic, plastic (ABS, polypropylene, polyphenylene oxide)
Poor	Require pre-treatment and copper plating first: lead, tin, zinc, cadmium

is 48–54 Rockwell (500–600 VHN) but this can be increased by heat treatment which will bring the finished article to a level of 60–70 Rockwell (900–1100 VHN).

Nickel plate allows previously unsolderable materials to be soldered; this is a significant advantage for stainless steel which can present a number of problems when used in electrical applications.

Metals that can be successfully treated this way are: stainless steel, carbon steels, copper or alloys, beryllium, titanium, magnesium and aluminium. If necessary it can also be used on nickel alloys.

Electroless nickel and copper plating can also be applied to some plastics, ceramics and other non-conductive base materials provided these are correctly prepared and properly pre-treated (see Table 9.2).

The only drawback is the cost which is about 50% more than electroplating.

9.2.4 HEAT TREATMENT

Heat treatment will not prevent oxides from forming or propagating, but it will delay it for a considerable time in normal working conditions. Providing a high enough carbon steel is used, the heat treatment is carried out in an oven and the finished article is polished (or 'blued'). The resultant item will be reasonably rust proof, but this is a temporary reprieve.

9.2.5 VAPOUR DEPOSITION PROCESSES

In theory any metal can be deposited as a coating (as can some non-metals such as silicon monoxide, cadmium sulphite and a few polymers) but in practical terms the actual metals used are restricted. For vapour deposition the coating material is heated in a vacuum and as it evaporates it is allowed to condense on the target (cooler) surfaces in line of sight. Limitations arise from the need for a vacuum chamber, with the related problems of component size, and the thinness of the coating produced. Although the coating is thin, it does have all of the properties of the coating material, and there is sometimes an advantage of such a thinness. Another consideration for the designer is to ensure that the assembly will withstand the vacuum necessary: if not then a chemical deposition method may be more suitable.

The main advantage of the vapour deposition system is that polymer coatings condense to provide a uniform thickness even on small sections or in crevices, where a liquid technique would be unsuccessful because of surface tension.

Vapour deposition can be applied to inner, as well as outer, surfaces. There is a limiting internal diameter which cannot be coated but this is easily established by one quick process trial.

The next four sections describe types of vapour deposition.

9.2.5.1   Ion Implantation

This is a vacuum chamber deposition process as in metallising, lens blooming etc., but which uses a high voltage glow discharge to prepare and activate the surface, and accelerate the coating material towards it. As a result a very high adhesion is obtained. Some of the applications are from the aerospace industry, such as aluminium coating of titanium alloys, silver coating on steels, and conductive or reflective coatings on non-metal substrates.

9.2.5.2   Sputtering

Sputtering techniques use a low pressure sealed chamber and operate by ion bombardment of an item. This is used primarily for coating machine tools and in electron microscopy.

9.2.5.3   Chemical Vapour Plating

This technique doe not require a sealed chamber, low pressure or vacuum, but operates by thermal decomposition of gases of the plating material onto the pre-heated surfaces of the target. Examples of some depositions of this type are with carbides or borides. Unfortunately, because of the comparatively high pre-heat temperatures required for the substrates (over 600°C) only some metal alloys can be processed in this way.

9.2.5.4   Glow Discharge

This is a technique which involves the polymerisation of organic monomers in a gas discharge to coat the whole surface of a component, or assembly, with a very thin polymer film. This method produces a pin-hole free film with no volatile inclusions. There are many applications including the deposition of polyparaxylyene onto finished printed circuit boards to give an insulating protective film. This is comparatively cheap, easy, low pressure, low temperature method. Table 9.3 lists the properties and advantages a polymer applied this way can provide, the details provided by Nova Tran Ltd.

Plasma coating is also used in medical applications, an example is plasma sprayed hydroxyapatite coatings on metallic joint prostheses.

Table 9.3 Properties of a vapour deposited polymer coating: Parylene*

Uniform thickness	The established process guarantees precise control of thickness and inherent uniformity, even under and around tightly spaced components. No bridging, thin-out puddling, run-offs or sag.
Tough, pinhole free	Coatings as thin as 0.10 μm are free of pinholes
Superior barrier properties	Physically stable and chemically inert polycrystalline material, extremely resistant to chemical attack and insoluble in most known solvents. Provides exceptional protection from moisture, salt spray, corrosive vapours and other hostile environments.
Impressive mechanical strength	Encapsulating microcircuits in this strong polymer film increases the pull strength of wire and lead bonds, face bonded chips and conductor bridges. Parylene contributes significantly to device integrity and provides abrasion resistance for toroid winding.
Thermal stability	Parylene coatings remain stable at continuous temperatures as high as 130°C in air or 220°C in the absence of oxygen. Has good mechanical properties from –200°C to 275°C.
High dielectric characteristics	The inherent conformity and uniformity, and total permeation of all exposed surfaces provide unique dielectric strength for parylene coated components and assemblies.
Environmental protection	Parylene provides superior corrosion resistance, pinhole free coverage, crevice penetration, dielectric and mechanical strength, and purity in conformable coatings.
Stress free film	Since the polymerisation of the film task place at room temperature, there is no thermal or mechanical stress in application, and performance parameters of coated subjects are basically unaffected.
Particle immobilisation	Assures circuit integrity, preventing mobility of loose solder, wire particles or other mobile debris left from manufacture. Pressed powder parts, ferrites ceramics, corrosive metals, glass and epoxy particulate can be positively stabilised.
Dry film lubricant	Inherent characteristics of Parylene make it a valuable asset as a dry film lubricant, particularly in microminiature applications such as stepping motors.
Biocompatibility	Biomedical applications such as hypodermic needles, blood pump rotors and stators, and implantable devices are being accomplished due to the totally inert and absolute barrier characteristics of Parylene.
Simple, economical application	One-step, room temperature deposition of Parylene assures a fast, economical process with assurance of no alteration of properties or damage due to heat or stress.

* Parylene is the tradename of a polymer coating by Nova Tran Ltd, Northampton, UK. Table © Nova Tran Ltd. and reproduced here with permission.

9.2.6   GALVANISING

Galvanising is commonly used to protect low carbon steel sheet; it is annealed, acid treated, cold-rolled to increase the polish and then dipped into molten zinc. There is a characteristic 'spangle' pattern that makes identification easy. Unfortunately adherence is not good and it can peel or flake off if sharply distorted or bent at a sharp radius.

Zinc can also be applied by electrodeposition which provides a uniform surface covering, unlike the traditional method where the edges can acquire a build up. Electrodeposition, however, produces a dull appearance if not post treated or specifically polished.

There are two distinct methods of protection. The first is as a physical barrier shielding the substrate from contact with a corrosive medium. The second is as a sacrificial anode, so that the galvanising will corrode in preference to the substrate, if the substrate is higher in the electrochemical series. Table 9.4 shows the electrochemical series. The duration of galvanic protection depends on the thickness of the zinc coating.

Table 9.4   The galvanic table of metals

Anodic (corroded) end
Magnesium and its alloys
Zinc
Aluminium
Cadmium
Aluminium/copper alloys
Iron/steel
Cast iron
Chromium/nickel/iron alloys (active)
Chromium/nickel/molybdenum/iron alloys
Lead/tin solders
Lead
Tin
Nickel (active)
Inconel (active)
Brass alloys
Copper
Bronze alloys
Copper/nickel alloys
Nickel (passive)
Inconel (passive)
Titanium
Chromium/nickel/iron alloys (passive)
Silver
Graphite
Gold
Platinum
Cathodic (protected) end

Galvanised wire is produced either by dipping or continuous electroplating. The cost depends crucially on the diameter.

9.2.7 TINPLATE

Tinplating is achieved by a hot-dip process using a vegetable or non-mineral flux or alternatively by continuous electroplating. Hot dipping can produce bad edge effects caused by the molten tin running down the sheet to form droplets which accumulate at the edge. Electrotinning gives uniform and adherent coatings of any desired thickness. The plate produced this way can have a coating as thin as 3 μm, which is about one third that of the thinnest possible from a dipped plate product. A little cold rolling of electrolyte tinplate gives a bright and smooth finish.

Tinplate is used for the manufacture of food cans because of its resistance to the action of vegetable acids and its non-toxic character.

9.2.8 PAINTING

Paint is normally applied in liquid form to the surface of items, sometimes before assembly sometimes after. The advantage of the latter technique is in the sealing effect at joints and split lines. Although usually liquid, paint may also be applied as a dry powder and converted to a protective film by a combination of evaporation, chemical reaction or polymerisation, often with the aid of heat. Table 9.5 summarises the methods of paint application, which the designer must consider with regard to holding, cover or overall protection; it is important to avoid bald spots.

Paint coatings range in thickness from 0.05 mm to 0.75 mm. Paint provides corrosion protection from a wide range of active agents, increases surface hardness if required, camouflages surface defects, increases or decreases the friction, can provide identification or a colour change. The required coating may be achieved in one coat or a combination of three or more different types may be necessary. Primers are used to improve adhesion to the substrate, to enhance the corrosion protection or to improve surface finish.

Top coat materials usually have a better surface finish, toughness or hardness than primers. They may have fickle process or application requirements. The quantity of parts to be painted has a great effect on the final production process chosen to apply the paint, since a custom built paint booth can cost over £10 000 just to do one job. Some items can be coated on a conveyor belt with no restrictions, other items may well require individual specialist work.

9.2.9 EPOXY RESIN ENCAPSULATION

Resins are thermosetting and inert, for encapsulation they cast easily with little shrinkage. They have very high adhesion to metals in particular but are

Table 9.5 Methods of paint application

Brushing	Liquid paint is applied with a hand held brush.
Roller coating	Similar to brushing except that a cylindrical roller is used to spread the paint over the surface.
Curtain coating	Application which is put on by passing the component(s) beneath a trough which has a bottom split of variable width, through which the paint is allowed to flow. The amount of paint applied varies by controlling the width and speed of component feed.
Dipping	The component or assembly submerged in a container then held to drip off.
Flow coating	A stream of paint is directed against the component by one or more nozzles. The paint is not atomised and the excess is allowed to flow away and drip into a container.
Air spray	Compressed air is used to atomise liquid paint and propel it towards the part.
Airless spray	Hydraulic pressure is applied to liquid paint forcing it at a great velocity through a nozzle. Once released the paint forms into small droplets which disperse onto the target surface.
Electrostatic spray	Electrical energy is used to charge air or airless paint-spray droplets and cause an attraction to the grounded workpiece.
Powder coating	Powdered paint particles are projected towards the component and adhere to its surface, principally by electrostatic attraction. The part(s) is heated to fuse the powder particles and create the coating. The powder may also be sprayed or suspended as a fluidised cloud into which the component is dipped.
Electrodeposition	Charged paint, in an aqueous medium, is electrically plated out onto the surface of the surface of the submerged part.

also suitable for non-metallic materials. Epoxy resins are heat resistant to 300°C with a dielectric strength of up to 550 Vmm^{-1}. The hardness is dependent on the fillers used, but even basic compounds can achieve a hardness up to 100 Rockwell. There is very little elongation on finished parts and they have a high resistance to the majority of solvents, acids, oils and chemicals.

Epoxy resin materials are stored and used as a two part combination that, once mixed, immediately begins to react and harden. The working time (in which parts can be manipulated) and time to cure vary greatly with the ratio of the mix. Care must be taken to ensure that a precise ratio of the two parts is maintained to achieve optimum properties and mechanical strength.

Heat is generated because of the exothermic chemical reaction on mixing. Generally the quicker the cure, the higher the temperature. External heat can also be used to accelerate the curing. Allowances may need to be made for this heat to be dissipated, but it is rarely a major problem.

Epoxy encapsulation is an expensive solution to coating or protection requirements. Another disadvantage is that the catalysts used can be harmful and require careful handling in the separate state. After curing the resin becomes inert and is safe.

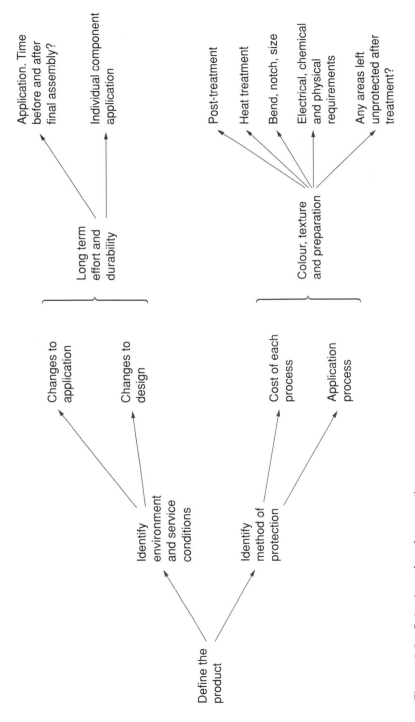

Figure 9.3 Selection of surface coatings.

9.2.10 *OTHER COATINGS*

Some coatings are difficult to classify. When items are lacquered this may be called an epoxy but it is more accurately described as a paint. Adhesives are sometimes used to coat or encapsulate small components. They can cover surfaces and exclude corrosive substances. For more details about adhesives see Chapter 8.

There are a number of other surface coating or modifying systems, such as thermal spray or overmoulding for example, but these are less relevant to corrosion protection. As a summary, Figure 9.3 offers a choice of surface treatments.

10
Biocompatibility

Biocompatibility is the ability of a man made material to exist in an in vivo environment for an acceptable period of time with no detrimental effect on the host.

All materials used in invasive medical devices have to be biocompatible, but there are degrees of biocompatibility depending on the application. Temporary skin contact is not as demanding an application as a permanent prosthetic implant. Conversely a collection bottle for postoperative waste products needs virtually no biocompatibility. There are many rules and regulations regarding levels of biocompatibility and the target values to be met or exceeded. Some I shall elaborate on in detail; for others I shall merely quote the relevant reference numbers. It is safe practice to aim to exceed biocompatibility requirements, which can be very costly. Generally speaking only very large corporations can afford to develop the products for the most demanding applications.

All medical device components and raw materials need to conform to the minimal standards laid down. With this in mind the majority of larger raw material suppliers carry out or arrange their own tests and issue detailed results to potential customers. You should use this information when claiming suitability for your specific application. If you can ensure that your manufacturing processes cannot contaminate the raw material, then the original certificate can follow the product right through to registration and sales.

The term biocompatibility covers a wide range or properties and Figure 10.1 shows a smallish view. Material properties that are relevant to biocompatibility include chemical inertness, toxicity, thrombogenicity and resistance to adhesions. Bear in mind that it is mostly the nature of the material surface that is important here, and surface properties may be different from bulk properties. It may well be that bulk properties are relevant to the function of the product (e.g. strength and stiffness of an orthopaedic implant) and surface properties are relevant to the interaction with the host (e.g. corrosion resistance). Hence there is scope for modifying the interaction by surface treatment of the material.

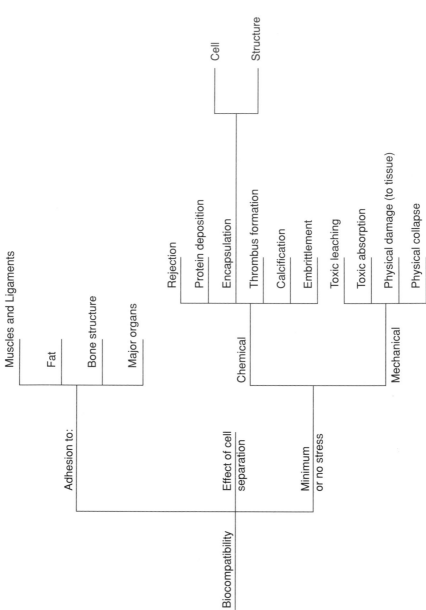

Figure 10.1 Aspects of biocompatibility.

Table 10.1 Medical Device Agency guidance on biocompatibility assessment

A   Data required to assess suitability
1. Material characterisation. This is specifically to identity the chemical structure of a material and identify any potential toxicological hazards. Residue levels. Degradation products. Cumulative effects of each process.
2. Information on prior use. Documented proof of prior use, particularly medical, which would indicate the material(s) suitability.
3. Toxicological data. Results of known biological tests which would aid in assessing potential reaction (adverse or not) during clinical use.

B   Supporting dossier
Then prepare a completed dossier of related information and specific assessments of the test results, this would contain the following.
1. Details of application: shape, size, form plus time in contact and use.
2. Chemical breakdown of all materials involved in the product.
3. A review of all toxicity data on those materials in direct contact with the body tissues.
4. Prior use and details of effects.
5. Toxicity tests as laid down in ISO 10993–1: 1992, (Guidance on selection of tests for Biological Evaluation).
6. Final appraisal of the above information and the toxicological significance. Presented conclusions of the data.

10.1   BIOCOMPATIBILITY REQUIREMENTS

To aid the assessment of biocompatibility requirements and classify the suitability of a product or material the MDA has issued guidance documents to be used at the initial material selection stages, see Table 10.1.

When determining or confirming compatibility at design acceptance stage, various tests should be undertaken. ISO 10993–1 lists these areas to be addressed:

- mutagenicity
- acute systemic toxicity
- oral toxicity
- cytotoxicity
- pyrogenicity
- sensitisation
- intravenous toxicity
- haemolysis
- irritation
- implantation

Over the last few years the emphasis of biocompatibility has changed and split into two directions. The first is biosafety, which involves the avoidance of harmful effects. The second involves the functional performance of the product in vivo.

Table 10.2   Testing categories for safety and function

Safety

1. Cytotoxicity. Split into a number of tests
   a) Cell damage by morphology.
   b) Sizing and cell comparison on growth.
   c) Assessment of cell damage and recording over a set time.
   d) Metabolism measurement.
2. Carcinogenesis. Bacteria examination involving the Ames test.
3. DNA synthesis. Methods of quantifying which may vary from microscopic visual examination and counting to FACS (flow cytometric analysis).

Function

1. Cell attachment. Introduction of materials or products to cell samples and assessment of adhesion to specific groups.
2. Cell growth. Actual proliferation within host tissue is critical especially when assessing the effect on prosthesis or implants. Cultures indicate acceptance or not.
3. Cell cover. The time and effectiveness of cells when attempting to adhere to and cover an implant.

ISO standards require in vitro testing when classifying biocompatibility and there have been developments in using cell cultures instead of live animals. Cellular and molecular biology methods of testing are becoming more refined, quantitative and widely accepted. Table 10.2 attempts to lay out categories for biosafety and functionality.

These lists and explanation of the need for testing and confirmation of biocompatibility are based on the 'Tripartite Guidance' drawn up in 1987 by the UK, USA and Canada to cover exposure time, exposure site and the finished device. Table 10.3 sets out the main points. See also Figure 10.2.

These guidelines were incorporated into the ISO standards, somewhat modified and expanded, resulting in International Standard 10993. The standard has twelve parts.

1. Testing for cytotoxicity by in vitro methods.
2. Degradation of devices and materials related to the biological testing.
3. National and International guidelines on the types and requirements of tests.
4. Immediate and proximity testing after implantation.
5. Interaction and effect on whole blood, the required tests and their selection.
6. Clinical investigations.
7. Reference materials and method of presentation.
8. Testing for carcinogenicity and reproductive toxicity.
9. Systemic toxicity and required verification.
10. ETO residuals after sterilisation.
11. Irritation and tissue sensitisation.
12. Animal input to testing. Positive actions to reduce involvement.

Table 10.3 Tripartite guidance on biomaterial testing

1. Any in vitro or in vivo experiments conducted must be done in accordance with recognised laboratory practices and results evaluated by competent recognised persons.
2. Any potential future changes in the chemical composition, manufacturing processes, physical configuration or intended use of the device must be re-evaluated with respect to those changes and differences which may occur regarding toxicological effects and subsequent need for additional toxicity testing.
3. The material, the final product form and any possible leachable chemicals or by-products (degradeable and age dependant) should be considered for their relevance to the overall toxicological evaluation of the device.
4. Prior to the selection of the material for a device the toxicological assessment, the full characterisation, formation, ingredients, impurities and method of processing should be considered.
5. Full experimental data, complete to the extent that an independent conclusion could be made, should be available to any reviewing authority, if required.
6. Toxicological evaluation performed in accordance with this guidance should also be considered in conjunction with any other information available from any known non-clinical testing, previous clinical studies or post-market experiences for a total overall safety evaluation.
7. Tests to be utilised in the toxicological evaluation should take into account the bioavailability of the bioactive material, the nature, degree, frequency, duration and conditions if exposure of the device to the body and specific tissues. This principle may lead to the categorisation of devices which would facilitate the selection of appropriate tests.

This ISO standard evolved and was reissued as ISO 10993–1.

There is a need to establish specific in vivo and in vitro tests to predict the biological effects and properties of materials to be used in contact with human tissue. Headings and explanations are listed in Table 10.4.

Quantitative results can be obtained by mixing material particles with solutions which simulate body fluids. Under various conditions the solutions are tested for chemical species resulting from reactions or leaching. It can be established whether there are substances present capable of inducing measurable degrees of systemic toxicity, sensitisation reactions, localised irritations and other unwanted responses. Tests such as the USP class VI plastic test ensures that there will be no adverse effect or reaction to test solutions exposed to filter constructions made from the tested materials, at an elevated temperature of 121°C.

One such test is for pyrogenicity, or the property of a substance that when injected can cause a rise in temperature of the host body or tissues. A filter must not contaminate the solution passing through with pyrogenic substances to be classed as non-pyrogenic. This can be determined by standard tests such as the Limulus Amoebocyte Lysate (LAL) test.

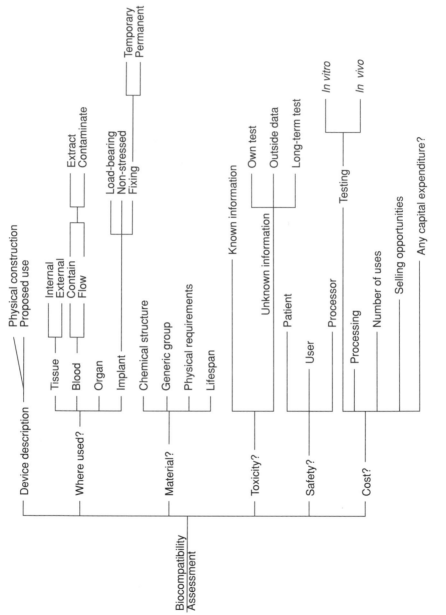

Figure 10.2 Information required for product assessment.

Table 10.4 Test headings

Immunogenicity	Method of assessing and detecting sensitisers which will determine the effect on the immune system to cause auto-immune disease.
Healing	Method to evaluate how a wound will react. Whether a selected material will enhance or provide beneficial aspects to the final would sealing and eventual healing, or create a situation where the damage is actually compounded. Animals do not provide significant quantitative results.
Compatibility	Method of establishing the blood contact effect and determining the haemolytic potential of materials. What happens simply to the blood make up when in short- or long-term contact.
Thrombosis	Method of assessing blood clotting, caused either by the introduction of a material (in direct contact) or by means of preventing the body's natural defences. The increasing or suppression of platelet production, some applying to thrombo-plastin.
Toxicity	Method of determining both the toxin and its effect, an unfortunately increasing problem as new chemical compounds are being put together and supplied without sufficient long-term data available.
Carcinogenicity	Method to evaluate and predict the long-term effect of materials on the human body. Animal tests are costly, time consuming and arguably only viable in showing what adverse effect a substance will have on that particular species, not humans. Also tumour effect, spread or containment is only restricted on a real time assessment basis.

10.2 BIOCOMPATIBILITY ASSESSMENT

The UK Medical Device Agency (MDA) has attempted to assist device manufacturers by issuing guidance notes on the assessment of medical devices and their necessary biocompatibility. Also relevant are the EC Medical Device Directive and European Standard EN1441 (Draft) on guidance for the analysis of toxicological and other risks.

All medical device manufacturers are responsible for assuring the biocompatibility of the materials used in their products and the MDA requires evidence of this assessment and the test results. The information required by the MDA is set out in Table 10.5.

A sponsor for an assessment from the MDA should compile the relevant data in the form of a dossier. The same dossier is used for quality assurance, design registration, obtaining the CE mark and MDA requirements. For the MDA, the dossier should contain the information listed in Table 10.6. BS EN 30993-1: 1994 regulates biological evaluation of medical devices, see Table 10.7. Table 10.8 illustrates an example of a CEN test.

Table 10.5 Medical Device Agency required information

Information requirements for biocompatibility	
Material characterisation	All information regarding formulation, component parts, residuals, degradation produces, adverse effects of a process. Sufficient to allow a chemical identity to be mapped and characterised with potential toxicological hazards more easily identified.
Prior use	Documented evidence of prior use for the same material(s) or their chemical components in similar situation. These can indicate suitability and reduce extended intensive testing.
Toxicological data	Results, verified and certified, on appropriate biological tests which will provide some degree of reassurance that any risk of adverse reactions is considered low.

Table 10.6 Compatibility dossier requirements extracted from Medical Device Agency requirements

Description of the device. Drawings, pictures or examples. Each component, generic type or trade name for material used. Who produced the raw material and the type of the patient contact (blood, fluid, topical or non-contact etc). Plus the duration of the contact.

Formulations for all materials used which will be in actual contact with human tissue. All chemical names and concentrations, compounds and methods of compounding for each and every ingredient. This will include additives, pigments, fillers, catalyses and processing aids etc. If in the final product there may be biologically active ingredients or reactive products, information on their residue concentrations should be provided. If any of the raw material data is not available to the processor then the base provider should contact the FDA direct. In some cases the compound/material formulation may already be held in the FDA data bank.

Review of toxicity data on each material in direct contact. This should contain, where relevant, data on residual monomers, heavy metals, contaminants, additives, pigments, catalysts, release agents and other chemical processing ingredients necessary to produce components. Where significant residues or biologically active ingredients are present, details of their migration, leaching or absorption should be supplied. Toxicity data does not always necessarily mean materials used within the medical device industry. Justification for such omissions should again be documented and supplied.

Previous experience of each material in related applications. Where ever relevant data from clinical use should be supplied. This should include details of use, number of applications used and their frequency, over what time period and any adverse reactions reported. Any patent material or novel applications should be broken down; the MDA may have the information already on file. All information supplied is treated as confidential and is not divulged.

Toxicity test reports. Testing of the device as a whole or/and as separate component parts still needs justification on the material selected. Justification for the materials selected must be documented. ISO 10993–1 (1992) part 1 gives the guidance on the selection of the correct tests, also includes details of which tests are required by device categories. Also EN 30993–1 is soon to be introduced to provide test guidance.

Table 10.7 BS EN 30993-1: 1994 Biological Evaluation of Medical Devices. © BSI

Part 1	Guidance on Selection of Tests.
Part 2	Animal Welfare Requirements.
Part 3	Test for Genotoxicity, Carcinogenicity and Reproductive Toxicity.
Part 4	Selection of Tests for Interactions with Blood.
Part 5	Test for Cytotoxicity: In Vitro methods.
Part 6	Tests for Local Effects after Implantation.
Part 7	Ethylene Oxide Sterilisation Residuals.
Part 8	Clinical Investigation (only ISO 10993).
Part 9	Degradation of Materials Related to Biological Testing.
Part 10	Tests for Irritation and Sensitisation.
Part 11	Test for Systemic Toxicity.
Part 12	Sample Preparation and Reference Materials.
Part 13	Identification and Quantification of Degradation Products from Polymers.
Part 14	Identification and Quantification of Degradation Products from Ceramics.
Part 15	Identification and Quantification of Degradation Products from Coated and Uncoated Metals and Alloys.
Part 16	Toxicokinetic Study Design for Degradation Products and Leachables.
Part 17	Glutaraldehyde and Formaldehyde Residuals.

Extracts from British Standards are reproduced with the permission of BSI under licence no. PD\1998 0481. Complete editions of the standards can be obtained by post from BSI Customer Services, 389 Chiswick High Road, London W4 4AL, UK.

Biocompatibility is not just a matter of arranging a few external tests and the correlation of suppliers' information. It requires the acceptance of a specific material for specific uses within and on the human body, whether that contact is short term immersion in blood or long term implants in bone. Many misunderstandings and mis-applications have arisen because of the acceptance of biocompatibility criteria for one set of circumstances, in a different setting or with modified materials.

10.3 ACHIEVING BIOCOMPATIBILITY

One way of modifying potential materials, which at first examination do not appear acceptable, is by surface treatment. Surface treatment can be by physical means or by the application of a coating. Many different surface coatings are possible, depending on the application and the tissues involved. Sometimes it is necessary to prevent the medical device from damage by the host, and sometimes the host needs protecting.

10.4 EXAMPLES

Much can be learnt from examining existing applications. Figure 10.3 shows the wide range of applications which need biocompatible materials to be able to function in the body.

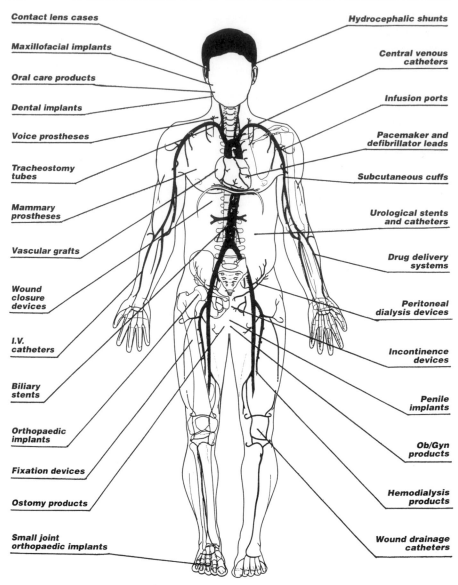

Figure 10.3 Anatomical range of medical devices.

Table 10.8 Example of CEN evaluation test. © BSI, extracted from BS EN 30993–1: 1994

Device categories			Biological effect							
Body contact (see 5.1)	Contact duration (see 5.2) A limited (< 24 h) B-prolonged (> 24 h to 30 days) C-permanent (> 30 days)		Cytotoxicity	Sterilization	Irritation or intracutaneous reactivity	Systemic toxicity (acute)	Sub-chronic toxicity (sub-acute toxicity)	Genotoxicity	Implantation	Haemocompatibility
Surface devices	Skin	A	X	X	X					
		B	X	X	X					
		C	X	X	X					
	Mucosal membranes	A	X	X	X					
		B	X	X	X					
		C	X	X	X		X	X		
	Breached or compromised surfaces	A	X	X	X					
		B	X	X	X					
		C	X	X	X		X	X		
External communicating devices	Blood path, indirect	A	X	X	X	X				X
		B	X	X	X	X				X
		C	X	X		X	X	X		X
	Tissue/bone/ dentin communicating	A	X	X	X					
		B	X	X				X	X	
		C	X	X				X	X	
	Circulating blood	A	X	X	X	X		X		
		B	X	X	X	X		X		X
		C	X	X	X	X	X	X		X
Implant devices	Tissue/bone	A	X	X	X					
		B	X	X				X	X	
		C	X	X				X	X	
	Blood	A	X	X	X	X			X	X
		B	X	X	X	X		X	X	X
		C	X	X	X	X	X	X	X	X

Extracts from British Standards are reproduced with the permission of BSI under licence no. PD\1998 0481.

10.4.1   PARYLENE

Parylene® is a xylylene polymer, poly(chloro-*p*-xylylene) marketed by Nova Tran. It is used as a coating which provides body tissue compatibility and promotes easy blood flow where in direct contact. It has minimal toxicity coupled with low moisture permeability and high electrical insulation. It can be sterilised by all methods and retains a transparent appearance throughout. Parylene functions as a barrier between the substrate and body tissues, and can act as a lubricant to aid insertion and liquid transfer.

Parylene is used to coat pressure sensors, cardiac assist devices, pins and plates for implants. It is also used to coat catheters internally, and externally on laparoscopy needles, mandrels, guidewires and growth stimulators.

Parylene is certified to maximum levels awaiting your input and use.

10.4.2   HAEMOGLYDE

Haemoglyde® is a synthetic polymer coating compound made from three monomer components. It is made by Portex and is used to reduce thrombogenicity and increase wettability. Basically it forms a slippy surface which prevents the adhesion of platelets. Haemoglyde is used extensively on the inner surface of chest drainage system catheters to enhance drainage, reduce the incidence of pericardial effusion and reduce occlusion. All these attributes lead to shorter hospital stays and reduce trauma to patients during their removal, which can be a harrowing experience since it is normally carried out under only local anaesthetic.

10.4.3   CATHETER COATING

A hydrophilic coating used on peritoneal and suprapubic catheters has been developed by Elemental Design. This coating is easily applied to PVC, PU and latex. A spin-off from this work is application as an antifouling coating for the hulls of boats and ships, protecting the external surface from marine growth and reducing the consequential drag (existing antifouling coatings are being phased out because they are toxic and are contaminating the sea: Elemental's coating is user friendly).

10.4.4   VASCUTEK VASCULAR GRAFTS

Vascutek vascular grafts are knitted polyester tubes used as vascular prostheses. They are used as arterial replacements in a number of clinical procedures. The standard products is supplied in metal laminated pouches. A gelatin impregnated version is also available for use where less porosity is required. These can be used even at high heparin levels without pretreatment. The product is supplied in various lengths and diameters designed for many procedures in peripheral vascular and cardiac surgery. One product, called Gelweave, has

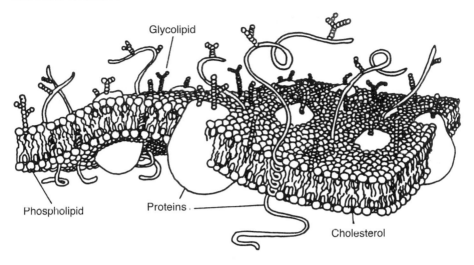

Figure 10.4 Representation of a biological membrane showing the basic structural unit made up from a lipid bilayer containing proteins and glycoproteins. Reproduced by permission of Biocompatibles Ltd. Thanks to Dr Yianni for information.

a 'floating yarn' construction which creates a velour fabric on the exterior surface of the graft, aiding incorporation into the surrounding tissue.

10.4.5 PHOSPHORYLCHOLINE

Phosphorylcholine an intrinsically biocompatible substance found in human cells (see Figure 10.4). It can be synthesised and used as a coating to improve biocompatibility considerably. This coating will not absorb proteins, has an overall charge and reduces the need for large dosages of anticoagulant drugs by making an antithrombogenic surface. Marketed and supplied by Biocompatibles Ltd, it is used in products for applications from cardiovascular care to lens manipulation.

10.5 SUMMARY

From the point of view of a device designer, the issue of biocompatibility of materials is simple (see Figure 10.5).

- Is it being used extensively now for the same type of application? If not, *test it.*
- Is it being used in a limited form for a similar type of application? If not, *test it.*
- Is it being used in any medical device for any type of application requiring biocompatibility? If not, *test it.*

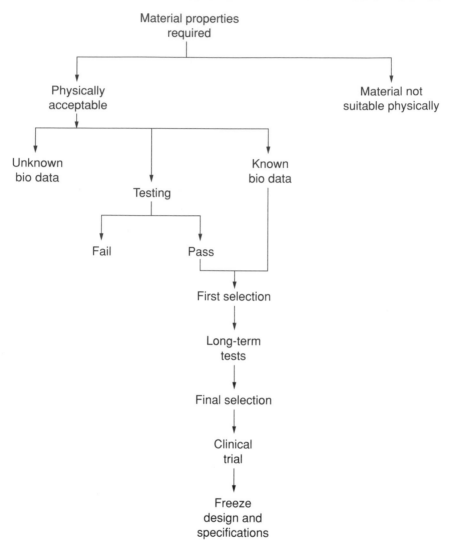

Figure 10.5 Decision tree for material selection and biocompatibility.

- Can the material manufacturer supply you with certified data on biochemical effects and toxicity? If not, *test it*.
- Has the manufacturer sent you data sheets stating non-toxicity, non-pyrogenicity etc. but still requires a disclaimer to be signed absolving them of any responsibility regarding your particular application? Yes? Then *test it*. No matter where the information comes from, if it cannot be validated, there are only two options for you. Either choose another material or instigate your own tests and build a large convincing design dossier.

11
Filters and Membranes

A filter is a sheet of material with pore sizes within a defined range used to separate particles or macromolecules from a suspension or solution. The word filter is also used to describe equipment for separating liquids from suspended solids, either for recovery of the solid, classification of the liquid or both simultaneously. The liquid flows through the pores in a cloth, mesh or granular bed thus the solid is filtered out. Filters are also used to clarify or clean gases before use.

These definitions of filters are not very informative when considering medical devices. There is no mention of the twenty-odd different types of filters and membranes, nor the forms the filters can take nor the range of applications.

First of all, filters are used in the context of medical devices primarily to clean and allow the passage of:

- body fluids,
- gases,
- treatment fluids, or for
- protective venting.

The mechanism or construction of the working part of the filter can be a non-woven fabric, glass fibre, foam, mesh, solids, perforated solids, paper or thin film. Materials can be plastic, man-made synthetic, solid organics, ceramics, metal or fibreweave. The characteristics of a filter are the most important factor when selecting for a particular application. Rejection or attraction (absorption) of the medium being filtered also determines selection, as does mechanical strength. There must be no chance of tearing, shear or burst, or that the filter medium becomes clogged by particulates.

Contamination of the filter barrier because of incorrect selection of the pore size compared to the particles to be trapped is one of the major problems. Figure 11.1 shows the size range of airborne particles, a few others like bacteria and viruses, plus the methods of separation and examination.

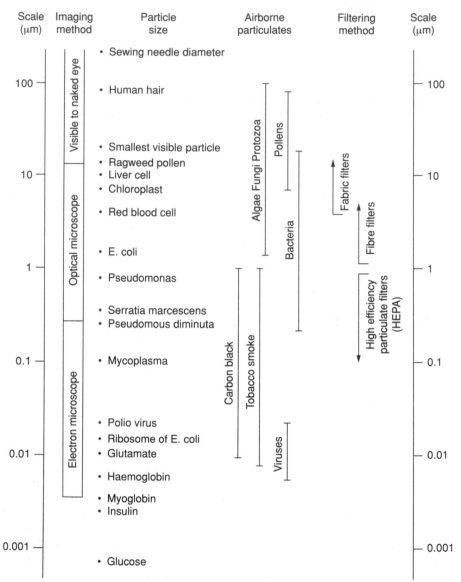

Figure 11.1 Size range of airborne particulates, biological particles, and filtration methods.

Table 11.1 Filter requirements and size of body components

Item	Size (μm)
Blood set filter	200
Human hair	120
Visual limits	80
DHSS maximum size filter	40
Industrial filter	15
Blood corpuscle	7.5
Small blood capillary	5
Lipid particle	4
Candida yeast	2
Spores	1.2
Bacteria	0.2
Viruses	0.1

Any particulate matter in the 5–15 μm range presents a risk of capillary occlusion.

11.1 FILTER SELECTION

When selecting the filter membrane of type of construction, first examine the problem; Table 11.1 shows filter requirements and the sizes of various body components. Couple these with Figure 11.1 and the pore size selection can be determined.

Here are some of the basic definitions and phrases used when discussing filters and membranes.

- Hydrophilic: tendency to absorb or bind with water, which results in swelling. Hydrophilic membranes can filter gases and liquids but can become clogged and then pass liquids through. Virtually any liquid will 'wet' a hydrophilic filter.
- Hydrophobic: antagonistic to water (repels). These membranes will not pass water or liquids with high surface tension but will allow gases to pass through. They are most suitable for gas and solvent filtration; see Figure 11.2.
- Oleophobic: these membranes will prevent liquids with both high and low surface tensions from passing, but still allow gases through.
- Pore size: defined as an aperture or cavity between particles, but simply put it is the average 'hole' size in the membrane or the gap in woven fabric. Additionally, pore size can mean the space between solids if porous materials are used, the path a liquid or gas will follow to pass through.
- Micromembrane: film or medium to filter gas or liquid with pore size in the range 0.1–10 μm; sometimes referred to as microporous membrane.
- Particle removal: when small solids are removed from gas and liquid normally 'the greater the removal rate the shorter the filter life'; obvious really.

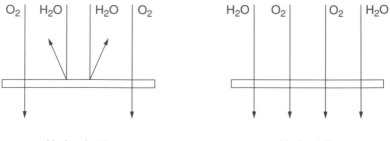

Figure 11.2   Hydrophobic and hydrophilic membrane types.

So with filters we have the ability to stop solids which are carried in either gasses or liquids and allow the carrier to pass through. The carrier can be contained and cleaned. We can pump liquids but stop any gas contained; alternatively we can pass gases and stop the liquid contaminates. We can choose whether to use the substances collected or discard them, the options are limited only by the technology.

Table 11.2 is a check list to aid in the selection of a filter, housing and membrane material. Providing there is a standard product for sale, costs for a high grade, certified filter can be as low as 50p each and if the housing can be incorporated into your actual design then the cost of a membrane or method of collection could be as low as one or two pence. At the other end of the spectrum, customised disposable filters can be 1000 times dearer at £10 each.

Of course there are other considerations, but as a general rule the check list should cover your first enquiry.

There are two main types of filtration to consider: sieve and depth. Sieve filtration prevents particles larger than the pore size from passing and traps them on the contact surface. Anything smaller than the pore size passes through. With depth filtration particles are trapped both at the surface and within the filter. This means that filter thickness, as well as the pore size, governs its performance. It also means that it can retain larger quantities of contamination before becoming clogged. The sieve filter requires surface cleaning, by varied means, but can be used for long periods. Advantages and disadvantages of these two methods are shown in Table 11.3.

When selecting the material for a filter the method of manufacture needs to be considered, as well as the compatibility with the liquid or gas with which it has contact, and the means of retaining the finished filter. What is its inherent physical strength, is it flat, plated, pressure sensitive? Table 11.4 lists the common materials used in filter construction and Table 11.5 shows the types of liquids, gases and contaminants the filter may have to deal with.

Table 11.2 Filter selection criteria

1. What requires filtering from what? What needs saving or protecting?
2. Disposable or reusable?
3. Life cycle once in use?
4. What size particles need to be stopped?
5. What flow rate of the gas or liquid passing through?
6. At what pressure?
7. Where will the filter be used?
8. What other liquids or gases will it come into contact with?
9. Does it need to be supplied sterile?
10. If yes, sterilised by which method?
11. Is there a requirement for post-sterilisation by the customer?
12. If yes, by which method and how many times?
13. What quantity of carrier medium (liquid/gas) will be used and for how long.
14. Any shelf time requirements or restrictions?
15. Is the filter incorporated into the product design assembly or is it to be a stand alone item?
16. Is there a need or reason for interchangeability?
17. Can a pre-built unit be used?
18. What restrictions are there on size within the device housing?
19. Any special feature needed in/on the filter housing to allow fixing?
20. What type of connections to be used to link the filter in?
21. How many per year required?
22. What target price for purchase? Is it flexible or negotiable?
23. Comparability of materials between medium/filter/housing/particle/carrier?
24. What is the end application?
25. What technical requirements are needed when using the device or filter? Is it user-friendly and fail-safe?

Table 11.3 Advantages and disadvantages of sieve and depth filters

Sieve filtration	Depth filtration
Advantages	
• Pore size definition.	• Good as a coarse pre-filter.
• No bypass.	• Cheap.
• Best suited for bacteria and similar.	• High flow rates at low pressure.
• Can be as small as sub-micron size.	• large contaminant retention.
• Easily tested and quantified.	• Not restricted to one particle size.
	• No surface cleaning required.
Disadvantages	
• Minimal particle tolerance.	• Contamination migration
• Relatively low flow rates.	• Dependent on pressure.
• Restricted range of materials.	• Easily damaged or blocked.
• Requires surface cleaning.	

Table 11.4   Common filter materials

Material	Form
Metals	
Stainless steel wire	Random and woven mesh
Zinc	Sintered sheet and block
Polymers	
Polyethersulphone	Sheet, film, laminate
Polysulphone	"
Polymide (nylon)	"
Polyester	"
Polyethylene	"
Acrylic	
Modified	"
Copolymer	"
PTFE (Teflon)	"
Cellulose acetate	"
Polypropylene	"
Expanded polyurethane foam	"
PVDF	"
Combinations of those shown above	"
Others	
Ceramic	Sintered or block
Paper	Woven, laminate, pleated
Woven textile	
Cotton	Woven, compressed
Silk	"
Linen	"
Fibreglass	Random and woven

Table 11.5   Liquids, gases and particles in contact with medical filters

Intravenous lines
   Drug delivery
   Fluid infusion/irrigation
   Blood transfer
Chemical transfer
   Acid
   Alkali
Urine
Blood
   Serum
   Plasma
   Blood substitute
   Whole blood
CO_2
Air/oxygen
Medication in gas form

11.2 FILTER PROPERTIES AND TESTING

The filter assembly must be tested and accepted before being used in any medical device. The medical and biocompatibility requirements are dealt with in Chapter 10. There are high levels of testing requirements and accredited certification. Testing to USP (United Stated Pharmacopia) class VI (suitability for long-term implants) and LAL (limulus amoebocyte lysate) tests require filtered extracts to test the filters.

Basic efficacy testing of filters comprises physical measurements of flow pressure, pore size, effect of immersion and efficiency. The following tests are standard.

- Bubble point: this test measures the level or amount of pressure needed to push a liquid (normally water) away from a wetted pore; this determines the pore size and type of barrier it can be used for. There is a visual test of when the first bubble is observed and obviously the lower the pressure needed then the larger the pore size. Microscopic examination is also carried out and the pore physically measured using a cross-hair Vernier scale. The bubble point test to ASTM F316–80 gives a result in p.s.i.
- Water breakthrough: this test measures water transfer through the largest pore of a dry hydrophobic membrane, and rates the membrane as an aqueous barrier. It is also described in ASTM F316–80 and gives a result in p.s.i.
- Water flow: to quantify the necessary pressure, porosity and filter surface area. This test provides a figure which is used for comparison. It is described in ASTM 317–72 and gives a result in millilitres.
- Air flow: used to measure how much gas can be passed through and at what pressure; measures porosity, area, pressure etc. The ASTM 317–72 standard test gives a value in $l \, min^{-1} cm^{-2}$.
- DOP test: the efficiency of a filter is determined by passing a measured amount of dioctylphthalate aerosol particles (0.3 μm diameter) at a set pressure through the filter. The standard test is regulated by ASTM D2986–71, giving a result as a percentage. The number detected determines the rating.

Figure 11.3 illustrates the tests described above.

11.3 FILTER MATERIALS AND CONSTRUCTION

Filter materials must be constructed and sealed to the highest standards since they are one of the most demanding products for sale to original equipment device manufacturers: the filter must perform 100% to specification. Construction, the method by which the whole filter assembly is held together, can generally be described by three groups:

Bubble point test

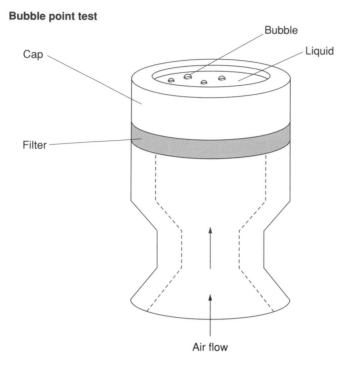

Water breakthrough test

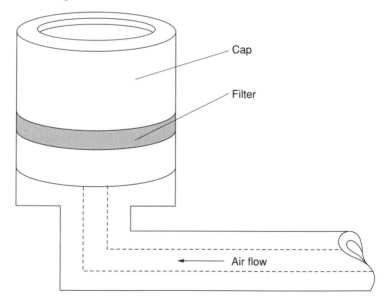

Figure 11.3 Tests of filter properties.

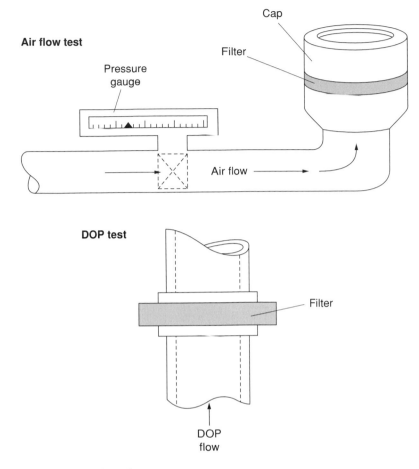

Figure 11.3 (*continued*)

- physical restraint;
- bonded; or
- energy directed.

11.3.1 PHYSICAL RESTRAINT

With physical restraint, normally a screw cap holds the membrane in place after pre-assembly within a defined space or cartridge. A different application of this method is a bolted down plate or container, which is very simple but sometimes not effective in terms of space and cost. Physical restraint is unlikely to give a hermetic seal. Compressive crimps are another alternative, by turning over a container lip and deforming the edge.

11.3.2 BONDED

There are many versions of this joint, but commercially it is restricted to three types: adhesive, solvent or epoxy. The epoxy resin type is specifically separated from the adhesive heading because it is not normally used just to bond or hold the parts together, but more as a sealant with gap filling properties.

11.3.3 ENERGY DIRECTED

By this I mean a generic term to cover ultrasonic, RF welding or heat sealing: all 'direct' energy in one form or another to close and contain the filter medium into a container. Elaborate pathways and energy directors are necessary for these constructions but once designed and correctly developed confidence in the finished assemblies is 100%.

Table 11.6 lists some of the more general guidelines which should be adopted when constructing filters. If you are purchasing the finished article, these rules can still be of use when establishing a quality check.

11.4 APPLICATIONS

Practical examples prevent any confusion or misunderstanding and this section shows how diverse the market is.

The materials mentioned previously are used in many other disciplines and industries, Table 11.7 shows just a few for comparison. The following examples are all products now on sale from various filter manufacturers.

- i.v. filter: this has a 0.2 μm pore size for bacteria retention and a gamma stable membrane contained within a clear plastic housing. It will withstand pressures up to 45 p.s.i. and has automatic venting to prevent airlocks. Product by Gelman.
- Drug filter: the transfer of digoxin immune fab (ovine) is a treatment for digitalis intoxication that must be given through a 0.25 μm membrane filter. Product by Braun.
- Syringe filter: this has variable pore sizes and flow rates. There is a common housing with female Luer entry fitting and male Luer exit. The cross section and surface area can be increased to suit flow. Products by all the major companies: Arbour, Millipore, Gelman, Whatman.
- Suction filter: this provides protection for equipment and staff to prevent contamination of vacuum pumps, aspiration or suction systems. It stops aerosol biohazards. Product by Arbor.
- Insuflation filter: this prevents contamination or transfer of solids during the CO_2 insuflation of the patient. There are various connections due to the large number of different types of insuflation units on the market. Product by Rocket Medical.

Table 11.6 Filter construction rules

Adhesives
- Surfaces must be contaminant free
- Ensure compatible with membrane material (cyanoacrylate fumes during curing)
- Some surfaces may require pre-assembly treatment: cornici discharge, acid drip
- Check the adhesives class clearance for possible fluid contact: class IV, V or VI
- Application methods: how to transfer the adhesive to the correct areas

r.f. sealing
- Dielectric properties of the materials used determine the quality of the seal obtained
- Some constructions may require 'carrier' components to hold and seal the filter medium or membrane
- Suitable for high volume but materials which can be used are restricted.

Ultrasonic
- Energy directors critical, normally located on the top component and as close to the welding horn as possible
- Similar to r.f. above but any assembly work better by entrapment of the membrane between two other components
- High volume application
- Any long delays or extended energy input should be avoided to prevent damage to the filter by secondary energy transfer
- Cheap method once set up. Highly repeatable joints produced
- Nesting of components critical to ensure the correct seal produced
- Avoid 'far' welds, less damage to the assembled membranes and finished welds are considerably better

Heat sealing
- Housing materials should have a lower melt temperature than the membrane
- Allow a generous seal area
- Inspection normally easy since the seal itself is a visual indication of success

Potting
- Epoxy generates heat while the chemical reaction takes place, consider this for assembly contact areas
- Wicking is easier when a high viscosity product is used

- Blood oxygenator filter: this is a large surface area unit to allow for low pressure feed, with varied connections to suit different machines it has 99.97% DOP. Product by Gelman.
- Vent cap: a protection for and means of venting gases from air systems of blood transfer lines. There are varied pore sizes and classes to suit probable contaminates. Product by Filtertek.
- Ventilation filter: a plastic two-part assembly traps a woven electrostatic filter for 99.99% viral or bacterial efficiency. Product by Air Safety.
- Transducer protector: this method of protecting monitoring equipment prevents cross contamination and eliminates machine changes. It is hepatitis B retentive, and has low wave form degradation for more accurate pressure monitoring. Product by Gelman.

Table 11.7 Examples of filter use outside medical applications

Application	Comment
Venting of gases but repelling water over electrodes	Protection on outside lighting or headlights, domestic or industrial
Heat exchanger cover, ventilation in and dust etc., out	Becoming more critical and a requirement for microelectronics
Safety venting on pre-packed liquids and food	During transit or temperature changes pressure relief required without loss of fluid
High speed fluid transfer via small (micro) bore	Prevents blockage or entrapment of air in ink jet
Oxygen barrier on zinc–air battery	Prevents electrolyte loss but allows ingress of oxygen to allow the 'fuel cell' to operate

- Depth filter: this 20 μm filter is made of needle-punched non-woven felt media, made from intertwined polyester fibres. There is a mechanical entrapment method. Product by Lypore.
- Bacterial isolation: this autoclavable unit and filter sheet is made from cellulose nitrate fast-wetting laminated with polyester film. It has a 0.2–1 μm pore size that is biologically inert with < 1.5% leachables. Product by Whatman.
- Pharmacy filtration: this is for preventing contamination in hospital solutions, when mixing additives with manufacturer's solutions, or making up multidose dispense solutions. Product by Millipore.
- High flow particulate filter: this self gasketing, resin bonded, low cost, borosilicate glass microfibre tube can be used in high temperature and pressure applications and is generally held in an acrylic outer housing. Product by Micra Filter.
- Tubular filter: an insert moulded nylon mesh is contained in a polypropylene housing to give very high flow with a coarse filter function. It is used in an in-line suction trap for tissue sampling. Product by GVS.
- Porous ceramic: pore sizes from 25 to 1.5 μm are available, with additional coatings which take it down to 0.2 μm. This can be used for gross particle filtration down to sterilisation of serums. Porous ceramics are inert and have high purity. Product by Coors.
- Filter cartridge: a polyethylene sheet spiral wrap, with centre feed and saturation filter for use as a water purifier. Product by Porvair.
- Vent plug: a porous plastic plug, with the pore size varying between 25 and 80 μm depending on the application. Materials used vary but the main ones are polyethylene, PTFE or polypropylene. Product by Porex.
- Piggy-back i.v. filter: this is a 5 μm pore-size unit for particulate removal with high flow rates to prevent impedance of secondary infusion. Product by Gelman.

The **HEPA** Bacterial/Viral Filter
High Efficiency PArticulate filter

The Filtration Efficiency Challenge.

Independent in vitro studies [1][2] show that the Intertech HEPA Filter achieves **99.9999%** **filtration efficiency** with a bacteriophage **four times smaller** than the human immuno-deficiency virus (HIV) and similar in size to Hepatitis C.

HIV IMMATURE VIRUS   ØX174 BACTERIOPHAGE
Transmission electron micrographs of negatively stained particles x 100,000.

The HEPA Filter

The Hepa filter works not only as a very highly effective bacterial/viral filter but also as an HME. It can be placed at either the patient or machine end of the breathing circuit.

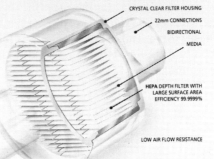

CRYSTAL CLEAR FILTER HOUSING
22mm CONNECTIONS
BIDIRECTIONAL
MEDIA

HEPA DEPTH FILTER WITH
LARGE SURFACE AREA
EFFICIENCY 99.9999%

LOW AIR FLOW RESISTANCE

The Aerosol Challenge results [1]

TEST ORGANISM	SIZE	FILTRATION EFFICIENCY
ØX174 BACTERIOPHAGE	27 nm	99.9999%

Relative organism size:

ØX174 BACTERIOPHAGE	27 nm
HEPATITIS C	27 nm
PAPILLOMAVIRUS	55 nm
HIV	110 nm

Additional Properties

- **Humidification (Moisture output):**
  22.8mg H$_2$O/litre meeting ECRI humidification requirements [3]
- **Hydrophobic:** Water repelling up to 50cm H$_2$0
- **Low airflow resistance:** 1.5 cm/H$_2$O at 50 lpm
  1.7 cm/H$_2$O at 60 lpm
- **Low deadspace:** Internal volume :90ml
- **Weight:** 47g
- **Connections (ISO)** ??mm ID/OD

  Also available Flextube & 15/22mm adaptor

The Mechanism

Filter matrix traps particles mechanically by Diffusional Interception, Inertial Impaction and Direct Interception.

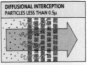
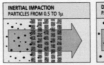

DIFFUSIONAL INTERCEPTION
PARTICLES LESS THAN 0.5µ

INERTIAL IMPACTION
PARTICLES FROM 0.5 TO 1µ

DIRECT INTERCEPTION
PARTICLES UP TO 1µ

ORDERING INFORMATION

CODE	DESCRIPTION	BOX QTY
002890	HEPA BACTERIA FILTER	20
002837	FLEX TUBE 165mm	50
	• 15mm PATIENT END • 22mm CIRCUIT END	
001679	15/22mm ADAPTOR	50

Supplied clean for single patient use.

References:
(1) Nelson Laboratories Inc. Virus Aerosol Filtration Efficiency Study. Data on file.
(2) Duberstein, Howard. Sterile Filtration of Gases: A bacterial aerosol challenge test. Journal Parenteral Drug Association. 1978: 32,4,192-198
(3) ECRI report. Heat and Moisture Exchangers. 1983: 12.7.155-166

Figure 11.4 Commercial bacterial/viral filter.

- HEPA bacterial viral filter: this filter achieves 99.9999% efficiency when used on bacterial air carried systems. It is fitted either on the machine or onto the patient side of a breathing circuit (see Figure 11.4).

11.5 SUMMARY

The information in this chapter on filters can all be found in manufacturer's catalogues or the data sheets provided on specific products. The information is there, so all it takes to specify a filter is some time and effort. Any minor difficulty or potential problem can be overcome easily by conversation with the manufacturers.

12
Fibre Optics

Fibre optic technology is expanding into many fields of operation including the medical devices industry. Developments which utilise the unique light transmission properties of fibre optic systems will be described in this chapter. More importantly, the principles of operation will be explained. Fibre optics is primarily accepted as a means of transferring information via a light carrier, but the opportunities are vast for other applications, none of which require more than white light at comparatively low power.

Once the principles and perceived limitations of fibre optics are understood, you may be able to conceive other ideas for new products. I will not attempt to describe telecommunications uses, which are well documented elsewhere.

As this is a very rapidly changing area of technology, you would be well advised to seek information and advice from the fibre optics manufacturers before you start trying to develop an idea into a product.

It was not until the 1950s that good quality optical fibres could be manufactured at realistic prices. Since that time a whole new industry has mushroomed. Developments are anchored to three key events. In 1964 Dr Kao proved theoretically that a clad optical fibre could provide communication values of 20 dB km^{-1}; the fibre would lose only 1% of light intensity over 1 km. In 1970 Corning Glass (USA) manufactured the first fibres to achieve the theoretical value of 20 dB km^{-1} but it took another five more years to transform this material into a commercially viable product. In 1976 the first experimental fibre optic telephone line was installed.

After this the whole industry opened up with other companies joining in to provide capacity and technology input. To illustrate what progress has been made, in about 1938 experimental surgical retractors were made from Perspex, connected to a light source and used to illuminate surgical incisions. These were not deemed viable owing to the high cost. By the end of the 1980s, fibre optics were being manufactured at low cost for non-communication uses at a volume of nearly 18 million miles a year.

12.1   GENERAL FIBRE OPTIC APPLICATIONS

This vast quantity of optical fibres, clad in a very thin coating was used for the following purposes.

12.1.1   TRANSFER OF LIGHT

Bundles of fibres are used to transfer light within buildings, to selected areas like alcoves or hidden recesses. Sometimes fibre optics replace conventional lighting by providing low level lighting in infrequently used corridors: one bright light source can feed ten outlets (250 W divided by 10 means not much cost to run).

12.1.2   SPOT LIGHTS

When items are on display fibre optics can concentrate light to specific areas and remove the potentially damaging heat generated by conventional systems. Perishable goods need not suffer, and delicate assemblies or heat-sensitive electronics need not be affected or require additional costly protection. Fibre optic spot lighting is popular for paintings and other art objects.

12.1.3   DECORATION

In the mid-1970s fibre optic table lamps and pool illuminations were very popular. They did not provide useful illumination and were purely decorative.

12.1.4   DISPLAYS

In displays, large bundles of optical fibres can be used to produce multiple points of light: one, ten or a hundred fibres for each point.

12.1.5   ADVERTISING

In advertising hoardings, for traffic information or for warning signs the display can be changed to suit differing circumstances. Fibre optic systems can present one of several options from a menu of choices on a single display surface.

12.1.6   SENSORS

In safety sensors fibre optic bundles can act as both transmitter and receiver. Fibre optic sensors are ideally suited to hazardous environments and locations affected by pressure, magnetism, radiation or gases. Some fibre optic materials do not tolerate radiation but others perform adequately.

12.1.7 INDUSTRIAL

Industrial applications of fibre optics include the transfer of UV light for adhesive curing. Alternatively fibre optics can be used to remove UV. The optical fibres are unaffected by electromagnetic capacitance or interference, function in hot environments and are not damaged by the majority of corrosive agents or moisture laden environments. Glass fibres are more resistant than polymeric ones.

12.1.8 IMAGE TRANSFER

In image transfer bundles of optical fibres give more light transfer and a better picture than conventional means. Fibre optics are used in CCTV, endoscopes and laproscopes. Some newer systems now utilise sealed liquid cables to provide crystal clear images. The fibre optic systems are 30–40% of the price of the new sealed liquid types.

12.1.9 MEDICAL

There are a number of notable medical application of fibre optics. The most popular, and lucrative, are the endoscopes and laproscopes. The ability to obtain clear and true images by minimally invasive means is vital to the development of keyhole surgery. Fibre optic technology is also used in the provision of visual stimuli for some disabled patients. Optical fibres are made in which light can leak out along their length. This Sideglow effect is connected to a light source with colour filters and coupled to a music system to create an output of light and sound that encourages brain activity and response in handicapped individuals. Sideglow™ is a trademark of Eurotec Ltd.

Another medical application is the illumination by optical fibres of various vessels in the body to provide surgeons with visible warning of their presence. This can greatly assist with some surgical procedures. Rocket Medical Plc has patented such a system under the name Uriglow™.

12.1.10 TEMPERATURE MONITORING

Standard grade optical fibre temperature systems can monitor between –150°C and +450°C by means of distributed temperature sensing: more details at the end of the chapter.

As the cost of producing optically pure fibres continues to fall and new materials are developed to give better or cheaper performance, the fibre optic industry is in a state of flux and opportunities are opening up for many new applications.

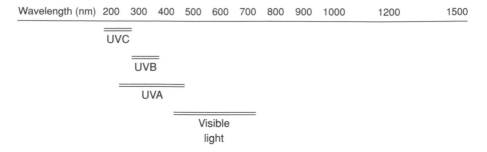

Figure 12.1   The visible waveband.

12.2   FIBRE OPTIC PRINCIPLES

Visible light is only a very small section of the electromagnetic spectrum of radiant energy, see Figure 12.1.

In the mid-1600s Willebrod Snell described how a beam of light changed direction when it passed from one transparent medium into another. In effect he was writing about refraction. Christian Huygens, another 17th century scientist, described light as an uninterrupted wave that could only travel in straight lines. These observations form the basis of optics and indicate how optical fibres work. If light is incident on the interface between two media at a glancing angle, it will not pass out of its medium but be totally internally reflected. Thus if a transparent rod is clad with a tube, light will bounce along the sides of the rod from one end to the other without being lost or absorbed at the sides. The greater the difference in refractive indices between the two materials, the more efficient is the light transport. Table 12.1 lists some refractive indices. The principle can be seen in Figure 12.2, which is a diagram of a plain rod within a transparent tube.

12.3   CLAD FIBRES

To overcome problems of surface quality, an optical cladding of lower refractive index is used to protect the core material. Thus total internal reflection is not impaired by dirt, scratches or surface imperfections, and attenuation is minimised. The development of cladding is the key to practical, inexpensive fibre optics.

Fibres clad as described are called step index fibres, because the refractive index changes in one step. The index profile of a fibre shows how its refractive index changes with distance across the diameter. It is not necessary for the change in refractive index to be sharp. If light is travelling through a substance that has a slowly changing refractive index then it will be refracted

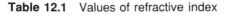

Table 12.1 Values of refractive index

Material	Refractive index
Air	1.00
Ice	1.31
Water	1.33
Silicone resin	1.41
Acrylic sheet	1.49
Crown glass	1.52
Polystyrene	1.59
Flint glass	1.62
Diamond	2.42

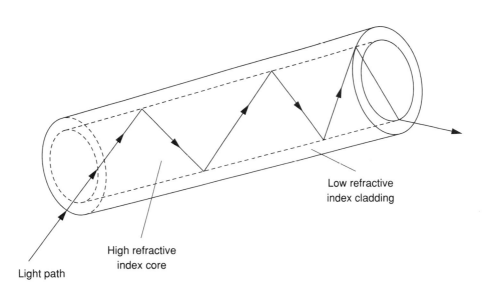

Figure 12.2 Lightwave path principle within an optical fibre with cladding.

along a curve. Graded index fibres have a core in which the refractive index is highest in the middle and decreases smoothly towards the surface. The further away from the centre a light ray strays, the faster it travels and the more it is refracted back towards the centre. As well as these two common fibre types (step index and graded index), there are others such as single-mode and elliptical.

When trying to get light into an optical fibre, you need to know which light rays will be trapped in the fibre and which will escape through the core–cladding interface.

12.4 MATERIALS

Material selection is critical for the application. Once the optical fibre has been made it may be coated for strength, abrasion resistance, colour coding etc.

12.4.1 STEP INDEX FIBRE

These consist of a core glass surrounded by a cladding glass with a lower refractive index.

12.4.2 GRADED INDEX FIBRE

These have a core whose refractive index decreases parabolically with the distance from the centre until it matches the index of the cladding.

12.4.2 PLASTIC CLAD SILICA FIBRES

These are made from pure silica fibres coated with a silicone resin and are usually of large diameter.

12.4.4 POLYMER FIBRES

Polymer fibres are made using the same principles as for glass fibres, except that the core is normally poly(methyl methacrylate) (PMMA) and it is clad with a thin coating of poly(vinyl chloride) (PVC).

12.4.5 SIDE EMITTING FIBRES – SIDEGLOW™

Unlike all other fibre optic applications, Sideglow is designed to emit light along its length rather than to conduct light to an end point. When used with a suitable colour wheel a very attractive sparkling colour change is effected along the length of the fibre.

Glass fibres vary in diameter from 0.025 mm to 0.6 mm. The thinnest ones are used in fibrescopes where their small size gives a high resolution. Fibres used for communications are typically 0.125 mm so that they can easily be seen and handled. The larger glass fibres are a recent development and are strong enough to be used without a sheath.

Plastic fibres are used for lighting and so are larger. They vary from 0.075 mm in bundles to 6.0 mm single fibres. Most fibres have sheaths, these are about 1–4 mm in diameter. Fibres are bundled into cables which may be a couple of centimetres across and include reinforcing braid.

The working temperature range of glass fibres is limited by the sheath material, PTFE sheaths are functional from –15 to +150°C, beyond that you have to use stainless steel, to 700°C. The glass fibres themselves have a range of –200 to +450°C for continuous use. Silica fibres can be used up to 800°C. Plastic fibres can endure 80°C continuously and 95°C for short periods. They become brittle below –30°C. Plastic fibres can be softened and bent to shape in hot water.

12.5 FILAMENT PRODUCTION

Fibre optic filaments are produced by a number of methods depending on material, costs, function and end use.

The simplest method is to place a billet of core material into a tube made from cladding material, then draw through a heated forming die, until the required size is achieved. The filament is coiled onto drums for storage or further processing to form the finished product. Because of the nature of the process, the two starting materials must be an excellent tolerance fit and have similar heat transfer and expansion properties. A simple sketch of the process is shown in Figure 12.3.

Another cheaper way to produce optical fibres is similar to plastic or metal extrusion, but using molten glass. By having two separate crucibles and gravity feed, coextrusion to form the required composite of glasses can give a noticeable improvement in quality compared to the previous method. To maintain quality and diameter, the two crucibles must be constantly monitored for temperature and volume, with the base materials constantly topped up. The sketch in Figure 12.4 clarifies the set-up.

The most complex filaments are the graded index fibres. These are made by depositing inorganic oxides onto the inside of a glass tube by chemical vapour deposition (CVD), to form glasses of known refractive index. By varying the blend of oxides as deposition progresses, the gradation in

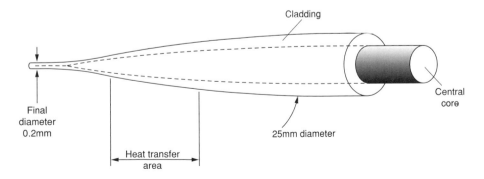

Figure 12.3 Simple drawing method for optical fibres.

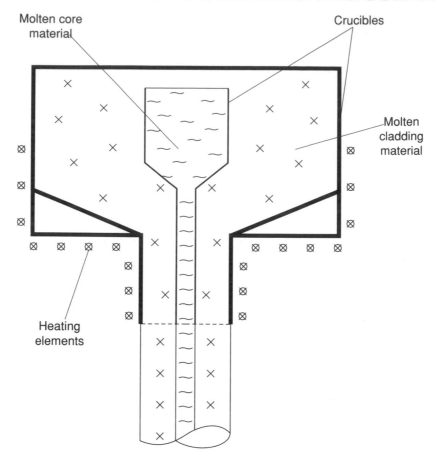

Figure 12.4   Co-extruding optical fibres.

refractive index occurs. The oxides used include boron oxide, phosphorous pentoxide and germanium dioxide. When deposition is finished, the whole assembly is compressed, by the application of heat and pressure, into and through a forming die and the fibre is drawn down to the required diameter.

Silica fibres are drawn and coiled by standard methods and coated with silicone resin. This method of manufacture is especially suited to larger sized fibres or rods. The only drawback is the difficulty of connecting or making joints with these fibres.

There are other methods or producing optical fibres but those already described are the more common ones.

12.6 FIBRE BUNDLES

The fibre optic cables used, especially in the clinical environment, can be one of two types of light transfer units. When using video imaging equipment in an operating theatre the connecting optical cable may be a cluster of hundreds of fibre strands bonded together with resin for strength, cut, trimmed, ends polished, fitted with ferrules and then covered in a protective sleeve or sheath. Alternatively, a liquid-filled flexible tube, sealed, polished and protected externally by a sheath can be used. As already mentioned, the sealed liquid tube gives better optical clarity but is the more expensive option.

The sheath, by the way, can contribute anything up to 60% of the cost of the finished item because of the extensive work involved.

Bundles of fibres are normally manufactured in a continuous process in which individual strands are grouped together and passed through a polymer extruding machine, sealed by the plastic in a tube form, cooled, sized and coiled. The larger finished diameter versions are sometimes cut to length as they reach the end of the production line. Figure 12.5 shows a schematic of the assembly process.

There are various coverings which are applied when extruding bundles but commonly PVC, silicone and LDPE are used to form the first covering. Subsequently protection oversleeves are added to meet specific demands such as resistance to abrasion, dust, heat or mechanical stress. Examples of the extreme conditions which fibre optic cables can endure are: sea beds, furnaces and jet engines. They can be crushed, dropped, coiled to a radius of curvature as tight as three times the thickness or protected by armoured coils which fit together like a suit of armour. If a light bundle is to be used in contact with the human body, then all toxicity and compatibility requirements must, of course be met.

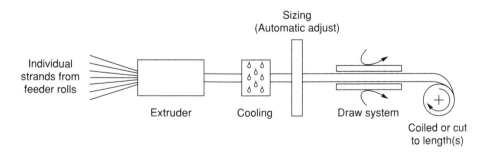

Figure 12.5 Optical fibre bundle manufacture.

12.7 MEDICAL APPLICATIONS

An example of using fibre optics in the medical field is the Biomedical Fibroptic Thermometer, manufactured by Luxtron. This has the following benefits.

- Stable fluorescent sensors unaffected by bending or moisture.
- Radio frequency and microwave-immune fiberoptic probes.
- Sensors unaffected by high DC magnetic fields.
- Fast response, low cost multi-sensor probes.
- User programmable high/low temperature limits.
- Analog voltage outputs for each channel.
- RS-232D serial interface port and data logging software.

Luxtron manufacture this high performance biomedical thermometer that offers exceptional accuracy and stability in demanding circumstances. The electromagnetic induction immunity and inherent stability of Luxtron's patented fluorescent sensor eliminates the problems encountered with conventional thermocouple or thermistor sensors.

The instrument has been designer primarily for use in electromagnetically hostile biomedical applications. Examples include the measurement of tissue temperature during clinical thermotherapy treatments using r.f. or microwave heating, electrosurgery, r.f. and microwave ablation, biological effects of r.f. and microwave radiation, and magnetic resonance spectroscopy or imaging. This instrument is medically approved as a device suitable for use in clinical applications.

Biomedical temperature probes for the above equipment are available in both single and multisensor configurations. Multisensor probes are offered in a four sensor linear array with several sensor spacing options and with four individual probes terminated with a common four fibre connector. Single sensor biomedical probes are available for special applications. All probe designs use moulded plastic connectors to ensure complete immunity to electromagnetic fields.

The company recommends that the probes be sterilised using ETO gas. These probes should not be autoclaved or gamma radiation sterilised because of possible damage that may be done, or effects on the clarity of the fibres.

Some examples of other applications are:

- in high voltage or r.f./microwave fields,
- inside microwave ovens,
- on live electrical circuits and power supplies,
- on tiny surfaces or samples,
- in plasma processing chambers, and
- with fast response on small masses.

The tiny non-electrical probes (as small as 25 μm tip) allow accurate contact and non-contact sensing of temperatures on integrated circuits,

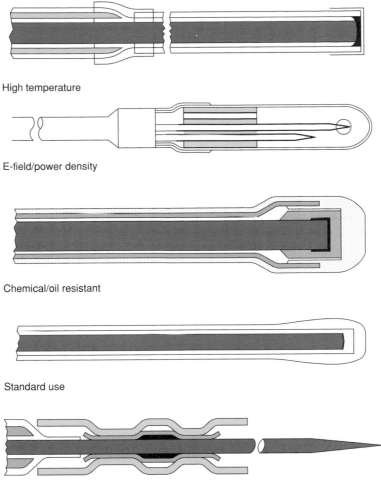

High temperature

E-field/power density

Chemical/oil resistant

Standard use

Micro-tip

Figure 12.6 Examples of fibre optic probe tips. Reproduced by permission of LUXTRON Corporation, a wholly-owned subsidary of Fairey Group plc.

hybrid components and semiconductor wafers, providing faster, more cost-effective thermal testing of electronic devices and packaging.

Small surface temperatures measured with improved accuracy are helping uncover design flaws and accelerate developments in a broad range of electronics.

With the widespread application of industrial heating of adhesives and similar materials and curing for composite materials, accurate temperature

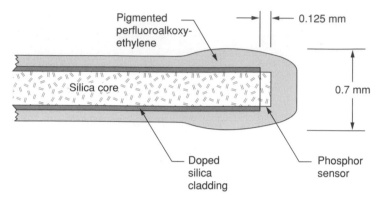

Figure 12.7 Cross-section of typical probe tip. Reproduced by permission of LUXTRON Corporation, a wholly-owned subsidiary of Fairey Group plc.

measurements are critical. Luxtron provided for the first time a means of interference-free control.

Examples of popular types of probes available for the temperature monitor follow. There are various application temperatures, ranges and lengths, feed throughs for vacuum and pressure chambers, as well as non-contact, detached-phosphor sensing kits. Replacement tips, heavy duty fibre sheaths and probe extensions are other options: see Figures 12.6, 12.7 and 12.8 for different types.

Because of this type of construction and their unique self-calibrations these fluorescent sensors lend themselves to custom probe designs. If requesting a quotation on such a probe the following information should be included.

- Description of the actual application.
- Temperature range to be covered with maximum and minimum values.
- Sketch of the area or apparatus to be measured (if possible).
- Details of the area or environment in which the probe is to be used.

This Luxtron patented technology is based on a temperature-sensitive phosphor sensor attached to the end of an optical fibre, which is connected to the instrument. Blue-violet light pulses are sent down the fibre causing the phosphor to glow red. The decay of the fluorescence after each pulse varies precisely with temperature, providing the basics for accurate temperature measurement at the sensor, up to an absolute accuracy of $\pm 0.1°C$.

The fluorescent decay time is measured by a multipoint digital integration of the decay curve. The same optical fibre transmits the excitation pulses and returns the fluorescent signal to the instrument.

Outer jackets on virtually all temperature probes shown are normally of PFA, a high-melting (320°C) member of the Teflon family (PTFE). Probes made of plastic clad silica or all-quartz fibres are also fabricated in cabled form with a Kevlar fibre wrap between two PFA layers.

a SIW–XX
Wide Range

Last 2.5 cm of probe is not Kevlar® cabled. Recommended for use with long SEC-type fiberoptic extension cables.

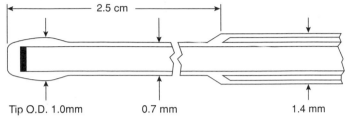

and Teflon® coated

b SFW–XX
Wide Range/Chemical Resistant

Sensors encapsulated with oil-resistant sealant. Probe is Kevlar cabled all the way to the sensor tip.
Not recommended for use with extension cables longer than 10 meters.

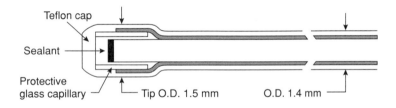

c SFF–XX
Wide Range/Fast Response

Last 1.2 cm of probe is not Kevlar cabled.
Not recommended for use with extension cables longer than 10 meters.

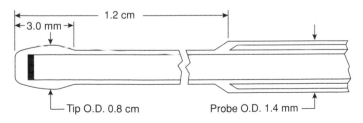

Figure 12.8 Various probes for fibre optic devices. Reproduced by permission of LUXTRON Corporation, a wholly-owned subsidiary of Fairey Group plc.

d   SIH–XX
High Temperature Range

Sensor located at the tip of a 10 cm alumina ceramic tube.

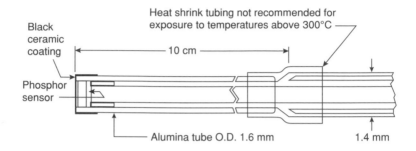

e   SEL–XX
Surface Contact Temperature Probe

Includes Teflon slip connector and two 10 cm-long replaceable probe tips.

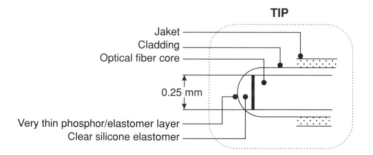

To order replacement probe tips for SEL Surface Temperature Probes, specify **SEL TIPS** which includes

8 replacement sensor tips
1 replacement slip connector
1 sensor cleaning kit

Figure 12.8   *(continued)*

Since many applications involve electrically hostile environments, the specially formulated black pigment used in outer jackets is electrically non-conducting, as are the rest of the materials. This minimises both the hazard of electrical breakdown in high voltage environments and conductive heating artefacts when the probe is used in r.f. or microwave fields.

The phosphor used by Luxtron is magnesium fluorogermanate activated with tetravalent manganese. This hardy material was originally developed as

f SMT–XX
"Microtip" Surface Temperature Probe

Includes one SSC-2 probe body with two 12.5 cm-long SMT replaceable probe tips, 3-axis micropositioner and probe holder.

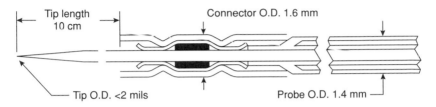

To order replacement probe tips for SMT Surface Temperature Probes, specifiy **SMT TIPS** which includes

> 4 replacement sensor tips
> 1 replacement slip connector
> 1 sensor cleaning kit

g SSP–XX
Remote Sensing Probe

Fiber end is polished for remote phosphor sensing. Last 2.5 cm of probe is not Kevlar cabled.

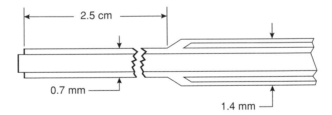

Figure 12.8 *(continued)*

a colour corrector for mercury vapour street lamps. It is prepared as a powder by solid state reaction involving firing in air at 1200°C. The resultant material is quite stable, fairly insoluble, and relatively benign from a biological standpoint.

Various binders and adhesives are used to form the sensor and attach it to the fibre tip or to a surface. These are typically silicone resins, or for higher temperatures potassium silicate, fired to produce a glassy matrix.

Table 12.2 lists the materials used in the probes.

All applications depend upon the creation of effective terminals for the introduction of light or a signal carrier beam.

Table 12.2 Materials used in Luxtron probes. Reproduced by permission of LUXTRON Corporation, a wholly-owned subsidiary of Fairey Group plc

Component	Fibre type			
	320 μm all silica	200 μm all silica	400 μm plastic clad silica	600 μm plastic clad silica
Fibre core material	Silica	Silica	Silica	Silica
Fibre core diameter (μm)	320	200	400	600
Fibre cladding material	Silica	Silica	Siloxane	Siloxane
Cladding/buffer diameter (μm)	420	240	550	700
Jacket material	PFA Teflon	PFA Teflon	PFA Teflon	Polyurethane
1st jacket diameter (mm)	0.7	0.5	0.7	0.82
Outer jacket diameter (mm)	1.4	1.4	1.4	5.5
Kevlar cabling for strength	Yes	Yes	Yes	Yes
Minimum bend radius (cm) mechanical limit	1.5	1.0	1.0	5.0
Minimum bend radius (cm) optical limit	3.0	1.5	1.0	5.0
Temperature range (°C)	−200 to 300	−200 to 300	0 to 200	0 to 80

12.8 TERMINALS

There are five requirements for fibre optic terminals.

- For communications use the ends must be ground and polished to allow the light to pass without interference. For illumination purposes a plain cut is sufficient.
- The ends must be perpendicular to the cable axis to avoid losses.
- The fibre strands must be close packed uniformly within the cable. Losses due to space between the strands vary from 6 to 15%.
- Light entry must be uniformly distributed across the cable diameter. Where cables are joined the diameters must match and the polished ends should be in contact.
- Cables should be made up in effective lengths with a minimal number of joints. No matter how well polished and matched the ends are, there will still be at least a 4% loss of light intensity (or energy) at each joint owing to Fresnel diffraction. Attenuation is inevitably associated with cable length and depends on core material, so these factors should be optimised for the application. Attenuation follows an exponential loss: in practice, if a length of cable has an attenuation of 50%, twice that length will lose 75%, three times will lose 87.5% and four times the length will lose 93.75%.

12.9 LIGHT SOURCE

For fibre optics the most powerful light source gives the best results, so go for the best your budget will allow. It is also important to choose a suitable wavelength. For example, in blood 150 W white light will give better results than 250 W red light. Filters can be used to reduce the heating effect of infrared wavelengths, which could be important if the end point is heat sensitive like a patient. Lamp suppliers generally carry a comprehensive catalogue of accessories.

You will need to consider several factors in choosing a light source. As well as budget there are the needs of the customer and their perception of value for money. Cheaper lamps may have limited life, so their suitability depends on likely running times. Other lamps have a warm-up time which may cause aggravation to the operation. Here are some examples:

Lamp	Power	Life
Xenon	100–1000 W	100–1000 h
Metal halide	100–1000 W	6000 h max.
Tungsten halogen (quartz)	50 W	4000 h max.
	150 W	500 h max.

Other considerations when selecting a light source are its cooling requirements and the effect of switching on and off repeatedly. The cooling circulation and restrictions or access of air to the unit must be investigated.

A summary of lamp requirements is as follows:

- Electrical: who, what, to what level, specific industrial or medical restrictions?
- Cooling: how fast, air flow, noise?
- Power: mains supply or transformer?
- Control: variable, fixed, remote, physical, digital?
- Wavelength: colour, intensity, stable over time or machine life?
- Lamp: price, life and power; ease of replacement, handling, size?

12.10 OTHER APPLICATIONS

There are many and varied applications for fibre optics, using either a single strand, multi-strand bundles or sealed bundles. Listed below are some working examples to highlight particular applications and as an indication of the diverse tasks for which fibre optics can be used. I hope that these examples will stimulate ideas for new medical products.

- Decorative: shop lights, directional displays, picture illumination.
- Electrically unsafe places: swimming pool illumination, spot lights, garden lights, fish ponds.

- Entertainment: discos, theatre.
- Information display: control panels, traffic information signs.
- Advertising: multi-messages from one source.
- Emergency use: safety signs, exit indicators during fire or power failure.
- Alarm system: loop of optical fibre to secure property or access area.
- Movement sensor: machine guards, intruder sensor.
- Heat sensor: replacement for conventional thermocouple, will also work in high pressure environments.
- Visual: extension cables for cameras or video (may require lens to be fitted), also used in conjunction with CCTV.
- UV adhesive: light cables for spot illumination of UV adhesives when selective bonding is required.
- Medical: Sideglow™ stimulation, with endoscopes, Uriglow™ illumination.
- Dental: intense light for curing adhesive filling materials.
- Communication: information transfer.
- Hazards: ideal for use in areas of high explosive risk with a spark free requirement.
- Industrial: fluid level sensor within tanks.
- Illumination: direct light transfer to a specific point.

12.11 BENEFITS OF FIBRE OPTIC TECHNOLOGY

To develop a new fibre optic product you will need to justify the project to investors or employers. To help you I have summarised the benefits as listed below.

- Electrically insulated from the working tip.
- Can be fitted with IR filters to provide cold illumination.
- The wavelength, i.e. colour, can be changed easily.
- Selective placement of light emission.
- By using lenses or shaped tips the light can be focused and redirected.
- The light source can be distant, removing or relocating heat, noise, and power requirements to a more convenient area.
- A single light source can supply many strands or cables.
- Excellent suitability for use in difficult or hazardous environments.
- Comparatively cheap optical cables permit disposable applications.
- Extremely thin strands afford access to difficult locations.
- Resistant to most chemical and body fluids.
- Applications other than light transfer, e.g. sensors, heat monitors, movement monitors.
- High visual impact with long distance remote viewing application.
- Long life coupled with low maintenance costs.
- Low susceptibility to damage.

13
Battery Selection

This chapter is intended to provide an insight into the problems of specifying a portable power supply for equipment, medical or otherwise, and then ensuring that everyone is safe. The final product may not be for clinical use, it may be part of the manufacturing process or an inspection tool for the quality control department, but if portable electrical power is required then batteries will be needed.

For mains power supplies you can consult the relevant technical standards: this chapter is about batteries.

A cell is a self-contained power source which relies upon a chemical reaction to provide a low-voltage, DC electrical current. A battery is an assembly of cells coupled to provide more voltage or current than a single cell. Batteries can comprise cells connected in series and/or parallel. In common practice single cells are sometimes called batteries, but this indicates a lack of understanding.

Batteries generally produce nominal voltages of 3V, 6V, 9V, 12V etc. If you have special requirements, battery manufacturers can provide custom batteries producing the voltage and current you need. This is, of course, an expensive option and generally you should design equipment to use standard batteries. However, there is a school of thought suggesting that it is profitable for a medical device manufacturer to supply customers with special replacement batteries not available elsewhere if there is a long-term need.

Battery performance is difficult to compare because the various chemical systems have different attributes. For example, the effect of temperature on current means that a zinc–carbon cell will not produce a useful current at –10°C but a lithium–sulphur cell will still function at –50°C. Elevated temperatures increase the rate of self-discharge in all cells but to varying degrees, reducing effective voltage and cell life.

There is a huge range of cells and batteries available, so to understand the choice it is necessary to classify the types.

There are many factors to consider when selecting a battery. Table 13.1 shows most of these factors.

I intend to concentrate on the three most common round batteries used and their electrochemical systems first. Then I will explain some of the other systems, assemblies and developments.

Table 13.1   Battery selection criteria

Voltage requirements	Current load	Terminations
Weight limitations	Environmental (disposal)	Service conditions
Duty cycle	Battery capacity	Storage
Dimensions	Mechanical requirements	Cost
Local/National/ International Standards		

Primary cells are used once and discarded. They should not be recharged. Secondary cells are intended for recharging, which can be done a finite number of times. The main text of this chapter concerns primary cells and batteries.

13.1 CELL TYPES

The three common electrochemical systems for primary cells are as follows.

- Zinc-carbon: cheap, wasteful, short life and on the way out. Most European manufacturers are either phasing-out production or have already stopped. Zinc–carbon cells are used for cheap ready power of limited capacity and current.
- Zinc–chloride: widely used, middle range on price and capacity, but losing popularity. Zinc–chloride cells are used for constant low discharge rate requirements like clocks, hazard lanterns and railway beacons.
- Alkaline–manganese: comparatively expensive, high capacity, roughly 55% of the market but growing. Alkaline–manganese cells are now used for virtually every application since the seal can be guaranteed and capacity lasts. Their prime use is for high-rate intermittent discharge like toy motors, flash units and back-up emergency power.

13.2 CELL CODING

To identify cells and their systems a letter-code is used with prefixes to indicate size and shape. The code applies to all electrochemical systems except the zinc–carbon or zinc–chloride systems, because being original these have no lettered code. Alkaline–manganese is coded 'L', other codes are 'A' for air depolarised, 'M' for mercuric oxide, 'S' for silver oxide, but the first letter of the electrochemical system does not always denote the code as 'C' for lithium shows. The size and shape information is given by 'R' for round, 'F' for flat or 'S' for square. Then there is a number to denote the height and width, or length. Table 13.2 shows the nominal sizes for the most popular round cells. Alkaline–manganese codes are quoted, so a battery marked

Table 13.2 Maximum dimensions for round cells

	Diameter (mm)	Height (mm)
LR01	12.0	30.2
LR03	10.5	44.5
LR6	14.5	50.5
LR14	26.2	50.0
LR20	34.2	61.5

LR03 is easily recognised as a round cell nominally 10.5 mm diameter × 44.5 mm height with an alkaline–manganese electrochemical system.

Trying to remember codes is tedious, so think of it like this:

L01/LR01 : short dumpy ones, for the camera.
L03/LR03 : little thin ones.
L6/LR6 : thin penlight ones, most common.
L14/LR14 : short fat ones, for a torch.
L20/LR20 : big ones for the radio.

13.3 TECHNICAL STANDARDS

All coding and size regulations are controlled by the IEC (International Electrotechnical Commission). The first regulations were published in 1957. Battery manufacturers produce their products to IEC specifications. This compliance ensures a standardisation of external dimensions which allows original equipment manufacturers to make compartments which will accept standard batteries or cells. Also consumers can be confident that they may purchase a replacement power source any time and anywhere quite easily.

The IEC also lay down minimum values for storage, discharge and application tests. Figure 13.1 shows some of the discharge rates of normal applications. Table 13.3 and Figure 13.2 show the discharge durations of popular applications and the expected life for different cells. You need this information to select a cell system which is appropriate for you application, saving your company and customers time, effort and money.

Methods of connecting batteries by external terminals are also tightly specified. There are flying leads, snap fasteners, radial sockets, 4 mm screw cap and many more standard terminals. Cells are often connected by simple direct contact. Figure 13.3 shows the IEC international standards for battery profiles and their positive and negative areas. Figure 13.4 gives an insight into the consequences of neglecting these standards and the problems to be encountered if all regulations are not checked.

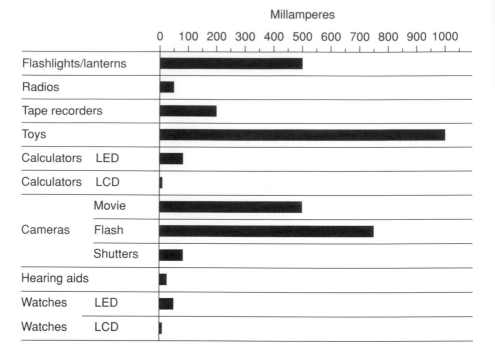

Figure 13.1 Drain rates for major applications: © 1992 Institution of Engineering Designers, first published in *Engineering Designer* Jan/Feb 1992 and reproduced with permission.

Table 13.3 Examples of drain variations: © 1992 Institution of Engineering Designers, first published in *Engineering Designer* Jan/Feb 1992 and reproduced with permission.

Drain rate (mA)	Alkaline–manganese (W.h in^{-3})	Zinc–carbon (W.h in^{-3})	Ratio
50	3.5	0.7	5 : 1
100	2.6	0.5	5.25 : 1
200	1.8	0.3	6 : 1
300	1.2	0.1	12 : 1

The IEC standards are under constant review with amendments to suit modern developments added regularly. To ensure no unfair competitive advantage is gained, representation on the IEC board from all major manufacturers in all European countries, is encouraged.

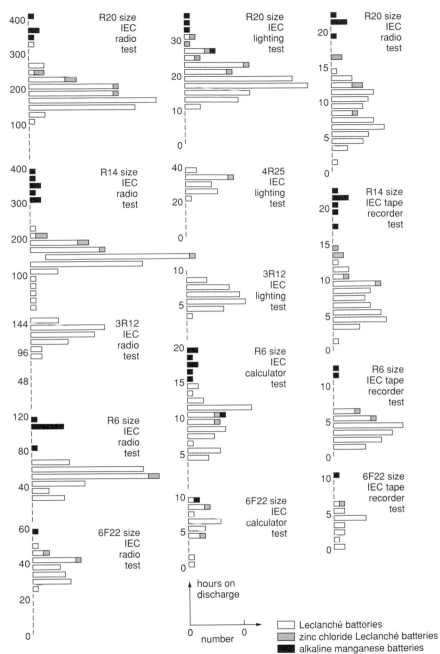

Figure 13.2 World survey of discharge durations on some important IEC application tests.

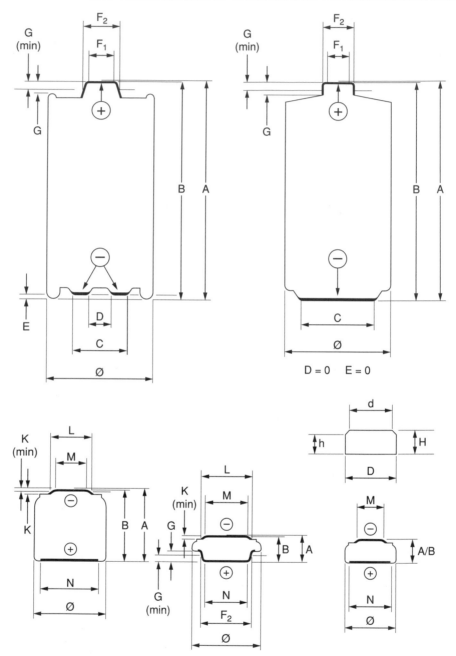

Figure 13.3 IEC profiles of round cells and dimensions specified by international standards.

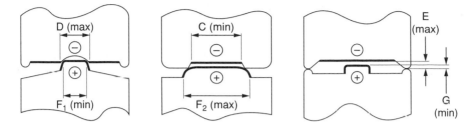

Figure 13.4 Some consequences of not adhering to the IEC terminal dimensions of cylindrical cells.

13.4 CELL OPERATION

An electrochemical cell converts chemical energy to electrical energy by chemical reaction. This normally takes place when the electrical circuit is completed. Within all cells there is an internal self-discharge taking place slowly while they are just standing, so in time a stored battery will lose its charge. This is why leading manufacturers now mark their products with a 'sell by' or 'use by' date.

The zinc–carbon and zinc–chloride systems work best at low current drain over long periods, say in a clock or radio. Alkaline–manganese cells are superior for high-drain short-term use, e.g. razor, or Walkman.

To calculate the charge available from your battery, the rated capacity should be divided by the current drain value. This drain is measured in milliamperes and when a current of 1 mA flows through a circuit for one hour the total charge passed is 1 mA.h. These rated values can be obtained from the manufacturers and are normally printed on the back of the packing for commercial and domestic sales. For example, consider a LR20 cell rated at 10 000 mA.h used in a circuit having a 7.5 Ω bulb at 1.5 V. The current would be 200 mA, and the cell would last 10 000/200 = 50 h. Describing cell capacity in terms of charge in mA.h, does not give the energy available. To do so the electromotive force or voltage must be taken into account. This is done by multiplying the charge in mA.h by the voltage, V, to give mW.h, a measure of energy. So our 10 000 mA.h cell has a voltage of 1.5 V and an energy capacity of 10 000 mW.h or 15 W.h.

Buying the best cell you can afford is a way of paying extra for no benefit. Consider Figure 13.1 to see the drains described. You could end up paying twice the price for less then twice the energy. So you need to do calculations to work out how much charge you need, what life you want and how much energy is required. Then you can select the cell or battery which is most appropriate. If you consult the manufacturer, they will gladly provide all the information you need and recommend a choice of product.

13.5   SAFE USE OF BATTERIES AND CELLS

Whichever battery system you select it should be treated with respect. All are packets of chemicals, each volatile and with the potential to harm the careless user. Cells can also damage the equipment in which they are encased, which could be costly to replace or repair. So here is a list of the do's and don'ts for safe battery use.

13.5.1   DON'Ts

- Don't slip one or two 'fresh' batteries into a set: this reduces the overall service life, creates the potential for mismatching cell types and most importantly can cause gases to be generated within the more depleted cells. Always replace the whole set. Gases will force out the corrosive electrolyte. Normally pressure builds up gradually and there is a slow leak of electrolyte, which is how cells are intended to function because if there was no leak, pressure could build up to seriously dangerous levels.
- Don't 'short out' batteries, especially alkaline–manganese or lithium, by direct contact across the terminals. The internal pressure generated can be a high as 800 p.s.i., enough to rupture the steel casing. Safety systems are built in to prevent rupture but there is always a slim possibility that the safety mechanism could fail. Remember that 50 million cells are manufactured annually in the UK.
- Don't 'arc' the two terminals, wrap the cells in conductive foil, or store in contact with conducting items. Store all cells in their packaging if possible, even loose metal straps could be enough to cause a spark. The heat from a directly shorted cell is enough to cause a fire.
- Don't mix cells of different systems. This can cause corrosion or rupture as one tries to force the chemical reaction to run faster within the other less capable one.
- Don't place batteries in their compartment the wrong way round; ensure that the plus and minus marks are correctly orientated. People misguidedly reverse cells to 'switch off' a device but this is hazardous. Incorrect placement of terminal contacts can, in extreme conditions, cause fire or explosion.
- Don't heat batteries to enhance their performance. This is most unwise.
- Don't try to open batteries to look inside. There may already be a build up of pressure inside with an amount of unused electrolyte; the potential is for damage to clothing at best or eyes at worst.
- Don't dispose of batteries in a fire. Because the seals to keep the corrosive electrolyte in are very effective, they also retain pressures produced when the cells are heated. If the fire damages the safety mechanism, there is potential for an explosion.

- Don't attempt to recharge primary cells. Although there are claims that this can be done to save you money, it is rarely successful, can cause internal pressure build up and force electrolyte out. If you want to recharge cells, buy those designed for recharging.

13.5.2 DO's

- Do remove batteries from equipment if it is not to be used for a long period of time. Batteries left in situ will eventually cause corrosion and ruin the device.
- Do consult manufacturers about their product and potential environmental changes.
- Do buy branded products. They are safer, conform to the IEC regulations, will fit the equipment and provide a steady reliable current.
- Do seek medical assistance: if exposed to leaked cell contents, if anyone swallows part or all of a cell or battery (especially relevant to button cells and small children), or if exposed to any fumes from a battery.

Figure 13.5 shows the same points as above in a more visual way, to help you to remember.

13.6 SAFETY BY DESIGN

There are safety devices within cells to prevent pressure build-up and explosion. As there are several electrochemical systems in use, there are various safety 'trips' appropriate to different cells.

For zinc–carbon and zinc–chloride cells the seal is a large, low tech, blob of molten bitumen–wax mixture (the wax modifies the viscosity). This seal is poured over the cell contents once compacted and covered with a support washer, just before the end cap is applied. The end cap seals with an interference fit on the inner contact rod. The end cap is pressed into the sealant and it is left to cool. The effectiveness of the seal is determined by the amount of sealant, the coding time, how far the cap penetrates the sealant, and the tightness of the interference fit with the rod. There is an additional 'top swag' or curl to pull over the outer sleeve which adds to the effectiveness of the main bitumen and wax seal.

Figure 13.6 is a detailed drawing of a commonly produced zinc–chloride cell, to illustrate the 'goo and wedge' concept. Although fairly crude, this is an effective seal for the pressures arising during use and abuse of zinc–chloride cells. To safely release over-pressure, the bitumen moves slowly and gives way. It has the flexibility to move without major problems occurring. After pressure release the seal can restablish because the bitumen and wax compound never completely solidifies. Figure 13.7 shows a more modern zinc–carbon cell, the construction is slightly different but the basic components

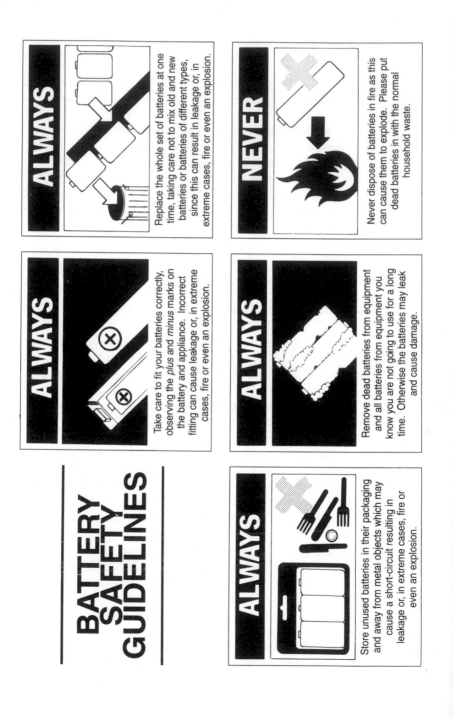

BATTERY SAFETY GUIDELINES

ALWAYS

Replace the whole set of batteries at one time, taking care not to mix old and new batteries or batteries of different types, since this can result in leakage or, in extreme cases, fire or even an explosion.

NEVER

Never dispose of batteries in fire as this can cause them to explode. Please put dead batteries in with the normal household waste.

ALWAYS

Take care to fit your batteries correctly, observing the *plus* and *minus* marks on the battery and appliance. Incorrect fitting can cause leakage or, in extreme cases, fire or even an explosion.

ALWAYS

Remove dead batteries from equipment and all batteries from equipment you know you are not going to use for a long time. Otherwise the batteries may leak and cause damage.

ALWAYS

Store unused batteries in their packaging and away from metal objects which may cause a short-circuit resulting in leakage or, in extreme cases, fire or even an explosion.

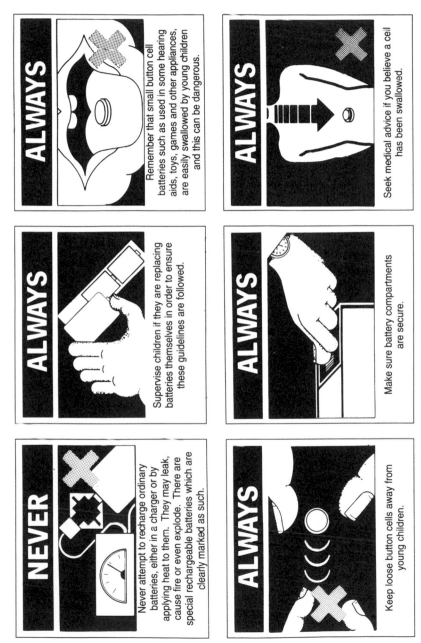

REPRINTED WITH THE KIND PERMISSION OF THE BRITISH BATTERY MANUFACTURER'S ASSOCIATION

Figure 13.5 Do's and don'ts for battery use. Reproduced by permission of the British Battery Manufacturer's Association.

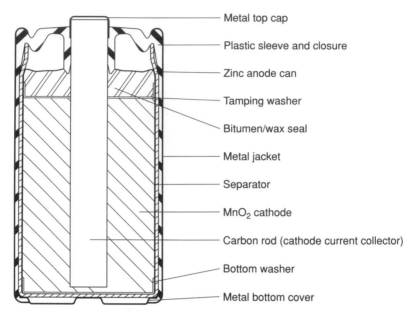

Metal top cap

Plastic sleeve and closure

Zinc anode can

Tamping washer

Bitumen/wax seal

Metal jacket

Separator

MnO$_2$ cathode

Carbon rod (cathode current collector)

Bottom washer

Metal bottom cover

Figure 13.6   Construction of a zinc–carbon cell.

and method of sealing still apply. The zinc–carbon system is also known by the eponymous name Leclanché (though strictly a Leclanché cell is a wet-system with Zn and C rods in NH$_4$Cl solution).

With alkaline–manganese cells the internal pressures are potentially significantly higher and can be generated more quickly. Internal heating can be significant if cells are abused. For these reasons different methods of sealing and safety release are required. The seal is formed by crimping the metal case and top cap together. The safety release device varies from manufacturer to manufacturer but is based on fracture of a plastic component.

Figure 13.8 shows the method of crimping used by a German company to close their version of an alkaline–manganese cell. It gives the side pressure so vital for a long term seal. Figure 13.9 gives a rough outline and general assembly of a pressure vent. Figure 13.10 is a detailed view of a more modern design, but showing that at the start of the newer types of cell systems the wax 'plug' was still favoured.

Figure 13.11 and Figure 13.12 show two top seal constructions with their respective venting systems; one is Japanese and the other is German.

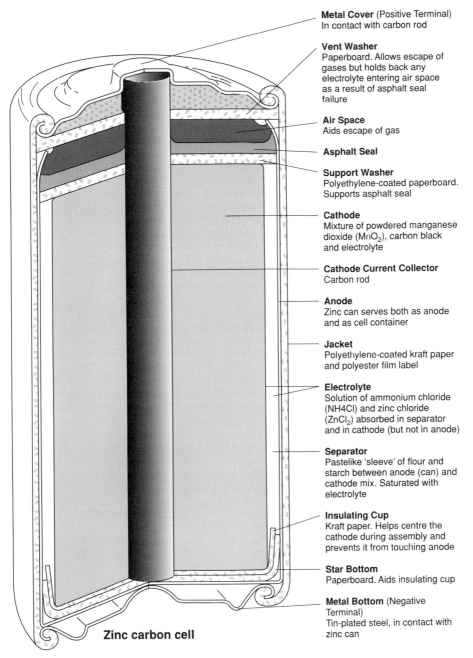

Metal Cover (Positive Terminal)
In contact with carbon rod

Vent Washer
Paperboard. Allows escape of
gases but holds back any
electrolyte entering air space
as a result of asphalt seal
failure

Air Space
Aids escape of gas

Asphalt Seal

Support Washer
Polyethylene-coated paperboard.
Supports asphalt seal

Cathode
Mixture of powdered manganese
dioxide (MnO_2), carbon black
and electrolyte

Cathode Current Collector
Carbon rod

Anode
Zinc can serves both as anode
and as cell container

Jacket
Polyethylene-coated kraft paper
and polyester film label

Electrolyte
Solution of ammonium chloride
(NH4Cl) and zinc chloride
($ZnCl_2$) absorbed in separator
and in cathode (but not in anode)

Separator
Pastelike 'sleeve' of flour and
starch between anode (can) and
cathode mix. Saturated with
electrolyte

Insulating Cup
Kraft paper. Helps centre the
cathode during assembly and
prevents it from touching anode

Star Bottom
Paperboard. Aids insulating cup

Metal Bottom (Negative
Terminal)
Tin-plated steel, in contact with
zinc can

Zinc carbon cell

Figure 13.7 Cut-away view of a zinc–carbon cell. © 1992 Institution of Engineering Designers, first published in *Engineering Designer* Jan/Feb 1992 and reproduced with permission.

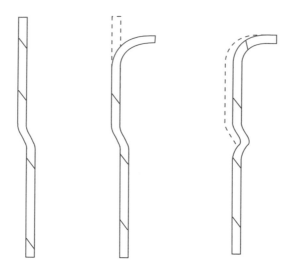

Figure 13.8   Detail of side crimp for an alkaline–manganese cell.

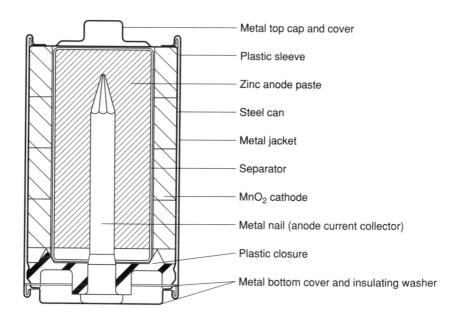

Metal top cap and cover

Plastic sleeve

Zinc anode paste

Steel can

Metal jacket

Separator

MnO$_2$ cathode

Metal nail (anode current collector)

Plastic closure

Metal bottom cover and insulating washer

Figure 13.9   Construction of an alkaline–manganese cell.

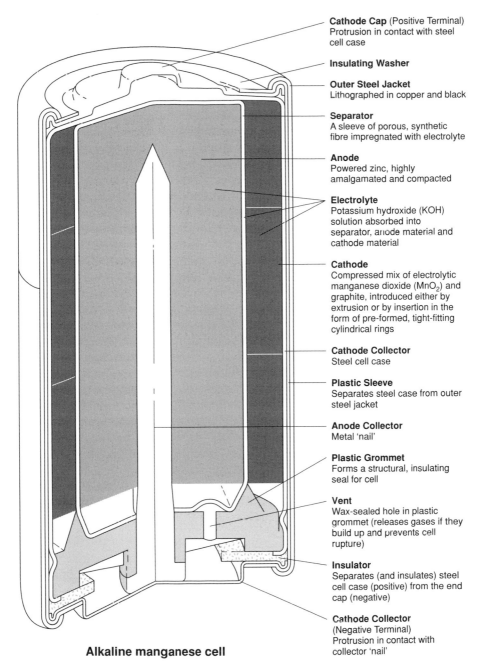

Cathode Cap (Positive Terminal)
Protrusion in contact with steel
cell case

Insulating Washer

Outer Steel Jacket
Lithographed in copper and black

Separator
A sleeve of porous, synthetic
fibre impregnated with electrolyte

Anode
Powered zinc, highly
amalgamated and compacted

Electrolyte
Potassium hydroxide (KOH)
solution absorbed into
separator, anode material and
cathode material

Cathode
Compressed mix of electrolytic
manganese dioxide (MnO_2) and
graphite, introduced either by
extrusion or by insertion in the
form of pre-formed, tight-fitting
cylindrical rings

Cathode Collector
Steel cell case

Plastic Sleeve
Separates steel case from outer
steel jacket

Anode Collector
Metal 'nail'

Plastic Grommet
Forms a structural, insulating
seal for cell

Vent
Wax-sealed hole in plastic
grommet (releases gases if they
build up and prevents cell
rupture)

Insulator
Separates (and insulates) steel
cell case (positive) from the end
cap (negative)

Cathode Collector
(Negative Terminal)
Protrusion in contact with
collector 'nail'

Alkaline manganese cell

Figure 13.10 Cut-away view of one of the first modern alkaline–manganese cells.
© 1992 Institution of Engineering Designers, first published in *Engineering Designer*
Jan/Feb 1992 and reproduced with permission.

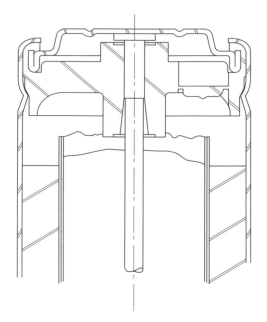

Figure 13.11   A German top-seal construction.

13.7 BATTERY SELECTION

When selecting cells or batteries for your products, seek advice from battery producers, but take more than one opinion. A custom power supply might be what you need, but beware of being tied to only one supplier. In general it is best to use standard cells unless there are overwhelming reasons otherwise.

Consider the following options.

- You can use existing standard cells or batteries. These are easy to replace, available off the shelf and there's little chance of equipment standing idle. You need to be sure that the voltage you require is available, the charge and energy needs can be met, the service life will be long enough and that the cells or batteries will fit in the space available. You should, of course, select the power source before defining the battery compartment.
- You could make-up batteries from standard cells to give greater voltage and capacity. This option is useful to meet special requirements. But will your company want to manufacture power packs? Will the combinations hold together and provide consistent voltages. What about product liability?

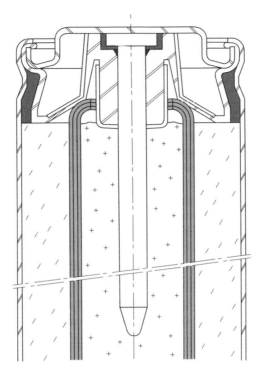

Figure 13.12   A Japanese top-seal construction.

• You could get a manufacturer to propose a custom power pack. First be sure that you can't meet your needs more simply, and then check out what contractural arrangements are possible. Become well informed before any negotiations and consult with more than one manufacturer if possible.

13.8   DESCRIPTIONS OF CELLS

Figures 13.6, 13.7, 13.9 and 13.10 show typical zinc–chloride and alkaline–manganese cells respectively. They have a basic structure in common and design differences arising from the different electrochemical systems. The common components are constructed as follows.

1. **Current collector**

   In the zinc–chloride cell the current collector is a carbon rod; sintered, extruded and ground. In the alkaline–manganese cell the current collector is a brass cold headed 'nail' welded to the negative contact.

2. **Moulded plastic closure**

   In the zinc–chloride cell the moulded plastic closure seals the end of the can by its central boss sticking into the bitumen-wax sealant and the outer sleeve closing on the outside. The plastic closure of an alkaline–manganese cell is secured by crimping the steel edge, see also Figures 13.8, 13.11 and 13.12.

3. **Negative contact**

   In the zinc–chloride cell the negative contact is a press-tool formed tin plate. In the alkaline–manganese system it is the same held by the crimp and insulated from the can by a plastic washer.

4. **Cathode**

   In the zinc–chloride cell the cathode is a mixture of powdered active ingredients, extruded loosely into the can. In the alkaline–manganese cell the cathode is compressed, formed rings of active ingredients, tightly fitted into the steel can ensuring full radial contact.

5. **Separator**

   In the zinc–chloride cell the separator is an outer sleeve of starch and flour, more recently a roll of porous fibre is used. For the alkaline–manganese system the separator is a 'packet' made from synthetic fibre constructed either in one part or in a two part cross form folded and pushed into the inside of the cathode rings.

6. **Outer jacket**

   The outer jacket of the old-style zinc–chloride cell was a metal tube plus an insulating paper or board barrier. Now it is commonly a four-layer insulating laminated board formed into a tube. The outer jacket of the alkaline–manganese cell is a metallised label over a deep-drawn stainless steel can.

7. **Positive contact**

   The positive contact for a zinc–chloride cell is a pre-formed metal cap in contact with the carbon rod. This is normally an interference fit to ensure contact and no arcing or intermittent contact during use. In the alkaline–manganese cell part of the formed stainless steel can is the positive contact. In some forms of cell a separate 'top hat' is welded onto a flat based can.

8. **Anode**

   The anode of the zinc–chloride cell is the zinc can, impact extruded from solid callots (pre-formed zinc slugs), trimmed and grooved on the same machine. It serves both as the anode and as the outer cell container providing strength and form. In the case of alkaline–manganese cells, the anode is powdered zinc, highly amalgamated and compacted. It is dispensed into the cell assembly in a slurry form combined with electrolyte.

9. **Electrolyte**

   In the zinc–chloride cell the electrolyte is $ZnCl_2$ absorbed in the separator and cathode. In the alkaline–manganese system the electrolyte is combined within the active ingredients of the anode and cathode, separated by the pre-formed packet described in point 5.

10. **Bottom washer**

 In the zinc–chloride cell is made of insulated kraft paper, which aids cathode insertion during assembly and insulates the cathode from the anode at the cell base.

11. **Tamping washer**

 In the zinc–chloride cell the tamping washer is made of laminated paper coated with wax or polyethylene. This compacts the cathode, aids assembly and supports the bitumen–wax seal.

12. **Sealant**

 In the zinc–chloride cell the sealant is a bitumen–wax compound, which is heated to 80–100°C and then injected to seal the inside of the cell. In the alkaline–manganese system a small amount of adhesive is used and placed on the underside of the neck of the 'nail' before insertion into the closure. Other types favour application to the outer diameter of the closure before final assembly, normally this type stays tacky for its lifetime: Figure 13.12.

13. **Plastic sleeve**

 Certain makes of alkaline–manganese cell use an additional outer can. This insulates the two conductive materials. Nowadays it has mostly been replaced by a label direct on the outer steel can.

14. **Vent**

 (A) Disruption of the bitumen seal around the centre carbon rod. There is a design on the market which is safe and better which has flexible lips moulded on the closure, these flex upwards but then reseal after the pressure is reduced, items 2 and 7 are significantly different. (B) The example shown uses a wax plug within the closure which 'pops' at a predetermined pressure preventing cell rupture. Many other more effective methods and variations are now on the market, two such can be seen in Figures 13.11 and 13.12 where thin areas of plastic mouldings are designed to give way as safe limits of pressure. Not only more reliable and consistent in performance but once tooling manufactured, cheaper to incorporate. An additional bonus is the reduction in the space they occupy which means the manufacturer is able to pack more active ingredients in to provide longer battery life.

15. **Air space**

 (A) This aids escape of gases generated and allows some movement of the seal without actually breaking it. (B) Accommodates any initial expansions of the anode after assembly and placement of the final crimped seal. Also acts as a reservoir for additional liquid electrolyte (sometimes added for special applications or discharge requirements).

Safety devices are designed into every cell to let any pressure which has built up above a set limit escape but at the same time keep everything else which is obnoxious in.

This had been, and still is being, done with wax seals, weakened sections, bitumen pitch, flexible closures and by other means, some more reliable then others. The vent must be strong enough to contain the gases which are normally generated during the working life of the battery. These gases are usually contained in each individual cell with no detrimental effect.

Figure 13.12 shows a Fuji cell construction which relies upon conventional adhesive and crimp to seal the completed cell. Top containment is by a flexible moulding with a solid centre section for the current collector, flanked by thin sectioned wings. Venting is via one or two weakening grooves, as the pressure builds up the wings flex and if inflated too far the grooves split and rupture. The gases are then allowed to dissipate through two small holes in the vertical sides of the top cap. Figure 13.11 shows how the Varta cell vents through a fully moulded component by means of a weakened thin diaphragm or disc. Again, once released the gases can escape through small holes in the top cap to the atmosphere.

Development is continually being carrier out on all systems to produce better, safer cheaper and more leakproof cells. These developments are also driven by the customer who is demanding batteries to meet more and more stringent requirements.

One example of the type of development under way for the bottom end of the market can be seen in Figure 13.13. This is an idea to use an adhesive for complete seal and vent on a zinc–chloride system cell, dispensing with the traditional methods of simple but physical mechanical containment. An additional benefit is that the closure could sit higher within the can creating greater internal volume, with the ability to pack in more material. Such a new development has to be tested to suit IEC regulations. These trials may take up to 12 months as the tests include initial discharge, storage, humidity, high drain, low drain, charge abuse (cell connected wrong way round to each other) and more as laid down by the IEC.

13.9 BATTERIES

Batteries are assemblies of cells connected together. For domestic use they are often constructed in a sandwich form as shown in Figure 13.14. This is a simple zinc–carbon flat cell stack, with similar construction even when the overall size increases as in Figure 13.15.

A very old method still used is similar to the original Voltaic Pile constructed by Allessandro Volta in 1800, although we have refined the materials and external sealing or containment. But his stack of discs made from zinc and silver, separated by pasteboard or leather which had been soaked in salt water, still provide the basis of the zinc–carbon battery.

The construction does change, however, when the cell system does. It is much easier to wire single commercial cells together and slot them into

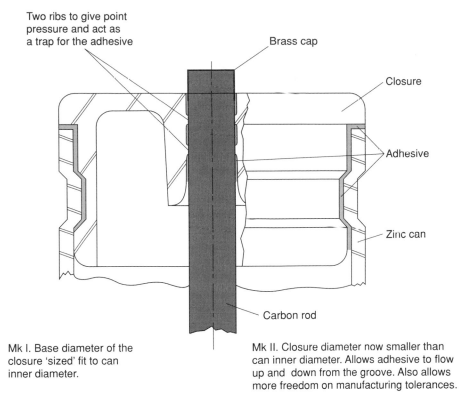

Two ribs to give point pressure and act as a trap for the adhesive

Brass cap

Closure

Adhesive

Zinc can

Carbon rod

Mk I. Base diameter of the closure 'sized' fit to can inner diameter.

Mk II. Closure diameter now smaller than can inner diameter. Allows adhesive to flow up and down from the groove. Also allows more freedom on manufacturing tolerances.

The adhesive was applied to the groove and inner bore. Once located over the carbon rod, the closure was pressed down and clipped into place by the preformed rill on the can. The adhesive thus sealed both at the carbon rod and zinc can interfaces.

Figure 13.13 New design concept: an adhesive seal and vent for a zinc–carbon cell.

a pre-formed carton or plastic shell, than to go to the expense of manufacturing specialist flat, rectangular sealed cells of, say, alkaline–manganese type, cells which can only be used in that particular sized battery. There is a version in which the chemical ingredients are packed into small 'trays' and the tops are either heat sealed or r.f. welded. These modules are then compressed together with spiked plates between, but this method is not extensively used. In Figures 13.16 and 13.17 the two batteries are constructed conventionally with six round cells and the contacts are welded together to supply the desired voltage. Note the wiring arrangement: flat strips of tinplate are resistance welded to the cell bases and arranged to give the 3 V, 6 V or 9 V stipulated.

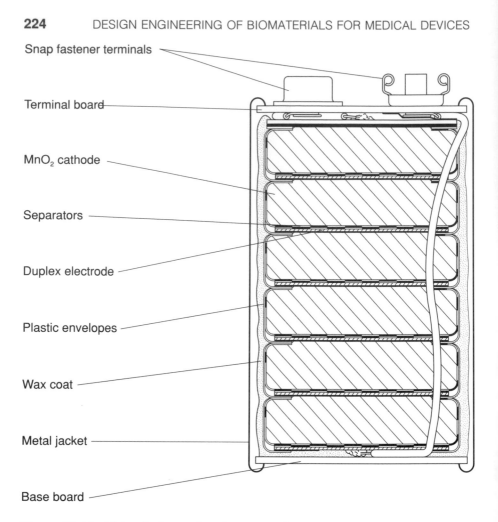

Snap fastener terminals

Terminal board

MnO$_2$ cathode

Separators

Duplex electrode

Plastic envelopes

Wax coat

Metal jacket

Base board

Figure 13.14   Flat cell zinc–carbon battery pack.

13.10   BUTTON CELLS

With the advent of the microchip, consequent reduction in power requirements and more reliance on smaller voltages, the 'button cell' has become
one of the most popular methods of providing a portable power supply.

Figure 13.18 shows the construction of a mercury cell and there are views
of silver oxide, lithium manganese and zinc–air cells (a favourite of mine)
in Figures 13.19–21.

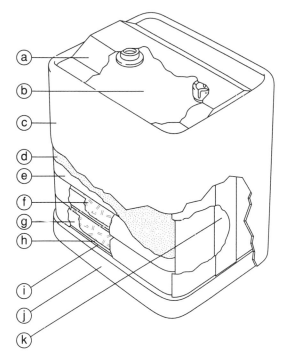

a Protector card
b Top plate
c Metal jacket
d Wax coating
e Plastic cell container
f Positive electrode

g Paper tray
h Carbon coated zinc electrode
i Electrolyte impregnated paper
j Bottom plate
k Conducting strip

Figure 13.15 Cut-away view of a zinc–carbon battery pack.

13.11 RECHARGEABLES

Rechargeable batteries and cells are available in the same sizes as the primary types but can be recharged and used again and again (500 times or more in ideal conditions). They cost more per cell than primary batteries, but less per unit of charge delivered. Rechargeable cells need more care and control when in use, and the working environments are not as flexible as for primary cells. To use rechargeables a charger is, naturally, required, usually this is built into medical equipment. Capital costs is thus increased, and you need expensive control systems and safety trips. For recharging access to a mains power supply is required on a semi-regular basis. The usual electrochemical

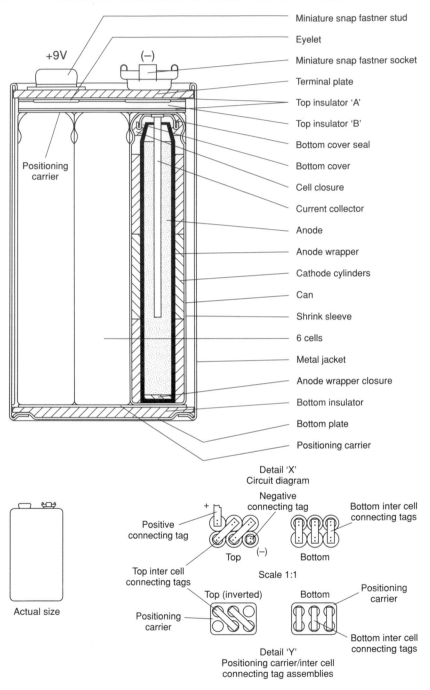

+9V

(−)

Miniature snap fastner stud

Eyelet

Miniature snap fastner socket

Terminal plate

Top insulator 'A'

Top insulator 'B'

Bottom cover seal

Bottom cover

Cell closure

Current collector

Anode

Anode wrapper

Cathode cylinders

Can

Shrink sleeve

6 cells

Metal jacket

Anode wrapper closure

Bottom insulator

Bottom plate

Positioning carrier

Positioning carrier

Detail 'X'
Circuit diagram

Actual size

Negative connecting tag

Positive connecting tag

Bottom inter cell connecting tags

+

(−)

Top

Bottom

Top inter cell connecting tags

Scale 1:1

Top (inverted)

Bottom

Positioning carrier

Positioning carrier

Bottom inter cell connecting tags

Detail 'Y'
Positioning carrier/inter cell connecting tag assemblies

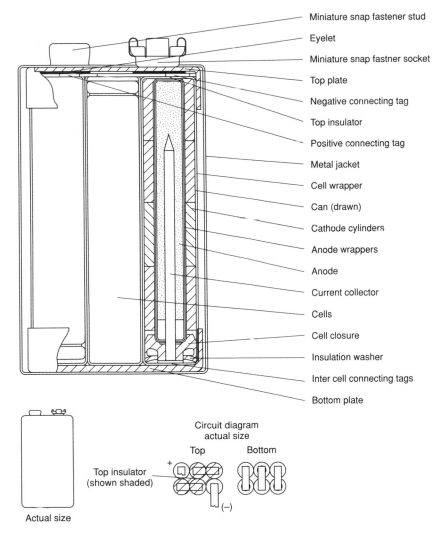

Miniature snap fastener stud

Eyelet

Miniature snap fastner socket

Top plate

Negative connecting tag

Top insulator

Positive connecting tag

Metal jacket

Cell wrapper

Can (drawn)

Cathode cylinders

Anode wrappers

Anode

Current collector

Cells

Cell closure

Insulation washer

Inter cell connecting tags

Bottom plate

Actual size

Top insulator
(shown shaded)

Circuit diagram
actual size

Top   Bottom

▲
Figure 13.17 Another design of alkaline–manganese battery.

◄
Figure 13.16 Section of an alkaline–manganese battery pack.

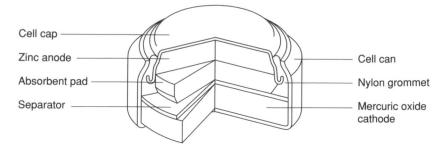

Figure 13.18 Construction of a mercury button cell.

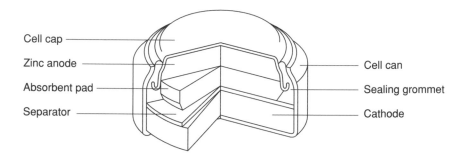

Figure 13.19 A silver–oxide button cell.

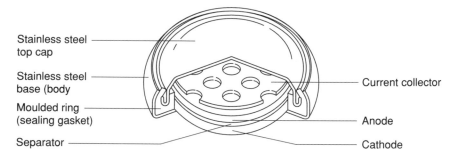

Figure 13.20 A lithium–manganese coin cell.

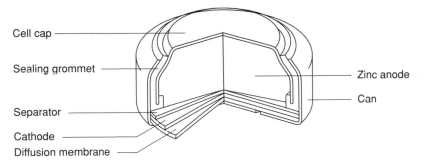

Cell cap

Sealing grommet

Separator

Cathode

Diffusion membrane

Zinc anode

Can

The zinc–air cell is sold with the air access holes sealed with an impermeable tape, which must be removed to activate the cell for use. Equipment using a zinc air cell must provide for air access to it.

Figure 13.21   A zinc–air button cell.

system is the nickel–cadmium cell, known as NiCads, and these self-discharge at an alarming rate if just left standing.

13.12   SUMMARY

There are many cell systems, battery configurations, voltage combinations, constraints, requirements, not to mention the different shapes and sizes. When selecting batteries or cells you should:

- use a standard sized battery when ever possible,
- check the contact regulations,
- design the electrical circuits so they use a standard voltage,
- consult manufacturers, specifying all the requirements and allowing them to recommend a cell or battery,
- use the experts: they will have already provided power sources to work under the sea, in space, in the wet, in the heat, in the cold, in sterile conditions. They can supply one-off or thousands, cheap or expensive.

Finally, there is now more and more a feeling that the environmental aspect of using equipment should be incorporated into design. Environmental issues are discussed in Chapter 28. The majority of battery systems contain either corrosive liquids or are toxic in their own right. The benefits of using them should be weighed against the problems of manufacture, obtaining the raw materials, the resources used to process them and their final disposal.

For contacting battery manufacturers there are quite a few trade magazines, buyers guides etc.

Part Two

Design

14
Training and Education for Design

We trained hard . . . but it seemed that every time we were beginning to form up in teams we would be re-organised.

I was to learn later in life that we tend to meet any situation by re-organisation, and a wonderful method it can be for creating the illusion of progress, while producing confusion, inefficiency and demoralisation.

Gaius Petronius AD 65

Now this may appear a strange opening to a chapter dedicated to training, education and the continued improvement of designers' skills and hence their company's products, but how often are designers frustrated by inappropriate managerial changes – too often!

Training is probably the single most complex issue affecting all industries today.

- What training should a new employee have?
- What training should this new employee have had before recruitment?
- How will the training be administered?
- By whom?
- For how long?
- What targets or methods of assessment are to be used?
- Internal or external tutors?
- What continued training should be planned?
- Over how long or no limit?
- Who, how, when to decide to stop or limit the training?

Get the picture: training is not something that should be an afterthought, it should be integrated into company development.

14.1 TRAINING PLANS

Training should be structured, documented and administered by one person. Depending on company size it should either be the responsibility of a director or at least a manager who reports directly to board level. Only this way can the importance be maintained. The employees are the most important assets of most companies: it would be unfortunate to lose them through incomplete training and frustrated use of their skills.

Training engineers, designers or technical managers has for a long time been left to chance. For many, many years the education system has concentrated upon analytical processes, formulae, theory and rigid interpretation of information obtained. There is a need, which is slowly being understood and acted on, to present students with a new form of creative target in their last years as college and first year(s) in industry. This is to be encouraged and expanded on as they progress through their employment.

14.2 CONTINUING PROFESSIONAL EDUCATION

Not only new or junior members of staff require training: in a rapidly changing world continuing professional education is essential for company competitiveness. Staff need to keep up to date with:

- market changes;
- technological advances in equipment;
- changing techniques for component manufacture;
- new, modified, or advanced materials;
- new, better, or faster manufacturing methods; and
- clinical developments.

All these factors affect the product: its development, its cost, its function and its use.

A product designer is normally originally an expert in one particular area, he or she needs to continually add to that store of knowledge to prepare and present the best new designs. This newly obtained knowledge is always changing, must be kept up to date, improved upon and be self-perpetuating. In Figure 14.1 a training plan for junior engineers is laid out; in Figure 14.2 a similar plan aimed at the more senior members of staff is shown.

When arranging training courses it is important to ensure that the course content is linked to existing on-the-job training and assessment. Strengths should be built up and weaknesses addressed if an external course is to be of benefit. One of the institutes actively encouraging senior design and engineering staff to continue to learn is the Institution of Engineering Designers. Another successful way of educating staff is to encourage senior members to publish papers on their design work (providing of course there are no

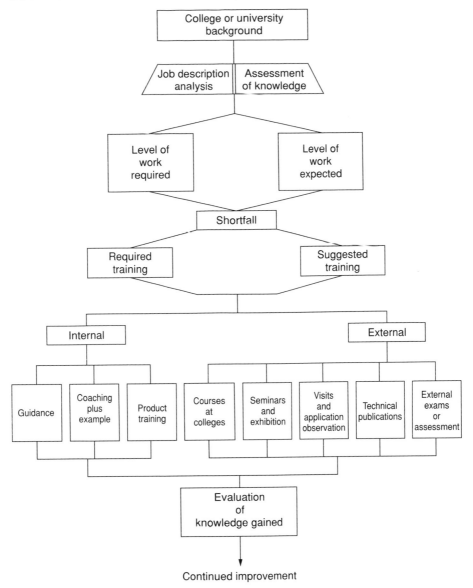

Figure 14.1 Training path for junior engineers.

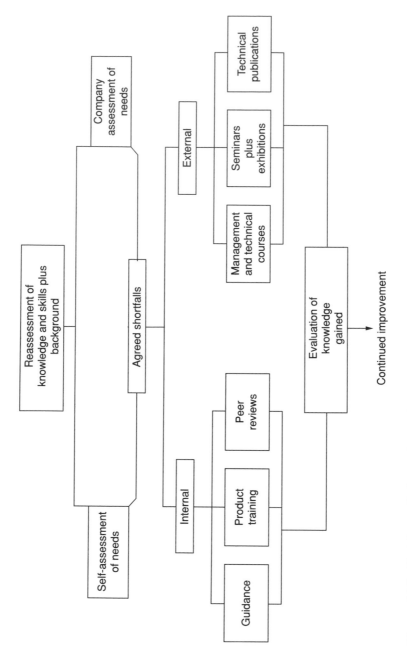

Figure 14.2 Training path for senior engineers.

commercial constraints or confidentiality barriers). This is beneficial in three ways.

- Younger or new designers can see the practical applications of ideas, materials and processes.
- The actual discipline of writing down and presenting thoughts and ideas allows the author to reassess the process or product developed. This is similar to an informal design review or brainstorming session with all avenues re-examined.
- The generation of new ideas often occurs when information is compiled and documented, or during the inevitable discussion that will follow presentation or publication of a paper.

Another beneficial aspect normally overlooked when discussions are held regarding designs previously undertaken, is the analysis of failures. Have the courage to discuss the problems and pitfalls that occurred during a product's development which resulted in the design going no further. By explaining the problems and the eventual solutions, others can benefit and learn. Such shared experiences can help form a formidable design team which will then be prepared to tackle anything.

Brainstorming is an excellent design tool and a method of finding solutions to specific problems. It can also provide insight to other concepts, ideas and ways of producing an acceptable end result. In an effort to control a brainstorming session some simple rules must be adhered to (see Chapter 15, Table 15.4).

You, as a design engineer or manager, need to establish three things to instigate and maintain good training.

1. Training needs:
   - Your company's needs: training must be relevant and productive, there must be a perceived and measurable return on the company's investment of time and money.
   - Individual needs: either your own or your staff's. Analyse the requirements or shortfalls within your department or division. Are you part of a team lacking a particular skill? How can this be remedied?
   - Type of need: decide if the requirements are technical, administrative or social. Remember talk to those involved; not everyone will require the same training nor at the same level, nor even feel the need for it!
2. Training resources:
   - External seminars, conferences and lectures.
   - Internal 'teach-ins' by experienced staff.
   - College courses – day school, night classes, block release or sandwich type.
   - Group sessions and discussions
   - Location of courses

- Who should attend? For how long? Over what time period?
- Who pays?

Remember that the above items are listed assuming you have staff, but still apply even if you do not. Consider all the points before applying for specific training you feel you may need. It will be more successful if you can anticipate and supply the above answers when requesting a course.

3. Monitoring and evaluation:
   - Once agreed, a programme of training which has been selected from information correlated and made suitable to meet all needs.
   - Monitor the effect of the training on company individuals.
   - Have the original needs been met?
   - Are any changes necessary for future use?
   - Is there any indirect effect, beneficial or not?
   - Continue to evaluate the effects.

   Remember my comments above; these points also apply to your own developments and education.

Once your employer is convinced about the benefits of continued education, and training has started, will everything run smoothly so you can sit back and relax? – no. For successful training there must be ample

Table 14.1   The importance of motivating designers

With motivation	Without motivation
Job satisfaction	Indifference
Goodwill	Internal politics
Authority	Apathy
Own decision making	
Team spirit	Disputes
Money	Feeling unappreciated
Salary/bonus/share option	
Product identification	Poor personal relationships
Loyalty	
Responsibility	Interaction with workmates/colleagues
Benefits	Actions not acknowledged
Flexitime/car/healthcare/leisure facilities	
Enthusiasm	Feeling alone
Status	Lack of cooperation
Within the company/among own peers	
Cooperation	Responsibility but no authority
Achievement	Absenteeism
Products launched	
Improved patient treatment	
Safer product	
Recognition	
Determination	

Table 14.2 Personality types

Influencer
Has firm fixed opinions
Is politically aware
Enjoys manipulating
Leader (or wants to be)
Eager to take command
Happy to expound own ideas

Affiliator
Enjoys close personal contact
Relates well to others
Enjoys working with others
Likes a cooperative set up
Dislikes criticism
Avoids confrontation
Annoyed by indifference

Achiever
Sets own targets (high but achievable)
Will only take moderate risks
Is innovative
Has high (self imposed) standards
Solitary worker (but can work within team structure, or with partners)
Requires immediate feedback
Is easily bored by routine
Enjoys change
Resents close supervision
Not motivated by money alone
Enjoys responsibility

---

motivation. Effective motivation depends on understanding personality types. Table 14.1 shows the importance of motivation and Table 14.2 indicates what motivates the three basic personality types.

Finally all engineers, in particular product design engineers, need to understand the need to gain more and varied skills so they can influence the development of future products. This can only be achieved by continued education throughout their career, education which will benefit everyone from the designer to the customer.

15
Design Process and Factors

Design is a complex and varied subject. Designers all follow different working practices, each convinced that they are correct. In a way they are, because success is determined by results, so if products are designed to budget and schedule all is well. The problem is that personally evolved modes of working are likely to be slow to develop and not flexible enough to adapt to the increasing pace of change in industry. On the other hand, if all text book recommendations on design were followed, very little would be achieved because of the burden of testing, documentation and proof that they demand. In this chapter I shall attempt to chart a middle way, based on my practical experience and drawn from the methods used in the companies I have worked for (companies which range from 50 person, one factory operations up to 5000 strong international concerns).

First I shall consider the designer themselves: what are the fundamental requirements that will ensure success? Success can be measured only by the sale of products. It does not signify if a great innovative design is devised, converted into a working prototype, manufactured at a low cost and design awards presented if no one will buy it. This does not denote success.

15.1 THE DESIGN FUNCTION

The product designer has two functions. The primary function is to devise new products, and the secondary function is to provide improvements to existing products. The designer may also supply technical back-up for their employer. To perform these functions the designer will need certain skills, listed in Table 15.1

Table 15.2 shows a skills table of different disciplines in the design sector of industry against the actual work that is normally undertaken and by whom.

Table 15.1   Skills required for design

Conceptual ability	The ability to visualise the completed product, the individual items, the interfacing, how the assembly will work, how single items can be manufactured. It is also necessary to understand how the product will be used, by whom and when. All needs to be understood before any detailing can begin.
Innovation	Not as inventor but as a means of using facilities, people, methods, materials etc. nothing new is ever invented it is merely shifted around towards a more productive use. So a full understanding and an open mind is essential, logical thought helps but sometimes restricts or narrows the options.
Confidence	If you know a design is correct and will work prove it, justify it, answer all doubts and questions. Then when there are no more solid reasons to prevent you completing the design process, do it.
Communication	No point in being the world's best design engineer if no one knows about it, or worse they all know something of your work but cannot understand it. Learn to transfer your ideas simply, by whatever means available: drawings, CAD, 2D/3D renderings, written specifications, reports, models or prototypes, any or all.
Technical knowledge	Perhaps an obvious statement but probably the one which should be shouted the loudest. Start with the basics at college, gain more by working, add to it by courses and teach ins and keep on learning. Right up to the last retirement day. Acknowledgement that you can never know it all and the need for continued information is paramount.
Experience	To enable a comprehensive understanding of the workings of a manufacturing company and in turn understand the requirements in providing a suitable design, experience should be obtained of these disciplines or departments:

Engineering	Marketing/Sales
Production/Manufacturing	Economics
QA	Design/Development
Electrical/Mechanical/	Materials
Hydraulic/Pneumatic	Legal/Patents
Mathematics	Chemistry/Physics
Personnel	Accounts

15.2   THE DESIGN BRIEF

First the designer needs a product to design: where does the idea come from? How does the designer know what functions and features are required? In the medical devices business this comes from a design brief, usually supplied by the marketing department, and obtained from purchasers, users, customer

Table 15.2 Job title and tasks done

	Artist	Industrial designer	Product designer	Production engineer
Create	✓	✓	✓	
Innovate		✓	✓	
Draw	✓	✓	✓	
Material		✓	✓	✓
Model	✓	✓	✓	
Analysis			✓	✓
Manufacture			✓	✓
Cost			✓	✓
Quantify and calculate			✓	✓

feedback and market awareness. In more detail there are really only four sources of information, and ideally the product brief should be a synthesis from all four.

- Observations made by marketing personnel on hospital visits etc. their predictions of what new techniques may be developed and what needs exist or may arise.
- Medical staff of all types – surgeons, physicians, nurses, therapists, radiographers etc. – all have ideas for product improvements, new instruments or new clinical procedures. In discussion with a medical device company these ideas can be evaluated and developed if appropriate.
- Manufacturers inevitably have an in-house programme of product development. Responses to customer feedback and new regulatory requirements can give rise to new products, enhancements of established products, and result in more sales.
- Competitor appraisal is often called parallel development, but in reality is it a matter of finding out what others are doing or are about to do, and trying come up with similar products either cheaper, better or sooner.

15.3 THE DESIGN PROCESS

Once there is a design brief, the process should follow the sequence listed here.

1. Analyse the brief and identify the main aspects.
2. Make a preliminary design for concept evaluation.
3. Consider material options and make a preliminary selection.
4. Conduct a feasibility assessment.
5. Build a prototype. Do lab testing and customer evaluation.
6. Involve quality assurance procedures.
7. Produce a fully detailed design.

8. Justify the choice of materials, manufacturing options and methods of assembly.
9. Document everything.
10. Quality staff conduct impartial design audit.
11. Make a pre-production quantity.
12. Arrange and execute clinical trials.
13. Assess trial results, modify or redesign if indicated.
14. Quality assurance assessment.
15. Write specification for finalised design – no changes hereafter.
16. Make or purchase production tooling and components. Complete paperwork.
17. Manufacture production quantities.
18. Product launch, sales and distribution.

Figures 15.1–4 give some graphic representations of the design process. Figure 15.5 illustrates the costs involved in producing a new product.

When drawing up a design, there are a number of do's and don'ts the first of which is positive thinking. Table 15.3 shows some of the ways to enhance creative thinking. One common method is brainstorming, Table 15.4 sets out some ground rules and should help you start up the technique. Figure 15.6 and Figure 15.7 show line and critical path diagrams of product development. Figure 15.8 highlights the contributing factors influencing a design. The design engineer must consider, evaluate, document and justify all actions to be taken. Figure 15.9 shows the items influencing a brief before design begins. Table 15.5 is a question and answer page featuring pitfalls occurring during development and ideas for their solution.

15.4 DESIGN PRINCIPLES

When you devise a design there are a number of principles which should be followed to arrive at a product with the necessary attributes at minimal cost.

- Keep it simple. All other things being equal, the design with the fewest components, simplest assemblies and fewest manufacturing operations will be the easiest and cheapest to produce. As a bonus, such products are inevitably the most reliable.
- Utilise existing components and materials. The use of ready-made components and mass-produced proprietary items will simplify purchasing, stock control, prototype production and manufacturing. Using components that you already use for other products avoids tooling investment and manufacturing problems. The same ideas apply to the selection of commonplace materials.
- Copy or modify existing designs. If there are similar products in your range modify these. If your workers are familiar with the shape or

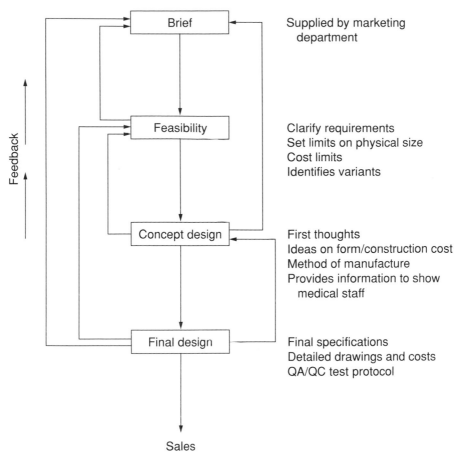

Figure 15.1   A flow chart for the design process.

assembly method, training and process control will be easier and capital investment in manufacturing capacity will be minimised.

- Open tolerances. This is very simple: the tighter the tolerance the greater the cost, so wherever possible increase the tolerances.
- Use easily processed materials. Provided the physical properties are acceptable, always favour a more easily manipulated material. There are normally significant differences in process times, cutting speeds, handling and machining, which are reflected in both costs and adaptability.
- Talk to suppliers: components could be changed to suit your requirements, new variations could be made available or new grades of materials produced – all at the supplier's expense. Many designers rely on the expertise of suppliers to complement their own experience: no one expects a design engineer to know everything.

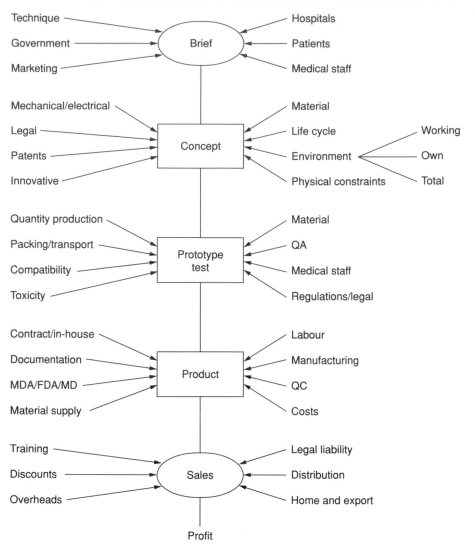

Figure 15.2 Factors that influence design.

- Avoid secondary operations: try to adopt a 'right first time' approach so that parts are handled and processed once. If a component needs, say, machining, then heat treatment, then machining again the costs are bound to be high.
- Optimise design and manufacturing to suit the production quantity. The contact aerial electrode shown in Figure 15.10 is most appropriately machined from stainless steel to produce 100 per year at a cost of £5 each,

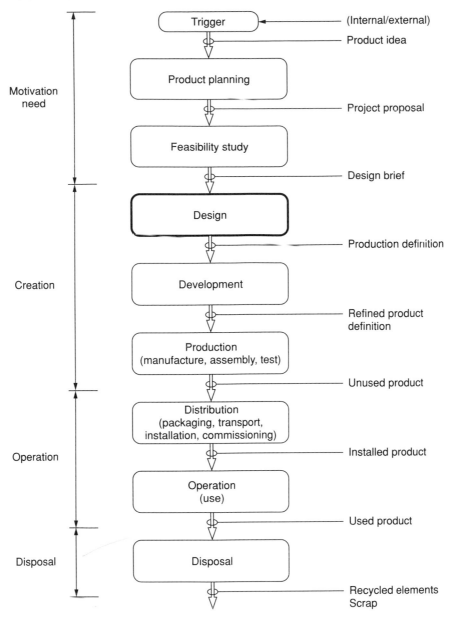

Figure 15.3 The product evolution process.

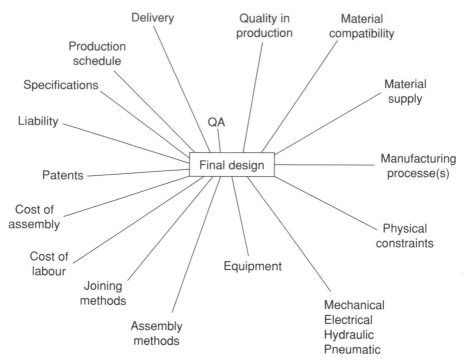

Figure 15.4   Factors affecting design through manufacturing.

Table 15.3   Attitudes in design

Negative thinking	Positive thinking
Accepting one single answer	Wide experiences of other disciplines
Repetitive behaviour	Brainstorming
Relying on old training	Lateral thinking
Not enough prior knowledge or information	Good prior information
Restricting yourself before the event	Assessment of all suggestions
Insistence on using existing methods	Comparison against previous products or competitors
Conformity, falling in line to fit in	Open discussion
Fixed methods	No-blame environment
Scared of appearing foolish	Compliment innovation or creative options
Not questioning all actions	Do not criticise
Agreement too early	Constructive comments
Desire to please directors or similar	
Critical workmates or office peers	
Rigidly adopting the logical approach	
Not allowing enough time for a full appraisal of the design	

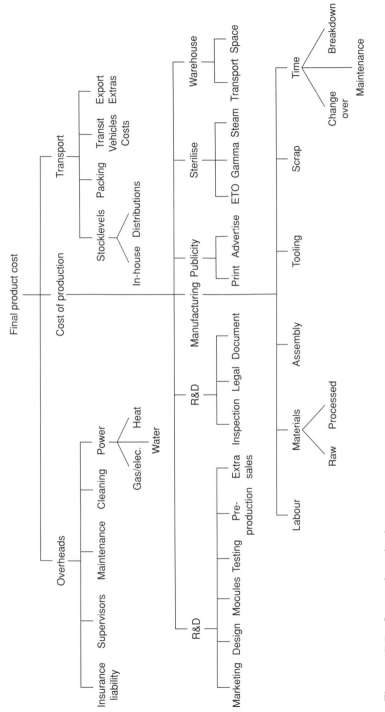

Figure 15.5 Costs of production.

Table 15.4   Brainstorming rules

1. Team of about five: over seven and the group fragments, under four and ideas stagnate.
2. Multidisciplinary membership: varied backgrounds and skills are an advantage.
3. No leader or controller; just someone to take notes.
4. No seniority regarding speaking, ideas or ownership of any eventual solution. Everyone classed as equal, no pulling rank.
5. One person presents the problem, information and requirements and then steps back.
6. Everyone should contribute. Go round each person for a solution to the problem. Aim to collect ten ideas before discussion. Note each idea briefly, use a flip chart or sticky notes. Let each person make a proposal or pass until no more ideas are forthcoming or an agreed time has elapsed. Aim for quantity initially, quality comes later.
7. Then assess and discuss each idea for a fixed time. Comment positively, never criticise, compare or ridicule.
8. If there are lots of ideas, set time limits.
9. Encourage unusual 'wacky' ideas – try to make the session fun: it will be more productive.
10. Allow combinations of concepts, encourage evolution of ideas without going into fine detail as this slows down the process.
12. Be prepared to contribute 'off-the-wall' ideas yourself if things start to stagnate.
13. Include someone to ask naïve questions – yourself playing a fool if necessary.
14. Brainstorming is suitable for the following sorts of problems:
    - ideas for new products,
    - specific problems with a product,
    - improvements to existing products,
    - production problems,
    - plant layout.
    Brainstorming is unlikely to help with:
    - technically complex, interrelated problems,
    - problems required detailed information,
    - problems with a single solution,
    - non-quantifiable problems,
    - speculative solutions.

but if the volume increased to 10 000 per year, it could be injection moulded in ABS polymer and plated with a conducting metal at a cost of about 25p each. Other manufacturing routes considered and costed for this product included: cast stainless steel, zinc investment casting, zinc die casting, same for aluminium, glass plus copper conductor, copper tube and plating conductive polymer.

See discussion of this example in Chapter 26 and Table 26.1 in particular, and compare the electrode example in Chapter 1.

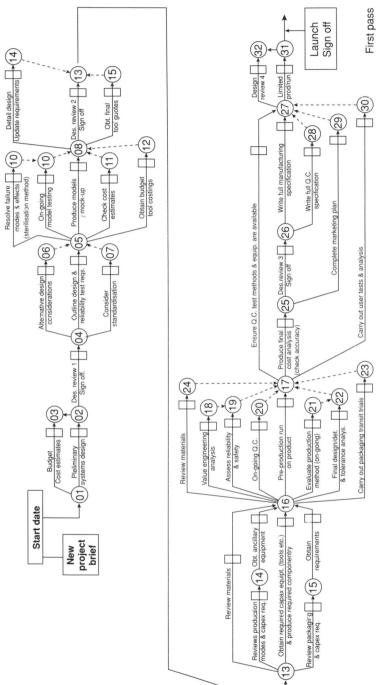

Figure 15.6 A flow chart for product development. © 1991 Rocket Medical Plc, reproduced with permission.

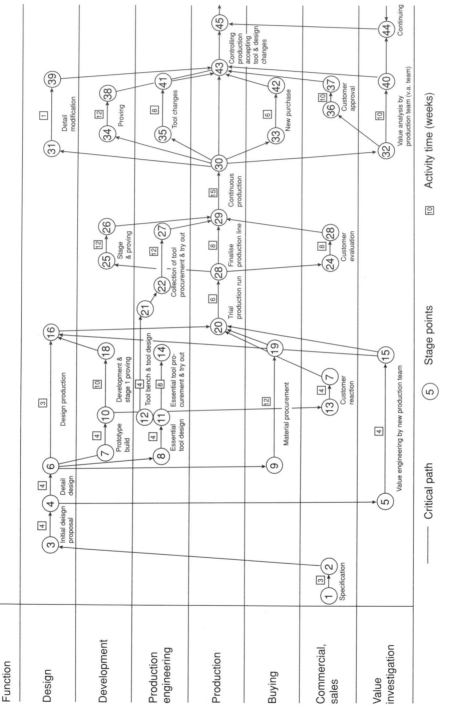

Figure 15.7 A critical path analysis of product development. © 1991 Rocket Medical Plc, reproduced with permission.

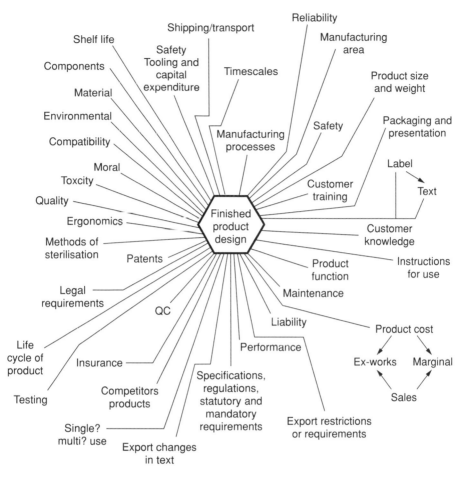

Figure 15.8 Design considerations.

15.5 ERGONOMICS

Figure 15.11 and Table 15.7 show anthropometric norms for male and female bodies. The data shown are for typical Europeans with allowance for clothing included.

Ergonomics was not considered important until recently, but it is now recognised as a critical part of any design brief: how will the unit be carried, will it fit a 'standard' hand, is the control panel user friendly etc? When an operator has to manipulate a product, all movements and forces should be assessed. The ergonomic analysis of the interactions between personnel and medical devices should be standard policy for all relevant products.

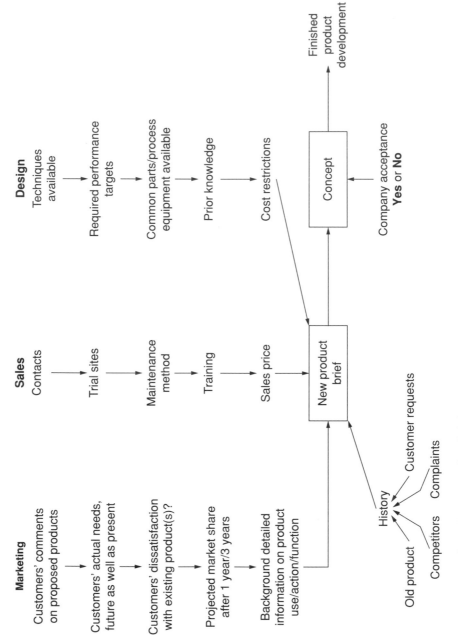

Figure 15.9 Compiling a product brief.

Table 15.5 Problems and solutions during product development

Problem	Solution
No formal strategy or development schedule	Make one and fix the dates yourself
Too top heavy and elaborate project schedule	Cut out the padding
Too ambitious on either timescales or deliverables	Seek advice on priorities and what's needed when
Unsure of the next action or stage	Reassess the schedule and do the next timed stage
Completing non-viable actions and trivial jobs	Be critical. Talk through the work with someone, let them act as a sounding board. You will find the solution yourself
Not transferring all the information successfully into a solution	Write up summaries and cross match
Building a large data bank of irrelevant and useless information	Unless specific discard it. If you have access now it can always be requested again
Lack confidence in your own designs	Do it, if they are correct then OK, if actually wrong find out well before anything gets built
Demoralised, discouraged, disheartened	Stick at it and plod on
Scared to talk through your design with others	Talk to everyone from the director to the cleaner. Rekindle their and your own enthusiasm
Lack of feedback.	Flood those concerned with messages and say the next ones will be copied to board members.

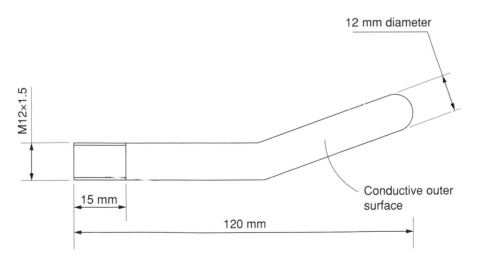

Figure 15.10 A contact aerial electrode.

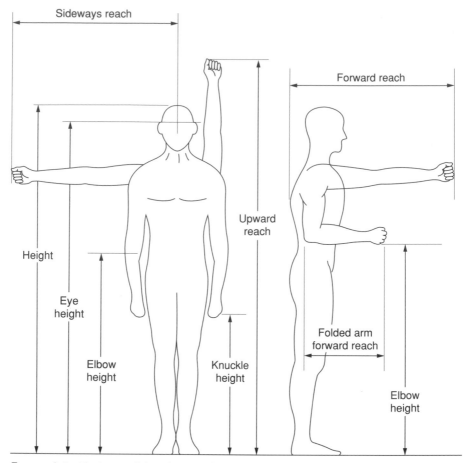

Ergonomic 'guides' are split into three sections: standing, sitting and sitting/standing with 22 separate dimensions for a full description

Figure 15.11 Examples of human body dimensions. Reproduced from *Handbook of Engineering Design*, R.D. Cullum (ed), Butterworth Scientific Ltd, Oxford, 1988.

15.6 CONCURRENT ENGINEERING

Concurrent or simultaneous engineering is an innovative approach to new product development in which product managers or 'champions' work with multi-function teams so that design, production, QA and marketing staff work together on a project from inception to launch. This is not really a new idea and this sort of method has been advocated by certain organisations for a number of years, but only recently has it become in vogue.

Table 15.6   Comparison of the use of in-house and outside staff for design and development

Advantages	Disadvantages
Use of in-house staff	
• Existing staff have the knowledge and background experience of your products	• Projects should be looked at as long term, staff in danger of being underemployed
• Project status can be checked at any stage and at any time	• If the work load increases beyond the capability of existing staff the use of overtime payments or short term contract labour may exceed the project's budget.
• Existing components and sub-assemblies are readily available for comparison/use or prototype construction	• If excessive overtime is necessary the work quality will drop
• Production engineering staff are on site and available for discussions regarding manufacture/machine needs. Any changes to the design can be immediate	• Existing staff may not have the expertise or particular skills for certain projects
• Easy access to previous products for comparison	• Additional product or process costs in training existing staff
• More than one project can be worked on for the same/less monetary outlay	
• Cheaper. Design and development costs are less when monitored in-house, also consultant fees apart from being large are also charged by the hour	
• Risk of commercial information leakage reduced if all contained in-house	
Use of outside contractors or consultants	
• Relieves any short term urgent staffing problems	• Critical and continuous supervision required on all stages
• Outside firms can bring either fresh thoughts to an existing problem, or new expertise and skills	• Cost
• Particular firms can be selected for their specialist knowledge on a process, technique or material	• Your own expertise and manufacturing skills become common knowledge
• Liability may be laid off or reduced if accepted by the contractor	• Your own staff become resentful and may not work fully with the contractor
• Also any delays can be covered by including penalty clauses	• Contractor's staff may change during the term of the contract and there will be a loss of knowledge
• Easier costing process. Set price for the design and development of a specific item against projected sales and profit.	• Delays as the contractor acquires product and market information

Table 15.7 Average available arm force. © 1988 Butterworth Scientific Ltd. First published in *Handbook of Engineering Design*, edited by R.D. Cullum

Workspace	Posture	Push (N)	Pull (N)
Restricted foot room and buttock space		3.8	4
Restricted foot room		4	14
No restriction		10	1.3
Hand support available		26.5	23.6
Buttock support		22.5	8
Thigh support		9.4	2.4

The objective of concurrent engineering is to provide higher quality products more quickly, no matter what the complexity. It is based on teamwork and cross-functioning of departments, and requires:

- strict attention to detail,
- a right-first-time philosophy,
- design audit and risk assessment to identify mistakes before they are implemented, and
- speeding up the development cycle.

The traditional method of product design took a step-by-step approach and each stage had to be completed before the next could start. The old method used an empirical 'try it and see' attitude: if it didn't work, think again. In concurrent design options are thought through carefully before being tried, and evidence of previous work is used to eliminate ideas that probably won't be successful. The stages of the design process are undertaken in parallel rather than in series as much as possible: see Figure 15.12 and Table 15.8.

15.7 CONTRACT OR EMPLOY?

There is a controversy about the extent to which companies can afford to keep all the departments and skills they ever need. The question is whether to employ lots of permanent staff and find suitable projects to keep them busy, or to maintain a core staff and buy-in expertise or manufacturing capacity as required. As this is an emotive issue I shall avoid the argument and offer a table of advantages and disadvantages for you to consider, see Table 15.6.

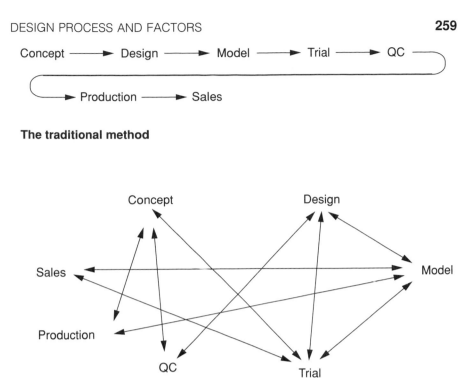

The traditional method

Concurrent method

Figure 15.12   Traditional and concurrent design processes.

Currently, received wisdom in management circles advocates the 'clover leaf corporation', in which one can imagine three lobes of staff resources. One is the core staff, people in permanent posts without whom the business can't function. These people are the ones in whom the employer invests in terms of training and personnel development, who receive attractive benefits and remuneration packages, and who are expected to be loyal and ever-harder working. The second lobe is composed of individuals on temporary or short-term contracts, a resource that can be switched on or off as fluctuating circumstances dictate. The third lobe is freelance workers, consultants and contractors who are used on a project-by-project or even hour-by-hour basis, and for whom there are no costs of employment or training.

15.8 STRUCTURAL DESIGN

When a design brief is first read a few obvious solutions will come to mind; on closer examination more features and functions are perceived but the problem remains that something will be left out or overlooked. To avoid

Table 15.8 Concurrent engineering techniques

Knowledge-Based Engineering (KBE)	Based on the product or components function(s), complete with background rules to ensure the functional specifications are matched. The KBE system uses both the geometric and non-geometric information that states and defines the design intent.
Just In Time (JIT)	Normally concentrated on production, JIT utilises a process or machine output to suit the whole system and not just one aspect. This leads to minimised work in progress, reduction in money tied up on stock and exposes QC problems earlier so allowing better response.
Quality Engineering (QE)	Normally any poor quality in production means additional cost to manufacturing and increased charges to the customer. QE tries to reduce this loss and extra cost by identifying potential errors during the design and production phases prior to work commencing.
Taguchi	A strategy for off-line quality control conducted at the product design stage of the manufacturing cycle (may also be utilised when deciding on process methods). Attempts to improve product reliability and manufacturability thereby reducing product development and 'lifetime' costs. Uses a series of factorial experiments and statistical techniques.
Poka-Yoke	Means 'mistake proofing'. First promoted as a concept by Toyota. Attempts to reduce costly QC inspection and statistical analysing by assuming that when a defect occurs it is the system not the operator at fault, so control earlier (and cheaper) is critical. Controls governed by the problem's severity.
Design For Manufacture (DFM)	DFM concept is to identify the aspects in a new product design which are easy to manufacture and focus on the ease of production and assembly. The process considers form, function, fabrication as well as the procedures of product design.
Product Delivery Process (PDP)	A process used by Xerox for development and production of products. Draws on all functions development, manufacture and marketing to produce correct product for the customers needs. A product's development is identified as 1) preconcept, 2) concept, 3) design, 4) demonstration, 5) production, 6) launch and 7) maintenance. An extended process seen as quality philosophy in development, as JIT is in production.

this possibility, one method is to build up a structured tree of the main functions. Figure 15.13 is one such tree. Table 15.9, Figure 15.14, Figure 15.15, Table 15.10 and Figure 15.16 illustrate a planned project development plan.

As an example of the design process, use the suggestions made earlier to consider a means of measuring accurately the volume of liquid in a container. The liquid is not constant in density and there may be solids in the container too. The level is rising and volume must be measured to ± 0.1 litre. The

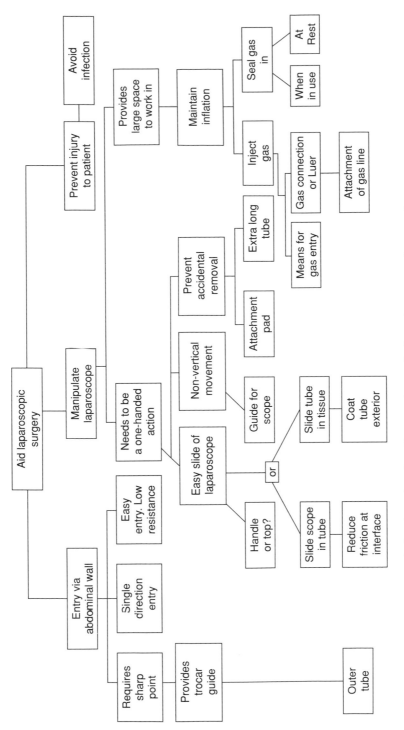

Figure 15.13 Structured analysis of product function requirements for a laparoscopic cannula.

Table 15.9   Product design and development

Product development should follow a system similar to this.
- *Conception*: draft specifications laid down.
- *Acceptance*: proof of concept being achievable by either calculation, sketches, computer modelling, or demonstration (on site, lab based or with a customer).
- *Execution*: working models prepared from the data obtained in the acceptance section. Complexity may mean a pre-production facility is needed. The models to be used by the marketing department to obtain customer feedback.
- *Translation*: when the product is in a form which can be made by staff within your own company and to a fully written specification.
- *Pre-production*: product produced in sufficient quantities to verify the application, design, specifications, method of assembly. Not until this stage should the development be classed as finished and specifications frozen.

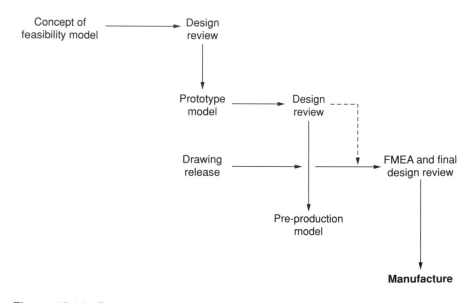

Figure 15.14   Design review scheduling.

container must be sealed and the container and contents will be incinerated on disposal: see Figure 15.17.

In this case the finished device used a load cell onto which the container (modified to a bag form) was hung. The liquid is weighed and displayed as a volume, any inaccuracy due to density variations is compensated for by using calibration data collected during product development.

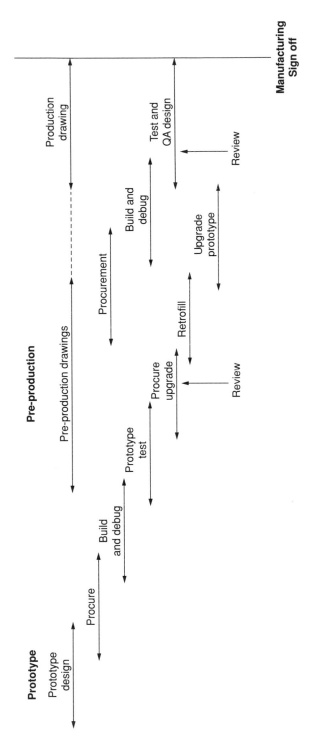

Figure 15.15 Prototype and production planning.

Table 15.10   Planning product design

1. Formal design reviews at set times or periods of actions ensure all departments are aware of actions taken and targets achieved.
2. Early on at the briefing stage, testing of any or all competitive products against the specified requirements. Compile full data with actual visit to view either the medical procedure or existing product. This is a design staff requirement. QC procedure involvement initially at the second development stage, then once final sign off in view and reassessed FMEA required.
3. Model or prototype of the design placed in the market for feedback prior to commitment on stage 2. The prototype should be constructed, within reason, regardless of cost.
4. Prescribe four set stages to the project development – sub-divided as shown in Figure 15.16.
5. Full commitment from all departments on spend once the prototype feedback accepted. Prototype may require some investment prior to manufacture. No retrospective actions once commitment made.
6. Ensure long/sufficient/enough time is taken on initial planning and writing schedule. QC visit – written in at this stage to ensure correct knowledge prior to first FMEA.
7. Build up enough time initially to fully assess requirements. Full abstract thought and consideration for new concepts of 'silly' ideas. Off-the-wall views, discussion with no formal requirement other than to consider options.
8. Planning schedule to be shown at each project meeting. Targets achieved and dates discussed etc. All present to agree on programme and any updates. Also awareness of existing ongoing projects which may allow the interchange of ideas and identifying potential pitfalls.
9. Planning schedule or equivalent to have the facility to record and display actual time worked as well as elapsed time. Major discrepancies will be highlighted and if possible eliminated. Can be noted with relevant comments, e.g. one year elapsed time but only three months allocated work time.
10. Each project to be minuted at the product meetings even if only 'on hold'. This will not only ensure nothing is overlooked but will comply with the MDA directive(s).
11. One person to be responsible for controlling the planning programme and the introduction or archiving of projects. Specific engineers to be designated and held responsible for updating and addition of notes regarding their own projects. The same engineer will compile and write the planned stages complete with agreed milestones.
12. FMEA to be introduced into the programme at stage two and reviewed at the end of each successive stages with a final update prior to launch commitment.

The steps above are shown in Figure 15.16 and should be used as a discussion document to suit your own system. Each stage can be expanded to include additional milestones. Each of the headings can be sub-divided if necessary to highlight the time allocated, also explaining specific steps particular to each project.

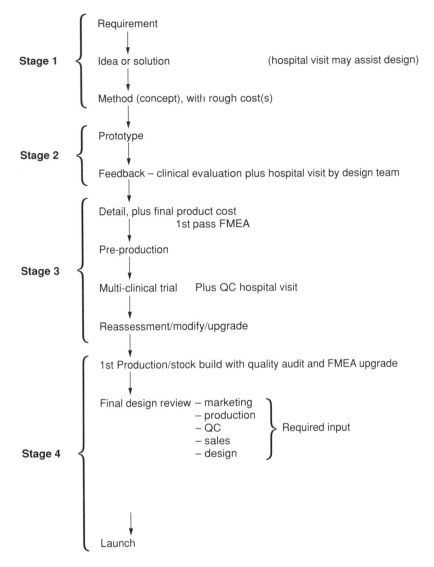

Figure 15.16 Stages in product design and development.

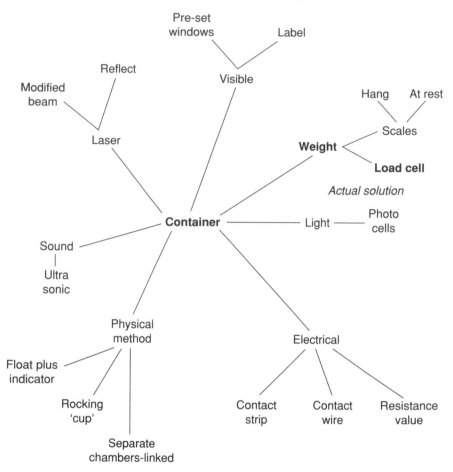

Figure 15.17   The design sequence: a case history.

15.9   SUMMARY

Here are some last thoughts for you.

- Do not cling to old formats; look for other concepts for a design. They may not work but the effort put in examining the ideas and justifying the final selection will pay dividends later.
- Keep up to date with processes, materials and other medical device advances – they can and will influence your own work.
- When progressing your final selection of the product's design, still be prepared to change, even at the eleventh hour if something better is suggested don't ignore it because it conflicts with your design.
- Keep an open mind and enjoy the challenge.

16
Microengineering

A few years ago I wrote a short article, somewhat tongue in cheek, regarding miniature medical devices so small that they could be inserted via a syringe directly into a vein. They would be self-powered, self-controlling and have a degree of intelligence (which would allow for self-correcting or variations from the original programmed instructions). The outcome would be a limited amount of 'real' non-invasive surgery within the body.

Further speculation for future additions to these devices would be cameras and radial cutters which could be guided (or assisted) through veins and arteries, cleaning and removing obstructions.

Although originally a flight of hopeful fantasy, a throw-away concept to prompt discussion or even start research, such devices are now as near a reality as is possible with today's technology and methods of manufacture. And the technologies are changing so rapidly that laboratory novelties are fast becoming tools for future development.

My speculations are becoming real through the new technology called microengineering which marries engineering, physics and a hint of vision.

16.1 DEVELOPMENT OF MICROENGINEERING
1978

Microengineering really started 20 years ago when engineers in many industries started to miniaturise equipment. The products were mostly gadgets or gimmicks but some good techniques for small component manufacture began to emerge. With the advent of the microchip these techniques came into their own.

The industrial application of photoetching, the LIGA technique, and electron beam manipulation started the ball rolling and gathering speed as each year passed. By the 1980s microengineering was poised to become a solution to an as yet unspecified problem.

Microengineering meant true precision engineering which could result in miniaturisation of optical, hydraulic, thermal and mechanical components and assemblies. The next step was to reduce the costs while maintaining the high quality and performance produced by the original laboratory samples.

These samples included motors the size of a match head, and gear wheels and cutters the size of a human hair.

At a similar time came the development of minimally invasive or 'key hole' surgery. The idea of using a very small entry wound, reducing trauma and avoiding long-term hospital stay, was attractive to medical staff and the public. These goals were achieved using smaller versions of conventional surgical instruments, made by existing methods. Costs were minimised as many surgical procedures became feasible as day case surgery. The second phase of development of minimally invasive surgery (MIS) involves the invention of completely new approaches to solve clinical problems and associated miniature medical devices.

Microelectronics and printed circuit technology led the way. Complex microsystems were initially available only in research institutions, but as applications became more numerous and the costs of production plummeted, microelectronics have become commonplace.

As microelectronics developed, it became apparent that a wide range of materials could be used in microsystems, and that material properties at a microstructural level were not necessarily the same as for bulk samples. New ways of working with materials at the microscale included the development of fibres of glass, carbon, ceramics and metals as well as polymers.

Manipulation of materials at a micro level required significant improvements in purity to produce defect-free structures with enhanced properties.

16.2   APPLICATIONS OF MICROENGINEERING

There now exists an industrial complex which has embraced most of the first world countries, creating microengineering benefits in many industrial sectors.

16.2.1   AEROSPACE

Microengineering of aviation and space components leads to weight reduction and fuel savings. Small and reliable sensors allow safety improvements by detection of faults.

16.2.2   LEISURE

Miniature optical systems have led to size reduction in cameras for domestic use. In sport, miniature cameras can be mounted on, e.g. mountaineers or formula one cars, giving observers a sense of participation. Microelectronics are used in monitors worn by sports or fitness enthusiasts to measure performance or health.

16.2.3 CONSERVATION

Microengineered machines and processes work more efficiently, faster, and use less energy, which means less pollution and lower commercial cost.

16.2.4 COMMUNICATIONS

Fibre optics, laser transfer and microwave transmission all fall under the wide umbrella of microtechnology. Miniature connections for chips and circuits allow cheaper, better, more efficient products, which in turn means more people are able to benefit.

16.2.5 AUTOMOTIVE

Miniature pressure sensors mounted internally and around the engine provide instant feedback for more effective fuel management and environmental control. Systems to monitor and control acceleration, exhaust, torque and suspension all aid the driver. Route finding developments using micro-electronics and LCD displays will provide a navigation set which could allow a trouble-free journey without the arguments about who got who lost. (These rows have recently been found to be a major contributor to 'road rage'.)

16.2.6 TEXTILES

Microengineering has produced miniature spinning nozzles which can produce fibres of narrower diameter. There is also a gain reducing hazardous manufacturing methods both in time and volume.

16.2.7 MEDICINE

MIS, mentioned above, can now be accomplished via ports 2 mm in diameter. Endoscopes exist to examine and record internal organs in virtually any part of the body (Figure 16.1). Manipulated catheters can reach the heart from an entry point in the groin. All these add to the trend for day care treatment.

Miniaturisation has led to lightweight portable versions of equipment formerly too large and heavy to move. This means that ambulatory monitoring or treatment allows patients to continue their daily lives during interventions that would previously have confined them to bed and hospital. Examples include ambulatory dialysis, gastric secretion monitoring and wearable artificial hearts.

Similarly, microtechnology has led to the design of implantable devices to assist the function of various organs or provide monitoring for diagnostic purposes by telemetry. Devices can be implanted which can be programmed or communicated with from outside by radio, so that routes for infection are reduced.

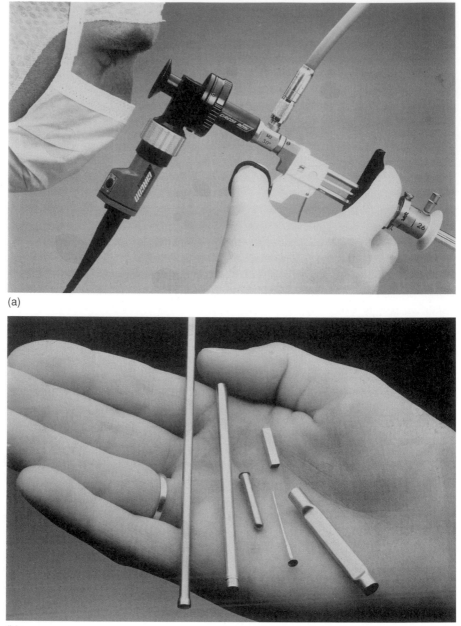

(a)

(b)

Figure 16.1 (a) Endoscopes are miniature telescopes. © Circon Corporation.
Reproduced by kind permission of Circon Corporation.
(b) Miniature tubular steel parts for medical products. © Judson A. Smith Company.
Reproduced by kind permission of Judson A. Smith Company.

16.3 MICROMANUFACTURING METHODS

Manufacturing of microcomponents can be undertaken either by high-precision conventional machines (e.g. milling, sparking, turning and grinding) or by new methods dedicated to microproducts. These new methods include micro injection moulding, laser machining, wet etching, electron beam cutting and UV masking. Table 16.1 shows some manufacturing methods used in microengineering, which refers to various illustrated examples.

With conventional methods the high precision and accuracy has been available for some time and the addition of magnified viewing techniques was not technically difficult. The real advances and interesting aspects of microengineering are the new developments.

16.3.1 LIGA

The name comes from lithographie–galvanormung–abformung, i.e. lithography, electroplating and micromoulding. This is probably the most advanced technique and certainly the one with the best potential for fabricating three dimensional microstructures. The LIGA system provides aspect ratios higher than 100, components with heights up to 1000 μm, very high accuracy in many different materials and enormous cost saving in mass produced items (Figure 16.2).

Table 16.1 Manufacturing methods for microcomponents

Method	Comment
Conversion systems which can be modified to produce items 1 mm or less in size	
Turning	Single point tools plus high speed machines, requires magnifying lenses
Milling	See Figure 16.3 and Figure 16.7
Electric discharge machining (sparking)	All metals
Grinding	Profile grinding via 100 : ratio, also useful for ceramics
Forming/spinning	Figure 16.1
Electroforming	Mainly restricted to nickel and copper
Fine blanking	Press tools, rubber pad pressing
Additional and new methods of microcomponent manufacture	
Laser micromachining	Suitable for ceramics and polymers
Microinjection moulding	Limited to polymer use, see Figure 16.5
Chemical etching	Figure 16.6 and Figure 16.10
Electron beam machining	Also suitable for nanolithography, beam spots down to 10 μm
UV masking	Layered boards and scaled 'masks'
X-ray lithography	Figure 16.4 and Figure 16.19
LIGA	Figure 16.2 and Figure 16.9

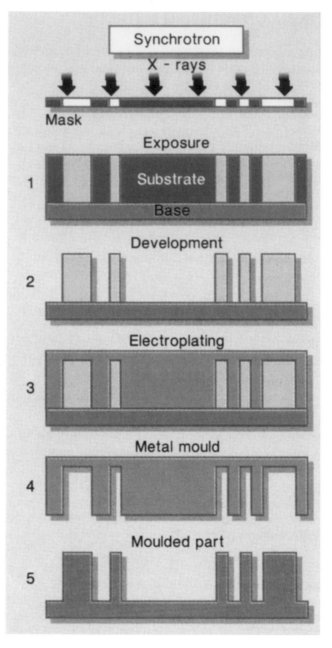

Figure 16.2 The LIGA process for fabrication of microdevices. From *Design Engineering*, Feb 1996: reproduced by permission of the Institution of Engineering Designers.

The shape or form required is set out in a mask, usually at 100 × scale, and either X-ray, electron beam, ion beam or laser energy is used to apply the pattern to the surface of a thick resist. The non-affected regions are removed (by various methods depending upon the resist used), and the gaps left are filled with metal alloys by electroplating, electroforming or electrodeposition. The resultant metal web is then either used directly (after cutting and separation) or it is used as the cavity for moulded components. The use of various materials at different levels or heights (steps) in the process gives versatility for the finished part.

The material most commonly used as a resist was PMMA but a new resist has been developed by BASF which is claimed to be 2–3 times more sensitive to X-rays and to require less critical control while being processes. IMM of Germany is currently working on a material which is expected to have 20 times more sensitivity than PMMA. This would enable direct deep X-ray lithography and components could be made direct.

Moulds made by the electroplating method are used to produce components in ceramics, polymers, glass and some softer metals. Ceramics normally require a secondary firing process once compressed or sintered into the moulds.

The LIGA technique was originally developed by Professor W. Ehrfeld at Karlsruhe Nuclear Research Centre in Germany. Further development of the process is being carried out by the Institute for Microtechniques in Mainz (IMM). UK interest groups and activities are being coordinated by the SERC Daresbury Laboratory, Warrington. Great interest exists in both the USA and Japan. The race to establish a practical, commercial system is now on. Which ever company first sets up commercial microproduction will control the introduction of microdevices for medical applications and all other industrial sectors.

16.3.2   MICROMOULDING

The Arburg injection moulding machine manufacturers have helped enormously in the development of this process and their *Allrounder 370C* can be used to produce items down to 1.5 g in weight. Even when multiple mouldings are made the feeder and sprue often contains more material than all the components together. See Figures 16.3, 16.4 and 16.5.

16.3.3   ELECTRON BEAM

Along with X-rays, ion beam and lasers, the electron beam offers a means of transferring enough energy to change the structure of the resist. The chosen pattern is left once the unactivated resist has been removed by solvent, water, laser or acid. The required pattern is laid out on a mask at 50 × or 100 × magnification, and focused down to provide an image which will allow X-rays etc, through only at correct pathways.

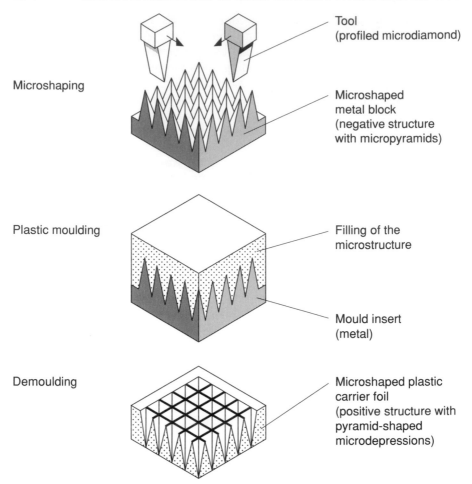

Microshaping

Tool
(profiled microdiamond)

Microshaped
metal block
(negative structure
with micropyramids)

Plastic moulding

Filling of the
microstructure

Mould insert
(metal)

Demoulding

Microshaped plastic
carrier foil
(positive structure with
pyramid-shaped
microdepressions)

Figure 16.3 By combining micromachining and plastic moulding, microstructurised plastic carrier foils can be produced at relatively low cost. (Original source unknown.)

16.3.4 UV MASKING

This is similar to the energy system described above but utilising ultra violet light to activate the resist (Figure 16.6). This system has the advantage of being easier to focus and uses a safer energy source.

Conventional X-ray intensifying screen   Microshaped X-ray intensifying screen

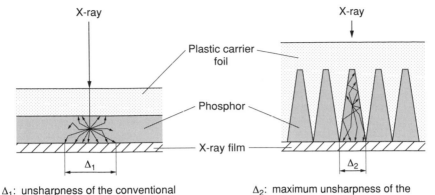

Δ_1: unsharpness of the conventional Δ_2: maximum unsharpness of the
          X-ray intensifying screen   microshaped X-ray intensifying screen

Figure 16.4 Microshaped X-ray intensifying screen. By locating the phosphor in microcells a significant improvement in sharpness is achieved. (Original source unknown.)

16.4 EXAMPLES

To highlight the possibilities of microengineering here are a number of items manufactured as either working prototypes or examples of the shapes, complex or simple, that can be made. I hope these will provoke your thoughts.

16.4.1 TURBINE BLADE

The first example shows a blade made by high precision machining. Subsequent fabrications have been made by different methods but this one, seen in Figure 16.7 was made on a CNC milling machine. Figure 16.8 shows a similar component made by laser machining.

16.4.2 GEARS

To the naked eye these look like tiny grains of sand but microscopic examination reveals gear wheels made from nickel. In Figure 16.9 the inner bore is only 50 μm diameter and next to it is a human hair for comparison. Eight teeth on a diameter 125 μm by 100 μm thick certainly indicate the sophistication of this new process.

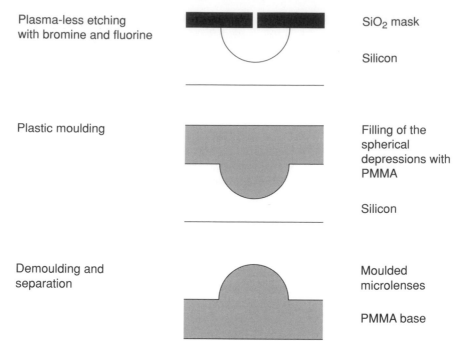

Plasma-less etching
with bromine and fluorine

SiO$_2$ mask

Silicon

Plastic moulding

Filling of the
spherical
depressions with
PMMA

Silicon

Demoulding and
separation

Moulded
microlenses

PMMA base

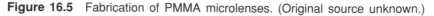

Figure 16.5 Fabrication of PMMA microlenses. (Original source unknown.)

16.4.3 FORCEPS

Using wire only 0.1 mm diameter and machining away grooves in one direction, microforceps have been made, some only 1 mm long. When inserted into a tube and drawn together these could be used for microsurgery.

16.4.4 MOTOR

Using similar techniques as with the gear wheels, a rotor only 100 μm diameter was constructed which ran in an electrostatic micromotor; this is shown in Figure 16.10.

16.4.5 PISTON

Attempting to put minute movement onto something like a circuit board is difficult, but now a method has been proven and awaits application. A small container with a single drop of oil inside is heated and cooled as current is applied and stopped. The effect is to cause the oil to become vapour and

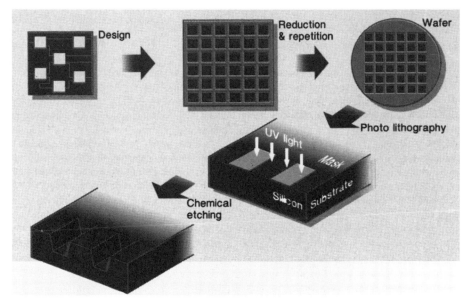

Figure 16.6 Photographic etching of semiconductors for manufacture of micro-devices. From *Design Engineering*, Feb 1996: reproduced by permission of the Institution of Engineering Designers.

then condense when cooling; this operates a small piston held in guides and exiting the container, giving physical lateral movement from a microcircuit. A sketch is shown in Figure 16.11.

16.5 PRODUCT EXAMPLES

While research has been supplying new concepts and samples the search for applications has been going on, and some of these products are now on sale. Here are actually working microsystems.

16.5.1 MICROMOTOR

Developed by IMM, this electromagnetic micromotor is only 2 mm in diameter. It has internal planetary gearing delivering approximately 0.1 μNm torque, and is capable of 10 000 r.p.m. on a spindle 0.25 mm diameter. There are plans to increase the speed and amount of torque to a target of 30 000 r.p.m. delivering 2–3 μNm. The components and assembly are shown in Figure 16.12.

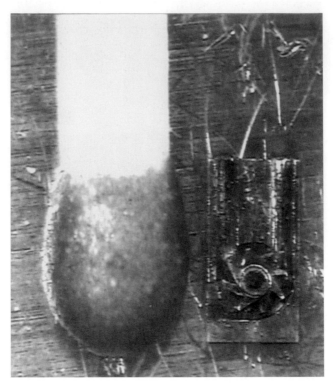

Figure 16.7   Brass microturbine prototype (seen next to a match) fabricated using precision machining. ©1995 IRC in Biomedical Materials: first published in *EPSRC Newsline* September 1995 and reproduced with permission.

16.5.2   MICRO-OPTICS

With the increasing use of fibre optics for communications and information technology the new LIGA system has been used to make housings to hold and join single strands of optical fibres. Ferrules constructed this way prevent damage to the fibres and subsequent loss of information. The assembly is dependent on micromoulded springs and wedges: see Figure 16.13 and Figure 16.14.

16.5.3   MICROPUMP

This is a simple diaphragm pump with dimensions radically reduced to 10 mm × 10 mm by micromachining. The pump is activated by a heater (PCB printed on silicon) with the power supplied by a strip cable. The polyimide diaphragm can deliver flow rates of approximately 150 μl min^{-1} and is designed for use with gases.

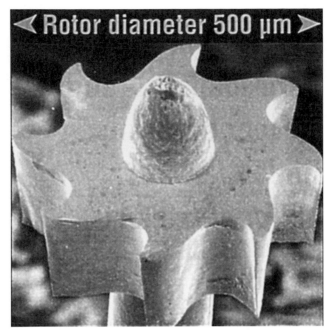

Figure 16.8 A nickel microturbine rotor from a laser micromachined mould. Reproduced from Lawes, R.A., Holmes, A.S. and Goodall, F.N. (1996) The formation of moulds for 3D microstructures using excimer laser ablation, *Microsystem Technologies*, **3** (1), © Springer-Verlag Gmbh and Co. KG. By kind permission of Springer-Verlag.

16.5.4 MICRO VALVE

Figures 16.15, 16.16 and 16.17 illustrate a self-contained system of switching valves 3 mm in diameter and only 1.3 mm thick. Within the structure are three micromembrane valves and a thermopneumatic actuator.

16.5.5 OPTICAL CATHETER

In late 1996 Research Medical of USA introduced a surgical catheter for removal of obstructions from the vessels in the lower leg, arms and other peripheral blood vessels. This consisted of a vascular balloon-tipped catheter with fibre optic viewing, lenses and a fluid irrigation lumen. Once inserted into a vein, the surgeon is able to view the progress as it travels towards the obstruction, (assuming the entire clot or occlusion is removed). This catheter was mostly constructed using modified, conventional products. To develop this approach further requires full use of microengineering expertise.

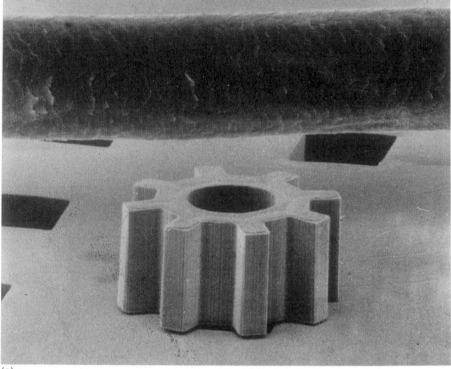

(a)

Figure 16.9(a) Nickel microgears: inner diameter 50 μm, thickness 100 μm. Human hair in the background. Reproduced by permission of Professor H. Guckel at the University of Wisconsin–Madison.

16.5.6 SENSORS

Catheters with mirrors, elastic spacers and a surface emitting laser mounted with a diode onto a silicone substrate then encapsulated in epoxy are used to monitor pressure while the patients are being operated on. The mirror moves, modifying the return signal reflected, when external pressure is applied to the catheter tip section.

16.5.7 EAR IMPLANT

Figure 16.18 shows a tiny implant for the inner ear to assist hearing. Additional information can be found in Chapter 27.

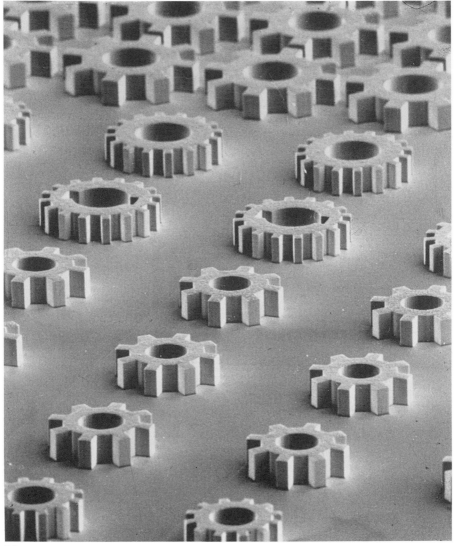

(b)

Figure 16.9(b) Nickel microgears: inner diameter 50 μm, thickness 100 μm. Reproduced by permission of Professor H. Guckel at the University of Wisconsin–Madison.

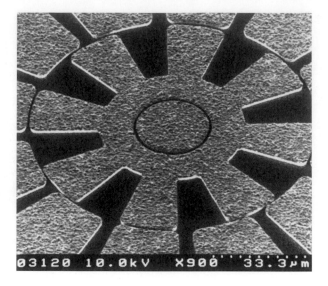

Figure 16.10 A rotor for an electrostatic micromotor: diameter ≈100 μm. © 1994 Institut für Mikrotechnik Mainz.

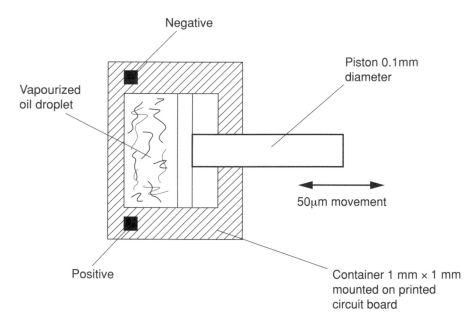

Figure 16.11 A miniature piston design concept.

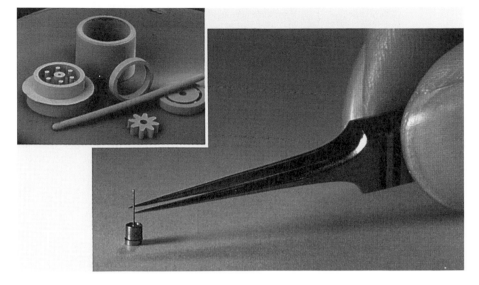

Figure 16.12 Parts for an electromagnetic micromotor: diameter 2 mm, torque 0.1 μNm. © 1994 Institut für Mikrotechnik Mainz.

16.5 FUTURE TRENDS

When miniature devices are created the ratio of strength to mass increases so the demands on material properties are less but the demand for material purity and homogeneity is more. Microengineering creates simplicity, whereas scaling down existing products creates the complex problems of model-making. With these advantages real advances can be made towards new forms of treatment. At Nottingham University research is going on with the view of delivering drugs to targets in the body by carrying them on 'nano-particles', particles so small (10 nm across) that one method would be to dissolve both the drug and carrier in a suitable solvent and then bring the two out of the solution together. The carrier could be a biodegradable polymer which would then release the active molecules in a time-dependent way. The main problem at the moment is manipulating the polymer carrier surface so that the drugs only reaches the correct tissue.

One area still being investigated as an ideal application for nano or micro-engineering devices is neurosurgery (Figure 16.19). Entry to the brain is not only complex but also emotive so the idea of lots of tiny tools being used to delve into the grey matter requires great care.

Finally as an idea, free for you to follow up and apply, in cleaning arteries of clots or dead tissue, why not use a multibladed turbine mounted on the end of a catheter, 1.5 mm diameter, driven by the flow of the patients own blood, used in a single direction (See Figure 16.8 and also Figure 16.20)?

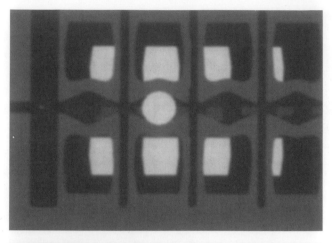

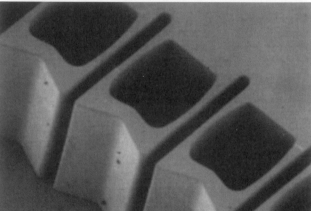

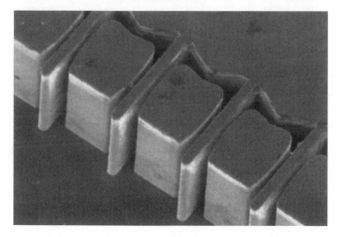

Figure 16.13 Centring a fibre using microsprings. © 1994 Institut für Mikrotechnik Mainz.

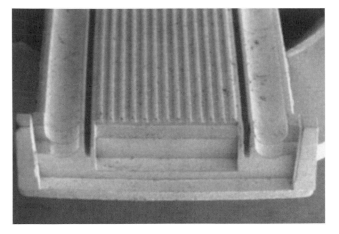

Figure 16.13 (*continued*)

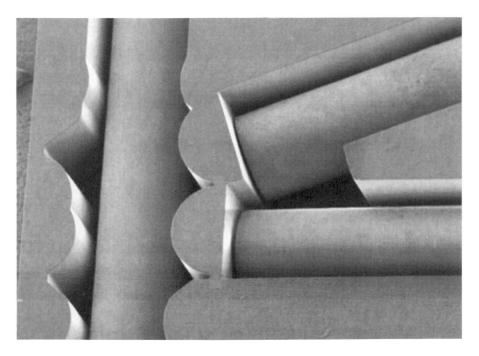

Figure 16.14 PMMA structure formed by deep X-ray lithography and guided optical fibres. Fibre diameter 125 μm. © 1994 Institut für Mikrotechnik Mainz.

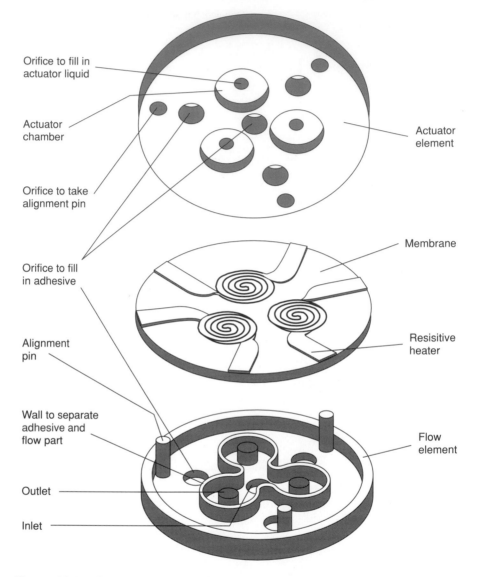

Figure 16.15 Diagram of a moulded microvalve system. © 1995 J. Fahrenberg: first published in *Microengineering* 5.

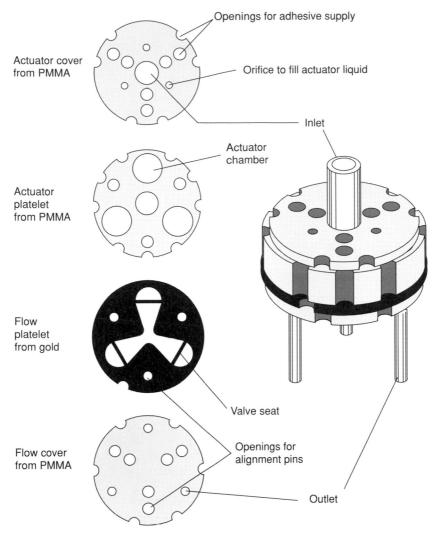

Figure 16.16 Diagram of the four platelets making up the valve system. © 1995 J. Fahrenberg: first published in *Microengineering* 5.

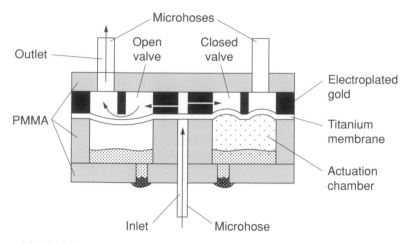

Figure 16.17 Diagram of the microvalve system showing the open (left) and closed (right) valves. © 1995 J. Fahrenberg: first published in *Microengineering* 5.

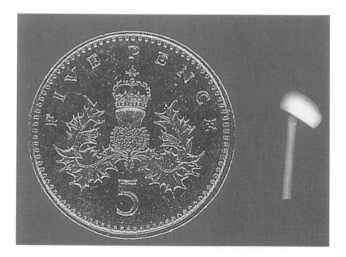

Figure 16.18 A HAPEX artificial bone for ear implants (made of hydroxyapatite-polyethylene composite). © 1995 IRC in Biomedical Materials: first published in *EPSRC Newsline* September 1995 and reproduced with permission.

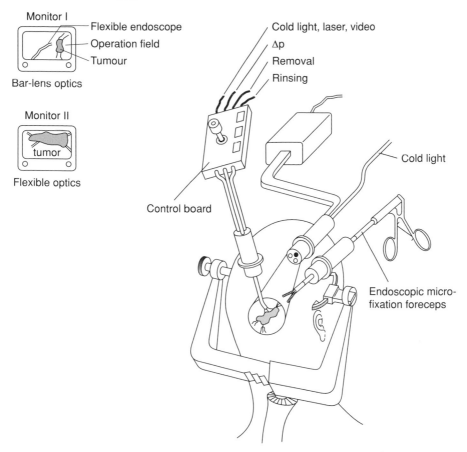

Monitor I — Flexible endoscope
— Operation field
— Tumour
Bar-lens optics

Monitor II
tumor
Flexible optics

Cold light, laser, video
Δp
Removal
Rinsing

Control board

Cold light

Endoscopic micro-
fixation foreceps

Figure 16.19 Neurological microsurgery. (Original source unknown.)

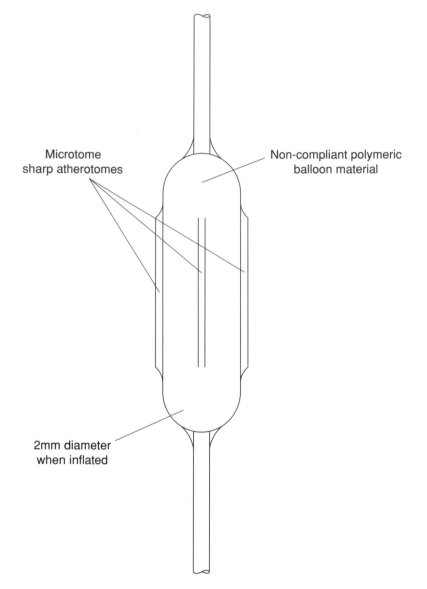

Microtome sharp atherotomes

Non-compliant polymeric balloon material

2mm diameter when inflated

Figure 16.20 Concept of a cutting balloon able to pass round a curve of radius 6 mm, to surgically incise plaque within arteries and relieve hoop stress. The deflated balloon protects the blade edges during insertion.

17
Prototyping

All new concepts for product design must be prototyped. This is a very bold and sweeping statement but over the years I have found it necessary. Without the assessment of a design in physical terms, certain flaws cannot be found and eliminated. A model or prototype allows such an assessment.

17.1 REASONS FOR PROTOTYPING

Creation and re-creation was a theme mentioned by Andrew Davis in 1996 regarding new musical scores but it also applies to any design. Without the re-modelling and re-evaluation of designs, the optimal product is unlikely to be manufactured. The success of a prototype or model can give the design team a welcome boost to their confidence.

In Figure 17.1 a design path to acceptance is shown: note the requirement for a minimum of two models. There are many reasons for the physical assessment of a design or feature, including:

- low confidence from production engineering,
- speculation on the methods (and costs) of manufacture,
- reluctance to accept change,
- unknown effect on the desired results, and
- need to convince sales (or customer) of the design's merits.

Figure 17.2 shows four different shapes proposed to meet the demands of a diathermy hook. Ranging from a simple curled wire to a complex form somewhere between a blade and a spatula, it was not until each type was made in scale size that surgeons could comment on which was the most effective, practical and acceptable. Shape D was found to be the most suitable, functional, and cost effective. It includes an innovative feature which aids the surgeon and could help the sales staff in selling the finished product. Figure 17.3 shows the final configuration.

Another valid need for prototype unit manufacture and testing before processing with a final solution is simply that there is no other way of establishing the 'right' answer. There may be no previous product, no scientific

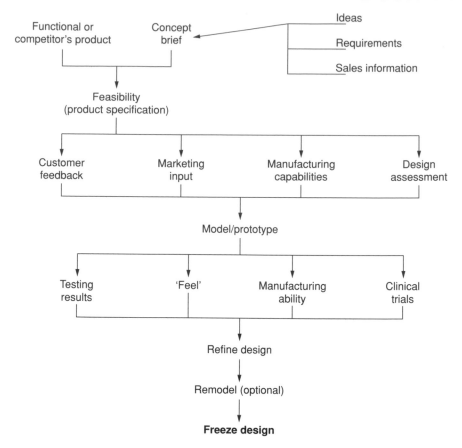

Figure 17.1   Design path for confirmation.

method of calculating a shape, just your innovative unknown, unproved design. In the sketches of Figure 17.4 the tip profiles for an electrode are shown: each one has merit, each one is justifiable, each one has a logical evaluation, but which one was the best could not be known until all were manufactured and tested. This was a necessary step to take before commitment of thousands of pounds on production facilities. It transpired that not only was the tip profile critical but also the overall length and angle of bend part way down the electrode. The finally agreed shape was number XVII when all parties acknowledged success.

The examples above illustrate the necessity of making models and prototypes; more good reasons are given in the design section of this book. Now I wish here to list the methods of prototyping, their uses and limitations, reasons for choice and rough comparisons of cost.

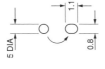

5 DIA 1.1 0.8

NOTES

1. 1mm dia stainless wire, which may be 'squashed' to this profile

2. Hook fitted to 27 dia, tube, (with 1 dia, bore) by crimp

3. Hook end must be domed and free from any sharp edges

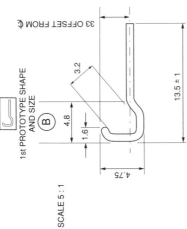

PROPOSED (A) 34 OFFSET FROM ℄ 2.75 4.8 2.4 Longer 13.5 ± 1 4.75

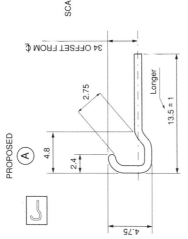

(C) 2.5 5 2.4 2.4 NORMAL HOOK FCR COMPARISON 1.8 DIA

1st PROTOTYPE SHAPE AND SIZE (B) 33 OFFSET FROM ℄ 3.2 4.8 1.6 13.5 ± 1 4.75

SCALE 5 : 1

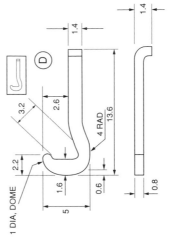

(D) 1.4 3.2 2.6 4 RAD 13.6 2.2 1 DIA, DOME 1.6 0.6 5 1.4 0.8

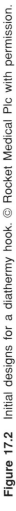

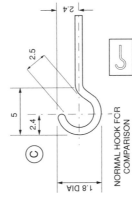

Figure 17.2 Initial designs for a diathermy hook. © Rocket Medical Plc with permission.

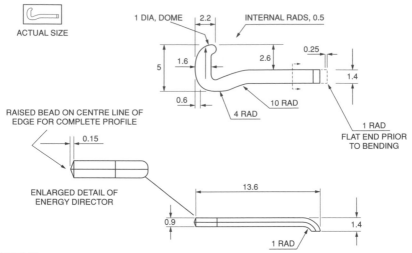

NOTES

1. Finished bent component is inserted into a 1.7 I/D tube. It is then held in place by crimping onto the flat 1.4 width.

2. Developed length $\left[\left(\frac{T}{3}+R\right) \times 1.5708\right] + 11.7 - 0.5 = \mathbf{13.3}$

3. In practical terms 13.5 with small upturn.

4. Component must be burr free and have no sharp edges.

Figure 17.3 Final design for a diathermy hook. © Rocket Medical Plc.

1. The simplest method is to use a modelmaker, toolmaker or similar skilled individual to fabricate, machine or build your item for assessment.
2. 'Soft' tooling can be used to provide an accurate sample of a moulded part; this is sufficient for comment, testing and a small pre-production run.
3. It may be possible to fabricate a model from similar parts, chopped and cut to suit. This should never see the light of day outside the design office as an assembly, but is acceptable enough for concept appraisal.
4. Consultants can be used to save time and effort in prototyping: leave the hassle to them (but you have to pay).
5. Rapid prototyping is held as the magic solution to all problems. Unfortunately this is not so, but the technique is still a very good option or 'tool' when used correctly.
6. In-house manufacture is another option: who better knows the project, especially if it's to be a modification to or evolution of an existing product.

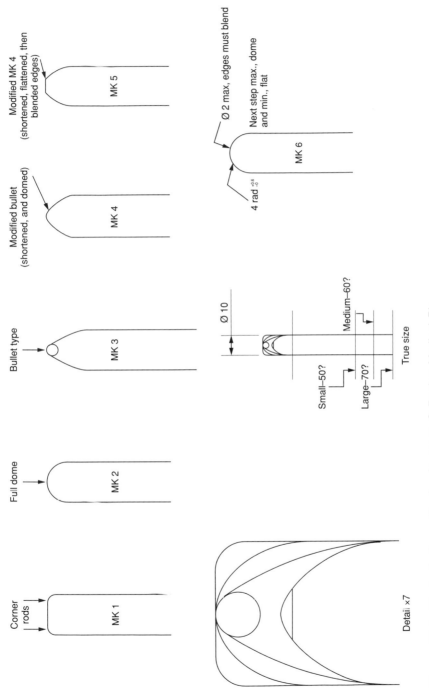

Figure 17.4 Electrode tip profile development. © Rocket Medical Plc.

7. Computer numerical control (CNC), computer-aided design (CAD), computer-aided manufacturing (CAM): these techniques can be helpful, but need to be selected and used appropriately.

All these methods can be seen in Table 17.1 for comparison and quick reference.

Table 17.2 shows traditional methods.

Table 17.3 shows computer-aided design and manufacture CAD/CAM techniques.

Figures 17.5 and 17.6 illustrate rapid prototyping.

Figure 17.7 shows soft or low volume tooling.

17.2   RAPID PROTOTYPING

Rapid prototyping systems consist of a target box or volume into which a focused laser beam fuses or cures a medium. The curing takes place on a linear path on X, Y coordinates to produce a slice of the required model: in effect it produces a solid cross section. By moving the whole table or box another slice of the cross section can be produced and fixed to the previous one, thus building the model layer by layer until a complete unit is finished. The layers are on average 0.2 mm thick and fused together by the same beam.

There are variations on the above method but they all basically work the same way, building layers. One method uses paper shapes cut by the laser and laminated together. The medium used to create the layers may be a liquid or a powder. The end materials vary in hardness, tensile strength, compression and brittleness. Unfortunately some physical tests are still not possible no matter which base material is used, although just arriving in the UK this year are powders which are 60% steel, 40% copper and when sintered provide a metal alloy which has similar mechanical properties to aluminium. This gives the potential to create moulds from 3D computer data, thus reducing tool manufacturing lead times and (more importantly) the facility to make comparatively cheap 'trial' tooling.

One other rapid modelling machine newly available is very similar to an inkjet plotter but deposits wax instead of ink. This builds the model in layers the same as stereolithography and selective laser sintering but is quicker, cheaper and now looking to replace the established systems.

Another development for the rapid prototyping machines is not as a product or model but a physical manistification of CT scanned information. If used correctly it would allow surgeons to practice on models of areas like the skull or heart before actually opening up the patient for real in the theatre.

Rapid prototyping techniques are evolving from methods of producing physical representations of a concept to ways of improving medical services and quality of life. Three examples of how this works are as follows.

Table 17.1 Prototyping methods

Method	Timescale	Cost	Comment
Rapid prototyping	Realistic turn round of 5 to 7 days. But beware of other scheduled work.	£1000 to £2000 for one 'shot'. May contain more than one component.	Number of systems available. All provide detailed components from rendered 3D drawings. Direct conversion of concept into physical reality.
Fabricate (from existing components)	Anything from one day to 3 weeks, dependent on delivery from stock.	With luck nothing (other than your time). Good relationships with suppliers normally mean free samples for assessment.	Quantities affect supply very much. Ideal for concept or visual model to see final idea in solid form.
(machined and assembled components)	Varies from one week to 5 weeks. Depends upon quantity, resource, complexity of parts and amount of money available to spend.	£10 to £20 per hour	Manual, auto or computer controlled production of parts.
Model maker	Depends upon the complexity and final function (visual v. functional use).	£20 per hour	If used for visual use only then non-functional parts will speed delivery. But if required for physical testing or even clinical trials then the methods of manufacture may change – as will delivery
Toolmaker Temporary tooling (Al tools, jigs and fixtures and precision machining)	Negotiate, anytime between 3 to 5 weeks.	Al mould tools from £400. Press tools from £500. Fixtures from £200. All depend upon the parts complexity.	Low cost tooling to simulate final items. Problem in initial acceptance of capital outlay and when change over to 'real' tooling. Quantities normally very good before the 'temporary' tooling needs replacement.

Table 17.1 (continued)

Method	Timescale	Cost	Comment
Production tooling	8 to 14 weeks	Varies between £4000 to £12 000 for basic 'small' items requiring mould tools.	Even at the design stage finished tooling may be the only way of assessing a finished product and the capital outlay must be considered to agree commercial viability.
In house	Immediate if you can swing the authority of arrange priority. Worst choice if not.	Zero. Lose it in over-heads.	Normally a good starting point (providing of course the necessary skills are available). But usually conflict of interests and the use of personnel cause this method problems. Provided agreement is acceptable early on in the procedure probably the best option available initially.
Consultant	Negotiate Short time = Cost Extended time = Problem	Anywhere between £50 to £200 per hour. Some space for negotiations when either a long term contract agreed or a fixed delivery price accepted.	1. Emergency route, facilities immediate to hand to cover for delays or time slippage. 2. Any additional design time can be built in. 3. Removes all problems from own site, state requirements, agree cost/targets then step back. 4. Very expensive. 5. Covers any temporary shortfalls in resource. 6. Provides expert personnel who may not be available in-house.

Table 17.2 Traditional methods of prototyping

Machining
  Milling
  Turning
  Grinding
Welding
  Brazing
  Oxyacetylene welding
  Electric arc welding
  MIG/TIG
  Soldering
Sparking
  EDM
  EDG
Casting
  Sand
  Vacuum
  Lost wax
Hand
  File
  Saw
  Form
Vacuum forming of sheet plastics allows large areas to be used as a base. Fabricate or enlarge to provide single items.
  Polyurethane expanded foam, easily manipulated, cut or made up to provide a visual representation.
  Wood, plastic, metal, resin all ideal to create a visual version of your concept. Even paper folded and stuck together may be acceptable.
  Control of the finished item is critical if the model or prototype is to be used for any kind of physical trial or quantitative tests.

1. As a 3D hard copy of the data set, a model can provide visual and tactile documentation for diagnosis, therapy planning and didactic purposes. It facilitates the communication between surgical team members, between the radiologists and surgeons. Even though radiologists are quite skilled now in interpreting 2D scans and 3D images the majority of other medical staff are not used to performing this type of interpretation, but because measurements can be taken more easily from 3D models they can be of great benefit in research.
2. 3D models can be useful in planning complex surgery which may involved using it in simulation of the actual operation. An example is facial reconstruction. Life sized models of a patient's skull are used to plan osteotomies (displacement of bone segments) prior to cutting tissue, by performing a surgical rehearsal on the mock-up. The critical aspect is the ability to predict the displacement of the bone segments while being able to measure consequential displacements in advance.

Table 17.3   CAD/CAM methods of prototyping

2D Drawing	Hand fabrication Machine Assemble	} Requires tooling and skilled personnel
2D Copy to 3D	Program write	CNC manufacture
2D Program write	CNC manufacture	
2D DXF file	Modify and transfer to 3D	Copy CNC
2D DXF file	Modify information	CNC (dependent on type)
2D DXF file	Modify or render	3D conversion SLA/SLS/LOM etc.
3D Render	SLA/SLS/LOM etc	May need 2D drawing later
3D Direct to CNC	May require 2D drawing later to allow dimensional check	

Only the last two methods do not require 2D drawings before component or finished item production, but they do require 2D versions at a later date to allow inspection, specifications etc, to be checked and recorded.

The SLA (stereolithography), SLS (selective laser sintering) and LOM (laminated object manufacture) rapid prototyping systems do need to be compatible with the original transfer system, consideration should also be made regarding the cost of software, interface, hardware and its frequency of use before contemplating purchasing your own system (of whichever type).

A CNC milling or machine centre costs about £40 000 plus software £5000.

3D software plus related machine console > £26 000 each 'seat' (some now down to £12 000)

Rendering 3D programs plus software and machine for SLA £300 000

Rendering 3D programs plus software and machine for SLS £200 000.

2D programs vary in price and complexity depending upon your needs but start at £1700 for software and computing hardware for the simplest.

3. With 3D models (accurate to 0.5 mm) of existing structures the design of prostheses is considerably easier. The model can either be used as a negative from which the implant can be manufactured before surgery or it can be used directly as a master for the implant construction.

Mirror images can be made to help plastic surgeons reconstruct faces, body areas and limbs to achieve symmetry. There are even developments in biocompatible materials which can be used immediately after production via stereolithography.

Probably the most interesting and possibly the application with the most potential is the concept of manufacturing customised implants from CT information and powders similar to those mentioned before, all done before the operation takes place.

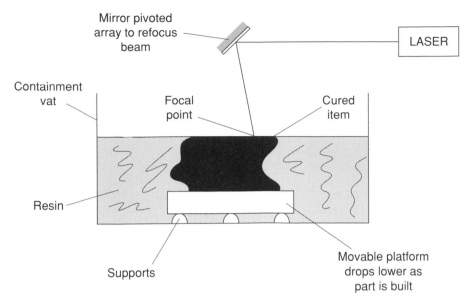

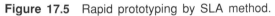

Figure 17.5 Rapid prototyping by SLA method.

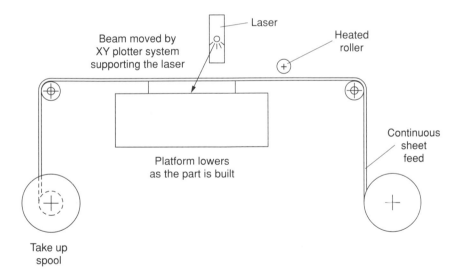

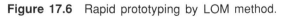

Figure 17.6 Rapid prototyping by LOM method.

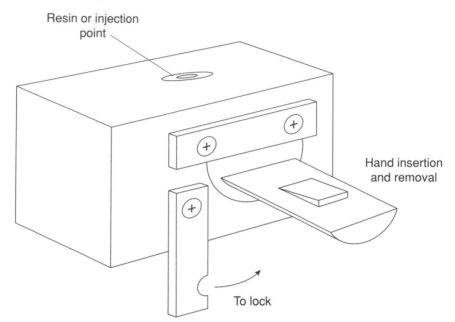

Figure 17.7   Prototype tool making by moulding.

17.3   COMPUTER-AIDED PROTOTYPING

Since engineering designs are now commonly produced on 2D or 3D drafting systems, single items for assessment are readily converted to systems like CAM (computer-aided manufacture). In some cases a stand alone system can be supplied which will machine 3D replicated from the 2D drawing – computer input direct to its own machining centre.

Other comparisons are shown in Table 17.3.

17.4   SOFT TOOLING

Toolmaking systems utilise the concept of 'soft' aluminium tooling for moulding, forming or casting. The basic idea being easy manufacturing, speed of cutting and all cores, inner parts etc, are hand laid and hand removed.

The labour content is obviously great, but since the requirement is only for very low volumes or even single parts there is no real problem. Problems do occur though when the same tools are used as production items, either deliberately as cheap quick solutions or as a just because of a carry-on attitude (until they collapse then we'll worry about it). I would advise you to

specify the tool life early on in the development programme and stick to the
dates and volumes agreed.

17.5   SUMMARY

Prototyping is a necessary evil of the development process: either it proves
the design or it is instrumental in disproving it and then has to be done again
(and again until all interested parties are satisfied). The only good aspect is
that once a product design is proven and accepted most obstacles and financial constraints are normally removed.

Although most people assume that prototypes are models of a product,
there may also be prototype tools which require assessment. Provided
allowances are included in your project plan there should be no problem.

Finally consider Table 17.1 on prototyping options. Do not narrow your
choice by always using the same system. Select the best option for your needs
at the time, not the fashionable one, nor the cheapest one, but just the best.
They are just tools: select the one to suit you, use it, then return it.

18
Sterilisation

The destruction of bacteria and other infectious organisms in industry, food products and medical devices must be carried out by a method which:

- does not damage the product or any materials contained;
- guarantees (within set limits) sterile surfaces;
- is economical for the user;
- is easily applied;
- is safe for those applying it;
- provides speed and turnaround to make stock readily available.

Once sterilised it follows that the product must be contained in suitable packing (see Chapter 21) to prevent recontamination; it is normally hermetically sealed. All these requirements apply rigidly to medical device products.

Before the final sterilisation process certain precautions are necessary to ensure that a clean product is supplied. The first requirement is for manufacturing to take place in a 'clean room': one with an environment controlled to EEC standards and codes of practice, with filtered air fed into the enclosed working environment. (The size or type of filtration is dependent on the classification necessary, but it is monitored and verified on a regular basis.) The FDA Good Manufacturing Practice (GMP) guidelines stipulate a clean room environment.

The second requirement of clean manufacturing is to clothe the operators in special suits to limit the number of particles which may fall and contaminate any assemblies or components.

Ensuring protection of the product from contamination during manufacture aids the sterilisation process (regardless of which method is used), since the larger the number or organisms present on the product surfaces before sterilisation, then the greater the statistical probability that there will still be live organisms left after the sterilisation process. This probability is recognised and there are acceptable levels called Sterility Assurance Levels or SAL. The usual level of acceptance is an SAL of 10^{-6} or one part per million non-sterile, but of course this is the minimum value. To quantify the SAL level, validation tests should be carried out regularly to prove the level of sterilisation on each product. It is not the process that is validated but each product, since size, shape, materials used, method of packing and the materials with which it is packed affect recontamination and sterilisation.

As an added insurance most manufacturers include indicators on the outside of either the packs or packing boxes to show that the product has been through a sterilisation process.

- Gamma indicators use dosimeters which change colour after a certain level of radiation has been absorbed.
- Ethylene oxide (ETO) indicator include bacteria; after sterilisation the indicators are removed and cultured to check that no bacterial growth occurs. If no growth is found after seven days, the load is certified. Each box or pack also normally carries an ETO strip which changes colour when exposed to the ETO gas.
- Autoclave indicators are similar to ETO indicators but with differences in the bacteria used.
- Electron beam indicators are similar to gamma indicators, and respond to radiation
- Cold sterilisation methods have no real reliable indicators. This is one of several reasons why the medical establishment does not favour chemical methods of sterilisation.

There is no 'best' sterilisation method since all the systems provide a method of killing potentially harmful organisms present on the product, but there are pros and cons of different methods which will affect your choice. Radiation has harmful effects on some materials, so this needs to be borne in mind.

Whichever method you choose the cycle must be validated to ensure that the organisms present on the product are being eliminated. Documentation is very important and no product should be allowed to be released for sale or use by the clinician without a full certificate of sterilisation.

18.1 STERILISATION METHODS

There are five commonly used methods for the sterilisation of medical device products.

- Gamma: exposure of items to gamma radiation.
- Electron beam: exposure of items to a high energy beam of accelerated electrons.
- ETO: exposure of the item's outer surfaces to a corrosive gas, ethylene oxide.
- Autoclave: exposure of items to steam at 130°C under pressure.
- Chemically: immersion for 20 min in a 'sterilising' solution such as formaldehyde, the items are used while still wet.

Table 18.1 shows the basic advantages and disadvantages of each sterilisation method.

Table 18.1   Methods of sterilisation

Advantages	Disadvantages
Gamma radiation sterilisation	
Complete product penetration	Some plastics degrade
Process in shipping package	Discolouration of some products
Immediate product release	Brittleness in some products
No residues	Large capital outlay (if in-house)
Proven use over 30 years	Limited use of some materials
Excellent process reliability	Isotope containment
Only one process variable – time	
Environmentally safe	
Guaranteed sterility assurance	
Economical	
Ethylene oxide (ETO) sterilisation	
Variety of materials possible	No hermetically sealed cavities
Process in shipping packaging	Elimination of CFC–12
Design expense	Flammability of 100% ETO
Historically acceptable method of sterilisation	Required aeration
	Usually quarantined 7–14 days
	Process variables: vacuum; pressure; temperature; time; humidity; ETO concentration
	Increasing regulations, documentation and inspections
	Residues left in some materials
Electron beam sterilisation	
In-line processing of product	Limited product penetration
Rapid dose rate	Complex dosimety
Utilises electricity	Shadowing effect
No toxic waste or by-products	Product heating
	Equipment maintenance and reliability
Autoclave (steam) sterilisation	
Cheap	May contain contaminants
Easy to control	Distortion (at 130°C)
Easy to monitor	Packing warping
	Vacuum pressure
	Moisture absorption
Chemical sterilisation	
Ambient temperature	Toxic fumes
Easy process	Possible allergic skin reaction
Quick	Spillage problems
Used within or close to theatre	Long term effect worries – unknown but some cause for concern

18.1.1 GAMMA

In gamma sterilisation items are exposed to a maximum of 5 Mrad of radiation at a prescribed wavelength. Although the agreed exposure for verified sterilisation in most countries is 2.5 Mrads, this apparent overdose is necessary to ensure that all items on the conveyor pallet passing the isotope receive at least 2.5 Mrad, since some will be shielded by others. The gamma beam penetrates about 200 cm into the products.

Very few parameters vary in the process. The majority can be controlled or checked and allowed for, e.g. density of packs, geometry of arrangement or source strength. This means that gamma sterilisation is a reliable process.

The radiation, see Figure 18.1, comes from a cobalt 60 isotope. Products are loaded onto carrier pallets and fed onto a conveyer which winds through a protective labyrinth and then go past the isotope. Figure 18.2 shows a typical plant layout.

The problem with gamma sterilisation is the selection of suitable materials, as many are degraded by the radiation. Glass changes colour to anything from transparent mild tan to black and opaque. Table 18.2 lists the materials most suitable and those best to avoid, and why. A substantial amount

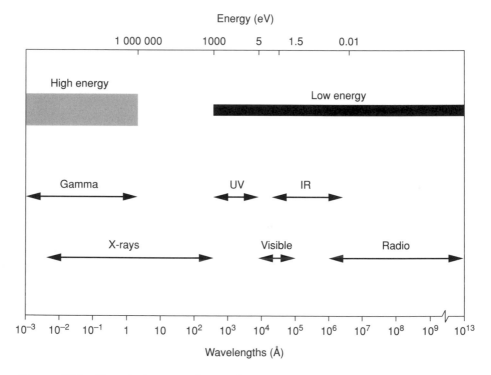

Figure 18.1 The electromagnetic spectrum.

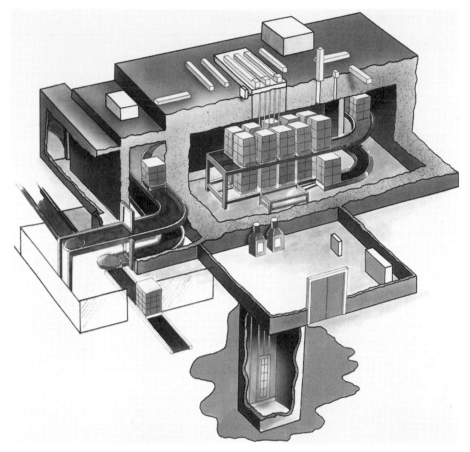

Figure 18.2 A gamma sterilisation system. © Gammaster.

of work has been carried out on the effects of gamma radiation on materials. Table 18.3 is a chart compiled by the UKAEA (now AEA Technology plc), for radiation from 1 Mrad to 500 Mrad.

18.1.2 ELECRON BEAM

This uses a line of sight system which generates a stream of electrons and directs them at a target. This target is located above a conveyer belt on which products pass. The machine is powered by electricity and is simply switched on or off when required. The main problem with electron beam sterilisation is that the beam only penetrates about 4 cm into the product. If correct and comprehensive validation is given and constant monitoring is assured then the amount of absorption or dose is certified.

Table 18.2   Materials for gamma sterilisation

Materials that can be used with practically no restriction

Styrene (the most stable common moulding material)
ABS (pigments may be affected)
Polyethylene: HDPE and LDPE
Polyester: PET, PETG, APET
Urethanes: aliphatic, polyester, polyether (esters may turn brown)
Cellulosics: cellulose acetate, propionate, butyrate
Polysulphone
Fluoroplastics (except PTFE)
Elastomers, silicone, kraton, EPDM
Polymides, nylon (some colour shift, may appear brownish)
Epoxy resins
Phenol formaldehyde (Bakelite)
Polycarbonate (embrittled at high doses)

Materials that require care in selection

Acrylic (PMMA) and PMMA copolymer with styrene. Anticipated temporary
    colour shift and modest loss of physical properties. After 60 to 90 days colour
    fades back to near clear.
PVC Available in radiation resistance compounds. Either in rigid or flexible form.
    Anticipate colour shift and odour with the normal grades (HCl evolved).
Polypropylene. Severe loss of elongation unless modified. Embrittled. Continues
    to degrade when stored in air after irradiation. May exhibit colour shift due to
    the presence of antioxidants. However, propylene can be stabilised. Several
    commercial versions now exist with no more than 20% loss of elongation out of
    400% available at break. Can be effectively modified for radiation.

Materials best avoided

Acetal	Embrittles, yellows
PTFE (Teflon)	Embrittles (but other fluoro polymers do not)
Cyanoacrylates	Loss of elongation and tensile properties. Work continues to upgrade radiation resistance.
Nylon and Polypropylene film	Exhibits more sensitivity to radiation and oxidation change.
Neoprene	HCl evolved.
Butyl rubber	Becomes fluid at low doses.

Other materials for reference

Metals	Are outstanding in their radiation stability
Glass	May change colour at relatively low doses, although stable forms are available.
Concrete	Very stable and used as shielding
Inks and paints	These can be predicted from knowledge of their base formulations. Certain unsaturated polyester based paints can be cured by radiation.

There is also a certain amount of product heating with the process. This
should be allowed for when packing the product and selecting materials. The
speed, ease and costs of electron beam sterilisation can be better than
gamma. Figure 18.3 shows a rough comparison of the cost advantages of
electron beam over gamma.

For heat sensitive items cooling may be needed to prevent damage. Local heating at a typical dose is about 6°C for water, 12°C for plastics and up to 60°C for metals with a typical 20 s exposure.

Treatments can be varied easily and quickly with the electron beam, even on a box-by-box basis, therefore reducing the required load size and cost. Also the microbiological effect of the beam is the same as for gamma radiation, so historical data can be used for reference. The same applies to material selection. The down side is the requirement for validation of sterility, so costs tend to even themselves out when comparing with other systems.

A limiting factor with the electron beam is the depth of penetration and therefore effectiveness of the sterilisation. If this is considered to be inadequate, then double-sided exposure using two overlapping doses may be a solution. Figure 18.4 illustrates a dosage validation graph.

18.1.3 ETHYLENE OXIDE (ETO)

This corrosive gas is flooded over a product, left to 'soak' and then extracted, achieving sterilisation. The product is loaded into a chamber, sealed and then the air is pumped out. The ethylene oxide is fed in at an elevated temperature of 45°C and left to impregnate the produce for about four hours. This process is repeated, sometimes up to five times, after which the gas is extracted.

Delays occur due to the time needed to validate each batch. The release of products is usually after 7 to 10 days. The packaging must be permeable to allow the gas to penetrate and have direct contact with all product surfaces. If an assembly has any sealed joints or inner areas the ETO may not be able to effect a full sterilisation.

If the permeability of the packaging is inadequate, it may be necessary to include special gas ports or filters. This is an additional cost and introduces concern about long-term storage and recontamination.

ETO is toxic and is a gas implicated in depleting the earth's ozone layer. There are inevitably traces of ETO present on the products after processing, and the safety of operatives must be considered. For these reasons there is considerable pressure to reduce or eliminate the use of ETO sterilisation.

18.1.4 AUTOCLAVING

The principle of this long established method is simple. Items are sealed in a pressure vessel and steam at about 130°C is introduced. After sufficient time for harmful organisms to be destroyed, the high pressure steam is evacuated, the items are cooled and dried and left sterile. This method is used in laboratories worldwide. An even simpler method heats items in a sealed vessel of water to above 125°C for 20 min.

Table 18.3   Radioisotopes Review Sheet G1. Reproduced with permission of AEA Technology plc

Radiation Stability of Materials

The stability guide shows only average observations. Not all mechanical properties change by the same amount, indeed in some materials tensile strength may increase whereas impact strength or modulus may decrease. Furthermore the stability is often influenced by the size and environment of the article being irradiated. The data are equally applicable to electron or gamma irradiation.

● ● ● ●	Satisfactory up to a dose of at least 5×10^8 rad (500 Mrad)
● ● ●	Satisfactory up to a dose of at least 10^8 rad (100 Mrad)
● ●	Satisfactory up to a dose of at least 10^7 rad (10 Mrad)
●	Satisfactory up to a dose of at least 2.5×10^4 rad (2.5 Mrad)
†	Very unsatisfactory, particularly at doses greater than 10^4 rad (1.0 Mrad)

Material	Stability	Comments
Rubbers		Stability influenced by the nature of the antioxidants present
Polyurethane rubber	● ● ● ●	The most radiation stable rubber
Natural rubber	● ● ●	Good stability
SBR Butadiene styrene rubber	● ● ●	Good stability
Nitrile rubber	● ● ●	Good stability
Silicone rubber	● ●	Usually polydimethylsiloxanes – methyl phenyl silicones more stable
Neoprene rubber	● ●	Hydrogen chloride evolved – beware of corrosion
Butyl rubber	†	Becomes fluid at comparatively low doses
Thermoplastics		
Polystyrene	● ● ● ●	The most radiation stable common moulding plastic
Polyethylene (high and low density)	● ● ●	melt flow index drastically reduced – stress cracking improved
Nylon 6 and 6:6	● ● ●	Hardens at high does (10^8 rad). Much less stable in film form
Polyester – Mular or Melinex	● ● ●	Turns brown. Much less stable in film form
Polyvinylchloride PVC and copolymers	● ●	HCl evolved. Turns brown. Polyvinlyidene chloride less stable
Polycarbonate	● ●	Tendency to become brittle at high doses
Cellulose esters – acetate and nitrate	● ●	Acetate slightly more stable than nitrocellulose (Celluloid)
Polypropylene	●	Becomes brittle, especially on storage (note 3)
Polymethylmethacrylate – 'Perspex' 'Diakon'	●	Turns brown becomes brittle and may crack
PTFE Teflon or Fluon	†	Acids evolved – much more stable in the absence of air

Table 18.3 *(continued)*

Material	Stability	Comments
FEP		OK. But can be problematic
ABS		OK. No problem
Polyacetal – polyformaldehyde and copolymers	†	Becomes brittle and loses strength
Thermoplastic Elastomer		Varied changes at high dosage. Advise gamma trials on material section at earliest point in design cycle
Thermosets		These materials are much more stable when filled with fibre
Epoxy resins	● ● ● ●	Very stable especially when cured with aromatic amines
Phenol formaldehyde 'Bakelite'	● ● ●	Good stability – sometimes colour changes
Urea formaldehyde UF resins	● ●	
Polyesters – styrene modified	● ● ●	Good stability – resins may be cured using radiation
Textiles		
Polyester – Terylene or Dacron	● ●	The most radiation stable textile material
Cellulose acetates – Dicel and Tricel	● ●	Loss of strength – acetic acid produced
Acrylic yarn – Orlon, Acrilan and Courtelle	● ●	Small amount of cross linking at low doses
Wool	● ●	Loses strength and solubilises. Silk is less stable than wool
Viscose Rayon	● ●	Much more stable than cotton
Nylon 6 and 6:6	● ●	Very sensitive to air. Degradation in air 5 × that in vacuo
Cotton	●	20% loss in strength at 5×10^4 rad and yellowing
Adhesives		
Structural adhesives – epoxies and phenolics	● ● ●	Araldite (epoxy based)
Vinyl type e.g.: polyvinyl acetate	● ●	Inorganic filters improve the stability
Pressure sensitive adhesives	†	Oxidative breakdown at doses $> 10^4$ rad giving excessive tack
Oils and greases		
Mineral oils and diesters	● ● ●	Viscosity increases and oxidation stability drastically reduced
Silicone oils	● ●	Viscosity increases
Natural oils	●	Drying oils polymerise – castor oil stable to at least 10^8 rad
Commercial greases	● ●	Soften and then harden. Resistant greases available commercially.

Table 18.3 *(continued)*

Packaging Materials
Most packaging materials behave satisfactorily at the sterilising dose of 2.5×10^4 rad. Polypropylene and coated cellulose films (Cellophane) are embrittled at 5×10^4 rad and should be used with considerable caution. Polyester film 'Melinex' or Mylar is the most stable with the exception of Du Pont's new experimental H 'A' is probably only suitable for doses up to 10^7 rad. Low density polyethylene and PVC based films produce odours on irradiation. The permeability changes produced in packaging materials on irradiation are very small and can be ignored.
Paper and Cardboard: Lose mechanical strength at low doses but are serviceable up to at least 5×10^4 rad.
Wood: Similarly loses mechanical strength but is stable up to at least 10^7 rad.
Cork: Is quite stable to radiation and doses of 10^8 rad produce small changes.

Printing ink and paint films
It is unusual to find colour changes in printed material although occasionally a change of shade may be found. The behaviour of paint films can be predicted from a knowledge of the polymers used in their formulation. The most stable coatings are made from phenolic and epoxy compounds. Halide coatings eg: PVC should be avoided. Certain paints such as unsaturated polyester can be cured using radiation.

Inorganic fillers, glass and concrete
There is little measurable change in inorganic materials at doses up to 10^9 rad, apart from slight colour changes. Glasses change colour at doses above 10^5 rad to give various colours from brown to violet. Radiation stable glasses are now available which show only small changes.
Concrete is very stable and is used as a shielding material.

Metals
These are outstanding in their radiation stability, and are largely unchanged at doses as high as 10^{10}–10^{11} rad.

Notes
1 Storage Effects
All plastics age on storage and this effect may be magnified following exposure to radiation due to either consumption of antioxidant during irradiation and/or the production of more oxidisable groups in the polymer structure.
An additional storage effect usually associated with plastics containing crystalline regions, e.g. polypropylene, is due to the presence of trapped 'free radicals'. These molecular fragments slowly diffuse from their traps and cause further chemical and physical changes. High temperature annealing removes these radicals but may also accelerate the ageing process.
2 Additives in Plastics
The stability of rubbers and plastics is very dependent on the additives in the system. The addition of antioxidants and plasticisers may have a very marked improvement on the radiation tolerance of a material. Many additives, e.g. antioxidants are consumed during the irradiation and it is advisable to add a larger initial amount to ensure that sufficient remains after irradiation to provide protection against thermal oxidation.
3 Dose Rate
Degradation reactions are not normally sensitive to rate of energy deposition. However, in those cases where oxygen assists in the breakdown of the material, e.g. Nylon and polypropylene, the rate of diffusion of oxygen into the sample may be rate controlling. In such cases samples irradiated at very high dose rate will show much less damage than those treated at low dose rate. The effects produced by γ-rays and fast electrons are similar and any observable differences are due to the differing dose rates used in irradiating with these two types of radiation.

Table 18.3   *(continued)*

4   Induced radioactivity
No hazard is caused by induced radioactivity in materials irradiated with ^{60}Cp γ-radiation or high energy electrons up to 5 MeV. This applies to most materials up to an energy level of 15 MeV.

(RLV) Wantage Research Laboratory, United Kingdom Atomic Energy Authority, March 1965.

References
1) R O Bolt and J G Carroll 'Radiation Effects on Organic Materials' Academic Press 1963.
2) A Charlesby 'Atomic Radiation and Polymers' Pergamon 1960.

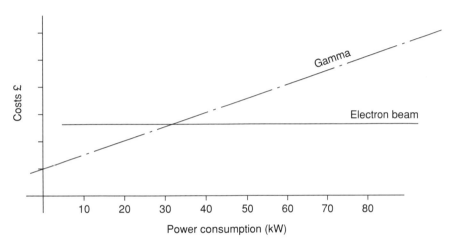

Figure 18.3   Comparative processing costs.

Problems with autoclaving are the retention of moisture in the products, and the need for expensive packaging to resist high temperatures and pressures for wrapped goods. As reusable devices are making a come back in hospitals, autoclaves are becoming more widely used again.

18.1.5   COLD (CHEMICAL) STERILISATION

Chemical sterilisation is not a very popular method but is nevertheless still in use. Because of the hazardous nature of the solutions used, theatre personnel are unhappy about using them; there is also evidence of carcinogenic problems. As previously mentioned, there is no proof of sterility after chemical sterilisation.

The method requires immersion of an instrument or appliance in the solution for 30 min minimum. Then the items are removed, the excess solution allowed to drain, and the items are ready for immediate use.

Personally I believe this method will be outlawed within the next few years.

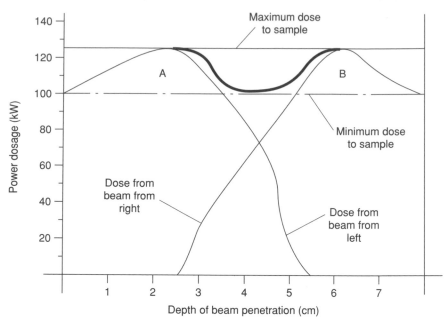

Figure 18.4   Dosage validation.

18.1.6 PACKAGING

Sterilisation is dependent for success on appropriate packaging, and there is no such thing as a universal pack because the packaging needs to be specific to the sterilisation method. Factors to be considered include:

- seal strength,
- permeability,
- physical and mechanical strength,
- heat resistance,
- clarity,
- ease of handling,
- cost, and
- even shelf life.

18.1.7 DOSAGE

The absorbed radiation required for gamma sterilisation varies from country to country, from as low as 1 Mrad to as high as 3.2 Mrad; the UK level is 2.5 Mrad. Because of these variations the designer must allow for the worse and accommodate the higher gamma levels especially because of new legislation introduced in 1996, which lays down requirements for validation, control, labels and levels of radiation for different types of product. Regulations include:

- EN 550: sterilisation of Medical Devices, Validation and Routine Control of Ethylene Oxide Sterilisation.
- EN 552: Validation and Routine Control of Sterilisation by Irradiation.
- EN 554: Validation and Routine Control of Steam Sterilisation.
- EN 556: Requirements for Medical Devices to be Labelled Sterile.

All these standards contain guidance sections to explain the requirements. There is a lot to read before popping a piece of tube into a poly-bag!

18.1.8 NEW METHODS

New technologies using plasma, ozone and chlorine dioxide are being developed as alternatives to the conventional methods already described. These may make a significant mark on the sterilisation market. The product's final performance and cost efficient production are the major factors that dictate the choice of which sterilisation process you select.

19
Standards

This chapter is all about the requirements laid down by various regulatory bodies and member countries in the EEC, and the rules pertaining to other countries and their own particular needs.

To manufacture and supply medical devices for use in any country worldwide there are standards to which you must comply. Design engineers refer to these standards and codes of practice continually because they provide an acceptable set of guidelines. Some standards are 'called up' by legislation and become legally binding, other are not, but still represent good practice. By adopting these regulations governments, ruling bodies and even the end user, enter into an accepted level of interchangability, standardisation and an agreed code of manufacturing.

Standards are influenced by many factors including, unfortunately, vested interests from national and international companies, and also from governments which may operate practices to protect their home markets. To overcome these vested interests, groups have been formed to protect the end users, the clinician and the patient. The International Standards Organisation (ISO) promotes the acceptance of global standards. These usually originate from collaboration between the ISO and member countries' national standards organisations such as the BSI in the UK, ASTM in the USA and DIN in Germany (BSI = British Standards Institution, ASTM = American Society for Testing and Materials, DIN = Deutsches Institut für Normung e.V.). Tables 19.1–3 give a summary of some of the international, European and national organisations.

In Europe there has been much discussion about the Single Market and the resulting removal of trade barriers between member countries. However, barriers remain while national standards exist. A process of harmonisation of national standards and development of European standards is being undertaken, but because of national interests and the need for cumbersome committees, this is proceeding very slowly. The same problems apply, maybe more so, on a global scale, to trade with countries like Australia, USA, India and China. Unless fear and national interests can be overcome, it seems that progress on international standards will continue to be much slower than technological changes, so standards lag behind product developments.

Table 19.1 International standards bodies

Standards making bodies	Certification schemes	Standards used
ISO: International Organization for Standardization, comprises national standards bodies of some 88 countries, promotes international acceptance of particular standards. **IEC**: International Electrotechnical Commission, the electrotechnical arm of the ISO, comprises national standard bodies of 43 countries.	**IECQ**: IEC quality assessment system for electronic components, international equivalent of the CECC. **IECEE**: IEC system for conformity testing to standards of safety of electrical equipment. **CB**: Certification Body, IECEE's certification system, originally developed for use with CEE. Comprises some 29 countries with others applying.	**ISO**: International Standard produced by an ISO technical committee. **IEC**: International standard produced by an IEC technical committee, represents an international consensus of opinion on requirements as accepted by the national committees. Any divergence between IEC recommendations and national rules will be indicated.

Table 19.2 European standards group (EC plus EFTA)

Standards making bodies	Certification schemes	Standards used
CEN: European Committee for Standardization, comprises national standards bodies of EC and other countries. **CENELEC**: Electrotechnical arm of CEN, comprises national standards bodies of many countries. **ETSI**: European Telecommunications Institute, standardisation body in communication policy.	**EMC**: EMC testing and certification coordinating committee under consideration within CENELEC. **LOVAG**: Low Voltage Agreement group for industrial equipment. **CCA**: Certification Agreement for low voltage equipment, components and electrotechnical appliances. **CECC**: 15 country agreement for certification and quality assessment of equipment.	**HD**: Harmonized Document, this is a standard ratified by the CENELEC board. **EN**: European Norm, a standard which automatically becomes the document used by member bodies.

Table 19.3 British standards group

Standards making bodies	Certification schemes	Standards used
BSI: British Standards Institution, national member body of ISO and CEN. **BEC**: British Electrotechnical Committee, national member body of IEC.	**BSI** Safety mark: a product certification scheme for products that conform to BS specifications. **BSI** 'Kitemark': an indicator on a product to show BSI satisfaction and accepted testing to show compliance with British Standards. **BEAB**: British Electrotechnical Approvals Board, UK notified member for participation in CCA and Certification Board schemes.	**HS**: Harmonized Standard, this is a published British Standard which is aligned with a CE Harmonized Document, (HD). **NS**: National Standard, not aligned with a HD, codes of practice, specs., test methods etc. Normalized Standard: a British Standard aligned with a European Norm.

To achieve a mutually beneficial end in Europe a new approach was needed. This started in 1985 with the EEC setting out technical and safety requirements (the Essential Requirements) in the form of directives. These directives are considered to be minimal requirements and member countries of the EEC strive to evolve their own legislation to suit the needs laid down in the directives.

Manufacturers are then free to make products which fulfil market needs as long as they remain within the framework of the directives. Examples of some directives are shown in Table 19.4

In 1993 the Medical Device Directive (MDD) was published. This was a direct development of the new approach described above, and was enthusiastically received by both the medical profession and the manufacturers. It was felt that for the first time the safety, function and application of a device could be determined by professional, caring engineers and doctors, and not by faceless bureaucrats. These directives were regulatory references not fixed rigid limits.

When a standard has been approved it is published and issued as a support section to the relevant directive, in the case of medical devices, the MDD. If there are no objections, the standard is then published in the *Journal of the European Union*. Acceptance and publication ratifies the standard as a Harmonised European Norm (EN). Although EN are not legally binding they are accepted by the industry and customers as a form of conformity

Table 19.4   Examples of EEC directives

MACHINERY: 89/392/EEC, 91/368/EEC.
Implemented in the UK by the Supply of Machinery (Safety) Regulations 1992
(SI 1992/3073), compliance period to 31/12/94.

EMC: 89/336/EEC AS AMENDED BY 92/31/EEC.
Implemented in the UK by the Electromagnetic Compatibility Regulations 1992
(SI 1991/2372), transition period for compliance to 31/12/95.

PRODUCT SAFETY: Under construction 9284/91, compliance period to June 1994.

---

with the essential requirements. If a supplier or manufacturer decides to introduce their own testing method or quality control procedure that differs from the 'recommended' method, this is acceptable if it can be shown that it matches or exceeds the requirements of the directive.

Working in this environment therefore allows a greater amount of flexibility and freedom but also places more responsibility on the manufacturer.

This is a short background to the immense volumes of paperwork put out by the regulatory bodies. My hope is to give you just enough information to allow you to obtain precise details and read up on the legislation specific to your project. Figure 19.1 shows one EC conformity route. These are the rules you must comply with to manufacture medical devices for sale within Europe.

1. The New Council Directive 93/42/EEC leading to the CE mark: manufacturers must be registered and audited by a Notified Body (an External Certification Agency that has been appointed by the Competent Authority which is the MDA in the UK) – see Table 19.5.
2. Manufacturers must affix the CE mark to all products up to 13 June 1998.
3. From 14 June 1998, CE marking and the requirements of the directive will be mandatory with penalties for infringements.
4. Devices must conform to either the requirements set out in Annex 1 of the MDD (the Essential Requirements) or Harmonised European Norms or European pharmacopoeia monographs.
5. The quality system requirements are addressed by the EN 4600 series on Quality Systems for Medical Devices (similar to BS 5750 and ISO 9000). CE marking requirements are:
   (a)   adherence to the essential requirements;
   (b)   audit to EN 4600 series;
   (c)   production of a CE declaration of conformity;
   (d)   technical documentation file;
   (e)   post-production monitoring system; and
   (f)   for class III devices an EC Design Examination.

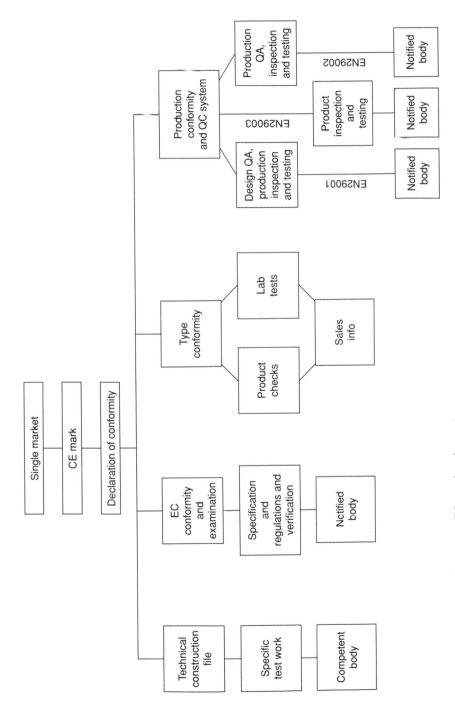

Figure 19.1 Example of one EC conformity route.

Table 19.5 MDA device guidance

Documents
* Guidance Notes for Completion of PCA 1 & PCA 2: 005375.
* Guidance on Biocompatibility Assessment: 005373.
* Guidance Notes for Manufacturers of Dental Appliances: 005379.
* Guidance Notes for Manufacturers of Class I Medical Devices: 005378.
* Guidance Notes for Manufacturers on Clinical Investigations to be Carried Out in the UK: 005374.
* Information for Clinical Investigations: 005376.
* Silicone Implants and Connective Tissue Disease: 005380.
* Framework Document: 005188.
* Business Plan 1994/95: 005187.
* Doing No Harm: 005189.

Bulletins
* Information for Manufacturers: 003992.
* CE Marking: 003993.
* The Vigilance System, Update on Directives: 003994.
* Conformity Assessment Procedure: 003995.
* The Notified Body: 003997.
* The Competent Authority: 003997.
* Information About the EC Medical Device Directive: 003998.
* The Citizen's Charter and Deregulation, A Code for Enforcement: 003999.
* The Classification Rules: 004000.
* Pre-Clinical Assessment Procedures, The Product Registration Scheme: 004005.
* Safe Supply of In Vitro Diagnostic Medical Devices: 005132.
* Standards: 005133.
* The Medical Devices, Electromagnetic Compatibility and Low Voltage Directive: 005856.
* Information About the Packing and Packing Waste Directive: 005857.
* Medical Devices and Medical Products: 005924.

Normally the detailed information can be found by contacting the Notified Body or the Competent Authority. Note that instead of auditing to EN 4600, there are other routes which can be taken such as batch by batch certification, product certification etc, but a full audit will reduce or eliminate the need for these and the information and systems will be in place.

For sales to the USA (potentially 250 000 000 customers) the following rules apply.

1. You must comply with, and audit to, the USA form and the Good Manufacturing Practice (GMP) standard set out by the FDA (US Food and Drugs Administration), before any sales of product.
2. For product market clearance there are two routes. Either the device selected requires a form 510(K) to prove substantial equivalence to a pre-arranged device (i.e. a device currently on the market that is acceptable and safe) to prove safety and effectiveness of the device (there is a short

form entry which should proceed through the regulatory department in 90 days) or a PMA (pre-market approval) for new devices that are proven not substantially equivalent under the 510 (K) route. This is a lengthy 3 year process, which is also expensive.

The following Draft International Standards have been released,

- 95/563336 ISO/DIS 12891-1 'Retrieval and Analysis of Implantable Medical Devices'.
- 95/563133 DC ISO/ 11737-2 'Sterilisation of Medical Devices: Tests of Sterility Performed in the Validation of a Sterilisation Process'.
- EC Packing and Waste Directive (MDA Bulletin 16) due to be enforced by December 1997 will significantly increase costs according to Alexander Watson Associates who are launching a multi-client study on single-use medical packing, sterilisation methods and waste management. The directive requires many types of packing to contain certain percentages of recycled materials and to be manufactured of recyclable materials.

Some standards are subject to constant review and revision, it is beyond the scope of this book to provide examples of individual standards. Consequently the importance of checking the latest revisions of standards and regulations relevant to any work that you do cannot be over emphasised.

20
Specifications

A specification is defined as a detailed description, including the dimensional drawings, qualities of the functional parts, construction, and materials quality, of a manufactured article. This seems straightforward enough, so why do specifications cause so much aggravation and trouble within any manufacturing environment?

The problem with product specifications in the medical device industry is that they serve several different purposes and consequently need to be written with different readers in mind: this is a challenging task for the design engineer whose literary talents may not be their foremost skills. However, forewarned is forearmed and an awareness of the problem goes most of the way to its solution. Product specifications should ideally:

- give the purchaser of the device all the information they need for appropriate use and safe and effective operation,
- inform suppliers exactly what is required of the materials or components they supply, the limits of acceptability, and consequences of failing to meet these requirements,
- define and describe the product as an in-house record of what, how, and why it is produced,
- satisfy the requirements of regulatory bodies.

In principle a designer works to a brief which contains the physical, chemical, electrical and medical requirements of a new product. To achieve or exceed these requirements a number of solutions must be developed from a vast number of suggestions. The final answers are the definitive specifications for the finished product: the materials necessary, the methods of manufacture, the assembly and function of the unit. Ideally this specification should become fixed, unable to be modified unless a proper assessment has been carried out. Then and only then should the specification be changed, so only then could a buyer, production manager or operator deviate from the original.

I may sound somewhat pedantic on this point but unfortunately over the years I have experienced well-intentioned deviations from a specification by people who wished to cut corners, save time, save money, make life easier or misguidedly just thought they were being helpful. The results were catastrophic each time, with the original designer or someone else being given the job of tidying up and trying to salvage as much as possible.

20.1 HOW TO WRITE A SPECIFICATION

Theoretically a specification could be compiled starting with a blank sheet of paper, but in practice there will already be an accumulation of information. A simple example of a specification is a data sheet; such sheets are normally used when purchasing a finished device or article. They lay down the tolerances, materials and performance requirements. Data sheets can vary from a single statement of need, to a volume of cross-referenced information which a supplier must verify and prove prior to supply. Sheets like these should not only be informative but also provide authority, by way of approval or checking signatures, to allow manufacture.

A full specification is a description vastly more informative than a collection of data sheets, it should describe design, operation, construction etc. Table 20.1 lists the information normally associated with a formal specification. (This can be used to indicate the information you require from a supplier of components.)

When describing the operation of a piece of equipment or assembly, for use in a specification, a number of points should be included as follows.

- There should be a list of what information is contained and where. This is particularly important if the document is large or is intended for more than one department.
- Details of priorities need to be included to ensure no conflict of interests.

Table 20.1 Basic information to be included in a product specification

---

1. Operation of device.
2. Design parameters.
3. Development.
4. Limits and areas of supply.
5. QA testing requirements, prior, during and after supply.
6. Packaging.
7. Delivery methods and timescales.
8. Delivery and performance penalties.
9. Payment methods, stages, targets.
10. Commissioning (equipment, capital plant).
11. Explanations of drawings and individual functions.
12. Standards, regulations which apply. Either straight text or the reference numbers.
13. Information transfer agreements.
14. Confidentiality agreements.
15. Detailed inventory of all documentation applicable.
16. Liability acceptance, in part/whole and by whom.
17. Individual, departmental and company responsibilities.

- A statement of consequences regarding any deviation from the specification is necessary.
- There should be formal notification that any changes or departures from the written specification must be documented, submitted and await reply. Any subsequent changes can only be accepted and implemented after a new specification has been numbered and issued.
- Also include a health and safety statement specifying who is responsible for whom and at what level.

For the information on design there should be two separate sections. The first section sets out previous work done, the results and aspirations. The second section describes the level to which a supplier can change or modify the product or his component parts. The supplier may wish to introduce something into the contract to protect their own designs.

The other points in Table 20.1 are either self-explanatory or do not need explaining, except for three points which, depending upon your job description, can be minor or crucial. These are assumptions, omissions and vagueness. When a specification is written sometimes the author assumes that a contractor has a high level of knowledge in that one area and so does not state the obvious. For example, specifying a builders plumb line implies two components: the plumb bob and the cord. In medical device specifications there should be no implied information – everything must be overtly stated and there should be no possibility of ambiguity. This is difficult to write when you are deeply involved with the product. You need to develop the skill of editing and reading your work from the viewpoint of an objective outsider. Ask all the naive questions you can think of, and check that the answers are there in the specification.

If possible (and this is something which the commercial departments get involved with) try to ensure some form of penalty clause into the specification. This will probably never be needed but it can ensure excellent service from suppliers and lets them know you are serious in your business dealings. Also it reinforces the importance of the products you supply as a medical device manufacturer to the clinical profession.

20.2 THE USE OF SPECIFICATIONS BY THE MANUFACTURER

Use of product specifications *within* the manufacturing company presents a whole new set of problems and additional requirements. These problems arise from the following:

- information needed for purchasing components, i.e. procurement,
- material specifications,
- production assembly requirements and sequences,
- quality control,

- internal production targets, and
- marketing timescales for new product launch(es).

Specifications must be adhered to and the person, department or group responsible should have the authority to enforce this compliance, sanctions can include production stoppage, financial penalties, bonus stoppage, etc.

20.3 SPECIFICATION CHANGES

Any changes should be introduced via a specification change request, checked and if correct agreed (and signed for) by members of internal, interested, interlinked departments. These are:

- design,
- marketing/sales,
- production,
- QA.

Until all departments agree the change should not be implemented.

On implementation, certain procedures need to be in place and be followed. Drawings, details or other information should be dated and the issue numbers applied. The record of why the change was introduced should be retained and the cancelled issue also retained for later reference.

A formal issue list should be maintained and those requiring copies of the revised specification must sign for and return old issues to the specifications department.

A list of all specification changes should be circulated regularly to confirm, inform and allow cross-checking. You may think this is appropriate only for large companies but believe me even small firms can get into terrible trouble because of lax record keeping.

Master copies of all specifications should be held by the QA department and copies issued recorded and dealt with by that department's personnel only.

Previous copies should be returned to QA for disposal.

All new copies issued should be stamped with the relevant date. Drawings should be named or coded in a central register with one person allocated responsible for its upkeep.

All drawings should include material details, dimensions and construction method. Drawings should be marked with the company's name and the draftsman's initials; they should be checked and initialled before transfer to the specification department where they should be finally signed off before issue. This final signing off should be from a senior level, QA manager or equivalent.

Once the immutability of specifications is accepted at all levels, then risks are minimised.

This is a very short chapter, with a very short message, but it is probably the most important in the book.

21
Packaging

Packaging is often left as an afterthought to a project, but for a good outcome packaging must be considered from the very beginning. It is necessary to integrate packaging into the design concept, so that the effects of the product on the packaging and the effects of the packaging on the product can be properly evaluated.

As well as needing to have something to contain the product, there are other requirements: EEC directives, labelling and marking, health and safety, sterilisation options and environmental considerations.

Packaging has many functions including the following:

- cosmetic appeal and sales value,
- means of handling during manufacture, transport and by the customer,
- protection from contamination during production,
- protection from physical damage in handling,
- protection during storage and sterilisation,
- maintenance of sterility, and
- identification at all stages of product life.

Figure 21.1 illustrates some of the above points.

Packaging methods are many and various. Consider some of the options:

- peel pouches,
- 'poly' bags,
- blister packs,
- vacuum packs,
- 'clamshells',
- vacuum-formed trays,
- heat-sealed containers,
- cardboard boxes.

The choice is vast, so you need to weigh up the pros and cons of each, as you do when selecting any option. But never forget that the packaging is the first point of contact with the user.

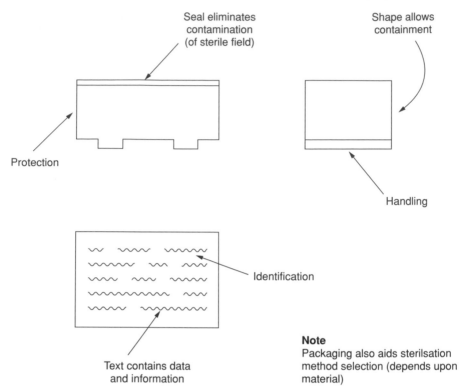

Figure 21.1 Packaging requirements.

21.1 STERILISATION

Sterilisation processes affect the product in question and also the material of the packaging. There are different packaging requirements for different sterilisation processes.

21.1 ETHYLENE OXIDE (ETO)

For ETO sterilisation the following packaging needs apply.

- The packaging must seal easily and form a cavity or channel for the ETO vapour to flow through.
- The package must be permeable to ETO vapour, air and moisture, which need to pass both in and out.
- Temperature tolerance up to 70°C is necessary, without any damage or degradation.
- The package must maintain seal at pressure and under vaccum during sterilisation.

- There should be no softening with vapour or liquid contamination.
- The packaging material must be resistant to the corrosive effects of ETO gas.
- Adhesives should be undamaged by sterilisation. Peel-packs must still peel after ETO treatment and storage.
- The pack must withstand the pressure–evacuation–repressure stresses of the sterilisation cycle.
- Materials must maintain their shape.
- Packaging should be appropriate to the timescale involved. A ten day validation time is necessary, but the time in the sterilisation phase may be up to three weeks if dual treatment is needed.

21.1.2 GAMMA

For gamma sterilisation packaging requirements are as follows.

- Radiation can cause accelerated ageing of material, which can be detrimental.
- Most materials undergo a colour shift; the degree of change determines acceptability.
- Many materials also experience changes in physical properties. Some materials become brittle and others distort. Suitable choice of material and design can minimise or allow for these changes.
- Plastic odour can be influenced by gamma radiation. If the package is porous, odour can disperse.
- Seals must accommodate changes in materials and adhesives.
- Packaging should resist the localised heating that may occur.

21.1.3 STEAM

For steam sterilisation the following apply.

- With steam sterilisation products are usually processed unwrapped.
- Any packaging or labels must be resistant to the heat and pressure conditions.
- The product and any packaging must tolerate the thermal cycling that occurs: ambient to 130°C.
- The pressure cycle varies from 30 p.s.i. wet to 45 p.s.i. vacuum.
- Porosity is vital. Steam must be able to penetrate and exit.

21.2 PHYSICAL PROPERTIES

With all packing, whether in the medical device market or not, there are requirements for degrees of rigidity and support for the product. The packaging material suppliers offer flexible, rigid and semi-rigid options.

21.2.1   FLEXIBLE PACKAGING

Flexible packaging for medical devices often consists of paper–film peel pouches. These cater for hospital applications which are sterilised on site. They have little cosmetic or visual appeal but are acceptably functional. The main reason for the selection of peel pouches is the ease of sealing and overall cost.

When original equipment manufacturers use pouches the normal plain paper and film materials are enhanced by the following methods.

- Surface treatment: where particular attention is taken when preparing the base paper and seals are formed with minimal fibre tear.
- Adding adhesives to polypropylene-based coatings on paper: these have become a normal pouch medium, though there is a tendency for permeability to be compromised by such coatings when coupled with the main flexible packaging.
- Triple layered or laminated sheets: these use a tough core material like nylon which reduces both tearing and splitting of the seal and covers.
- Reinforced paper: this combines paper with latex to improve strength, stability of dimensions and moisture resistance. It also increases the peelability of the pouch seals.
- Co-extrusions of different materials: combined copolymers and polypropylene to modify seals and peel characteristics.

Tyvek® is a trade name (Du Pont) for a bonded, non-woven paper made from synthetic polymer fibres like polyethylene. It was developed to meet the growing demand for a multi-purpose material suitable for all types of sterilisation. Tyvek is often used as one side of a pouch, giving strength and stability to the paper back. Alternatively the Tyvek can be used on both sides creating a virtually tear-free protective pouch, with overlapping chevrons to aid opening. Tyvek is also used for lids on semi-rigid assemblies. It is probably the best option for peelable lids but is comparatively expensive. The use of Tyvek has increased by about 8% per year over the last three years, which shows that purchasers recognise a need for tougher and better-sealed lids and will pay more for these features.

If costs are critical, particularly with disposables, or volumes are low then plain seals provided by paper lidding may well be the cost effective alternative. Paper can still provide an effective seal and peel strength with a suitable adhesive and can be reinforced if necessary. At normal speed the sealing equipment causes heating of the paper of at least 10°C. Figure 21.2 shows the peel method in which the adhesive is engineered to ensure that the seal splits and not the paper.

21.2.2   RIGID PACKAGING

Rigid packaging is solid, stiff and relatively expensive. It is used for prestigious presentation of costly or fragile items, and to enhance the value of a product through the customers' perception of quality.

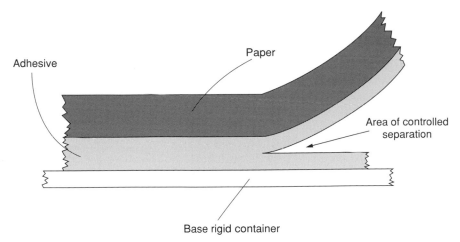

Adhesive

Paper

Area of controlled
separation

Base rigid container

Figure 21.2 Peel construction.

The cost of rigid packaging is high because of the amount of material used, the processing required, and the need for material stocks and storage.

Polystyrene containers padded with foam are used for economical packaging of fragile items. At the other end of the range, custom-made boxes moulded or fabricated from aluminium may cost as much as the product they contain.

21.2.3 SEMI-RIGID PACKAGING

This term describes duplex packaging with a relatively rigid container and a flexible lid or closure. It includes blister trays, shells, thermo-formed trays to fit dedicated profiles, clam shells and vacuum formed containers, all either sealed by paper or Tyvek sheets or placed and sealed in pouches. Two advantages are the ability to hold products securely and safely in place preventing damage and the ease of actual packing during manufacture. An additional advantage, which is somewhat difficult to quantify, is the quality of presentation that this type of packaging creates.

The materials for the 'lids' which close and seal the finished units tend to be the same and are explained in more detail later on in the text. The material for the rigid component varies greatly, generally determined by cost, clarity and size plus what type of sterilisation is to be used on the product.

The most commonly used material for formed trays and autoclavable packaging is polycarbonate. It provides a combination of features which make it the best suited for steam sterilisation, being crystal clear, tough, dimensionally stable during steam cycles, available in various thicknesses and easily thermoformed by either vacuum techniques or pressure forming. Although comparatively costly, polycarbonate does present a 'premium' product.

Polypropylene is used extensively for film and laminates with either foil or higher temperature grade thermoplastics, to allow autoclave use.

Polypropylene and poly(ethylene terephthalate) laminates are used in pouches for hospitals but are not suitable for dry heat treatment. Modified versions of high density polyethylene (HDPE) with rubber additives are used in controlled autoclave applications. Ultra high density polyethylene can be used without such toughening.

Crystallizable polyester (CPET) is thermally stable up to 240°C, and is well suited to gamma sterilisation. Crystallization is attained during the thermoforming stage using sheets in the amorphous state. (CPET is used for ovenproof and microwaveable food dishes.)

Poly(methyl pentane) (TPX) is another good heat resistant material with extremely low density and very good clarity, it also exhibits excellent chemical resistance and moisture resistance.

Polysulphone is a high profile material excellent for all types of sterilisation. It can be blown and added to other polymers as a film to form composite polymer laminates.

Poly(vinyl chloride), PVC, is a common tray material for disposable products, but there is a colour change during gamma sterilisation treatment.

Table 21.1 lists materials used in packaging films along with advantages and disadvantages.

For many applications medical packaging now uses laminates of different materials to provide features that would not otherwise be available. The growth in the use of such composite materials indicates that the customer is prepared to pay a premium for an enhanced product.

21.3 DISPOSABLES

During the last 30 years there has been rapid growth in the market for single-use or disposable medical goods. Consequently there has been an associated change in the consumption of packaging. In 1993, 20 000 tonnes of plastics was used for packaging disposables, a 50% increase over the previous five years.

Now the growth in medical disposables is under pressure from environmentalists, waste reduction and recycling requirements, European Directives and world standards, and available resource and raw material costs.

Environmental issues arise from the problems of waste disposal and the energy cost of manufacture and distribution. The consumption and refining of raw materials, both for the product and the packaging, causes concern. Solutions to these problems need to be found soon: the most promising approach to resolving the issues is the development of sophisticated methods of environmental audit, comparing the total life cycles of disposable and reusable products. A shift in economic systems would be required if the purchaser were to pay the true costs.

Problems arise from conflicts between the EC Medical Device Directive and EC environmental legislation. Article 30 of the European Treaty Market Law Review states that each country is free to fix its own Environmental

Table 21.1 Film materials

Material	Advantages	Disadvantages
Cellophane	Transparent	Cost
	Stiffness (dependant on thickness)	Sensitive to moisture Dimensionally unstable
Nylon	Tough	Cost
	Stable under temperature Impermeable	Permeable to H_2O
Polyester	Good surface finish	High cost
	Transparent	Difficult to form
Polyethylene	Variable sealing	Bad appearance
	Cheap	Difficult to print on
Polypropylene	Cheap	Static charge
	Very clear	Easily torn
	Good H_2O barrier	Poor gas barrier
Polystyrene	Clarity	Brittle
	Cheap	Easily marked
	Easily processed	
Poly(vinyl chloride)	Transparent	Colour shift under gamma sterilisation
	Cheap	Leachables
	Tough	

Protection Level but there is only a free market if environmental protection measures are applied universally.

There is political and social pressure to move towards recycling. Two scenarios can be envisaged: a total recycling system with nothing discarded, or a system which accepts a percentage of material lost and some recycled. My own view is that at present manufacturers cannot voluntarily move to recycling because additional costs would make their products uncompetitive. It may be that national or European legislation is brought in to require some recycling. It is to be hoped that this will be implemented throughout the European Community on the same date. If this seems likely, then you should ensure that your company has a say in the formulation of both the requirements and the introduction date. Manufacturers and environmental organisations should have objective discussions to decide recycling targets and methods of enforcement. If such measures are to apply universally, manufacturers should not have problems of vested interests.

Disposal can be integrated into the design of new products by the manufacturers specifying how a finished item is to be destroyed, depending on the materials involved. Biodegradable materials can be safely disposed of in landfill sites. If incineration is necessary, then it is safest to use materials with low burning temperatures and no toxic by-products. If it is intended to recycle used products, then collection systems need to be in place, and a destination for the materials arranged. If returning used products to the manufacturer, they need to be able to process the resulting mixed raw material.

The battery business has been forced into taking back spent batteries in some territories, but as there was little consultation the system does not yet have good administration or work well. On the other hand, the oil industry has very efficient waste oil cleaning and recycling systems operating, which evolved commercially because money is made and everyone can see and acknowledge the benefits.

European and International Standards are slowly producing coherent approaches to medical devices, especially for bacteriological barriers. Paper, plastic or rigid containers for transporting a safe sterile product can now pass recognised tests which are accepted over different borders.

Each country has its own version of good manufacturing practice but unfortunately not all agree priorities, and there are still some which operate protective policies which delay or prevent beneficial products from being sold in their territory. It has been alleged that FDA approval discriminates against imports, but this is specifically excluded by recent undertakings about processing all applications within fixed time limits.

Recent standards have emphasised environmentally sound processes, methods of manufacture and the elimination of harmful solvents from packaging. The advent of laminated plastic sheets has aided this but there are still further changes coming. These changes will affect not the end result, which is a sealed package, but the cost of manufacture.

Paper manufacture has had to change in response to requirements to reduce the use of bleaches of chlorinated compounds. Over the last 20 years the chlorine and sulphur contents of paper have been reduced by 30%, but they are still necessary to provide the strength and pure white appearance demanded by the user. Further reductions are anticipated.

There are no internationally accepted protocols for sterilisation, so validation has to be by practical methods and any changes to packaging materials would have to be assessed similarly. As some sterile products are stored long-term, checks of packaging integrity would have to be carried out at intervals of one, three and five years. This is a significant impediment to the evolution of new packagings.

The development of reinforced or laminated papers instead of plastic films is contributing to the reduction in harmful chemicals and evolution of more sound products. There is controversy regarding whether to use fibre papers uncoated or adhesive laminated reinforced papers. Three areas of current investigation are as follows.

- Eliminate toxic solvents from adhesives and use water-based emulsions.
- Reformulate hot-melt adhesives to modify dwell time and material compatibility, as well as making them more amenable to recycling.
- Elimination of toxic components from printing inks and development of new printing technologies.

22
Communication in Design

The function of communication, in whatever medium, is to transfer ideas and information from one person to others. A dictionary definition of communication is the imparting of facts.

In industry effective communication is critical, since the wrong instruction or wrong inference could result in millions of pounds wasted or lost. Over the years thousands of pages in hundreds of books have been written about communication, with little agreement except that the subject is complex. Fortunately, though, it is recognised that there are communication skills which can be learnt.

I shall not attempt here to instruct you in information transfer, but I hope to provide examples of what can go wrong and how these problems can be corrected.

We all spend much of our lives communicating, at work, at home and at play. Without care, means of communication which are effective in one setting may spill over into another where they are inappropriate.

Communication occurs in the context of the relationship between the parties, and the relationship can help or can hinder the effective transfer of information, the depth of understanding and the time taken. Between unusually close partners – Holmes and Watson, Jeeves and Wooster, life-long couples – unspoken communication and understanding may exist. But for workaday communication we rely on the spoken or written word, graphics and body language.

22.1 VERBAL COMMUNICATION

The problem with dialogue is how little information is actually given during conversation. Everyone knows how many times we need to repeat and check the information given, and how the important aspects must be reinforced again and again.

Whatever the faults of dialogue, it must be noted that the process involves cooperation between individuals, leading to understanding and consequent action. It could be argued that much information for daily living would be more effectively transferred by other means, but dialogue involves people in getting to know each other so that spoken communications improve in efficiency.

Of course, not all ideas are best conveyed in words, and dialogue gives the opportunity of including gesture and demonstration: try describing a spiral staircase, or how to tie a knot, in words alone. This illustrates that information is varied and thought should be given to the best method of communication before you begin.

The prime requirement of verbal communication is not speaking but effective listening. Misunderstandings more often result from failures of reception than transmission. Talking at cross-purposes is another common fault that you should guard against. Ambiguity can arise from a wrong choice of words, or using words with more than one meaning, as well as proceeding with unconfirmed assumptions. Closed questions, those that imply an answer or only admit 'yes' or 'no' replies, are much less useful for information collection than open questions, which give the respondent much more scope.

So, in dialogue:

- think first,
- define what you want to say or know,
- stick to one idea at a time,
- select unambiguous words,
- take care with phrasing, and
- confirm that you have correctly received or sent your message.

It is best not to assume what the other person thinks or feels. Use open questions to learn more, and closed questions to confirm what you have inferred.

I am assuming here that honest communication is the goal, but of course some people deliberately manipulate words to gain advantage. In theory, lying is not communication because the intention is deception rather than the transfer of information. Be aware though, that conveying partial information can mislead, whether intentionally or accidentally. In your design work it is important that everything relevant is overtly stated, or something that is so obvious to you that you don't mention it, could lead to a misunderstanding with someone else who sees things from a different point of view.

In speech be conscious of homophones, words with different meanings that sound the same, e.g. to, too and two. The converse are words with the same spelling that have different meanings. We discriminate by the context, e.g. 'in five minutes' and 'a minute particle'.

It is safest to assume some inefficiency in dialogue and to reiterate important points as well as seeking confirmation. This enables you to take a step-by-step approach, checking that one idea is established before proceeding to the next point of your argument, and importantly it helps all concerned to remember what has been said.

In speech more than in writing, you need to have some common ground with the participants. People with too little similarity of background, knowledge and opinion will not be able to communicate effectively. It is vital, too, that you address the right audience. Always ask yourself if you are speaking to the most appropriate person or people, and then you shouldn't need to wonder how to make them understand you.

Feedback to a talk, presentation or conversation is essential. Your colleagues need to know how you value their contribution if they are to be motivated team workers. Similarly you need to solicit questions after a presentation to check that you have got your message across.

22.2 BODY LANGUAGE

Regardless of the expertise of the speaker, the content of the talk or the receptiveness of the audience, if the body language is wrong the whole process is pointless. The way a person stands, how close they are, gestures and movements, as well as facial expression, all affect how the actual words spoken are understood. In addition tone of voice, stress and inflexion, pauses and volume, combine to modify the message.

An important aspect of body language is interpersonal distance. Everyone has their own personal space in which they feel safe. This volume changes depending on two factors: the topic being discussed and the relationship between the participants. If this space is invaded then all communication ceases. There are differences between people and cultures: Europeans tend to defend their immediate areas, but middle eastern people tend to allow closer association. Table 22.1 shows the distances we tend to accept in the UK and northern Europe. This is simplistic, of course, but you could try mixing the distances and settings to see the sparks fly!

Finally, eye contact is an essential contributor to dialogue. In conversation the listener usually watches the speaker. When the speaker pauses and breaks the eye contact, it is time to swop roles. If the listener wants to prompt the change over, they will look away. If you keep talking to someone who is not watching you, you have probably lost their attention. Holding a gaze for too long is normally seen as challenging behaviour.

Table 22.1 Working contact distances

Distance (m)	Comments
2–3	Desk distance, area for normal business working. Allows a formal approach without being offensive.
1–2	Either a more informal working environment between people, or a large casual social gathering.
0.5–1	Personal discussions and involvement. Close talk of a private nature.

In remote verbal communication, as by telephone, the eye contact and body language are absent, and the words and cues used will be modified. People who have strong verbal skills may be more effective communicators when they can concentrate only on speaking and listening, and they will have a good telephone manner. Those who need additional information from gesture, body language and eye contact will be less comfortable on the 'phone.

22.3   GRAPHICAL COMMUNICATION

'A picture paints a thousand words', they say, and for some purposes visual images can communicate more effectively than written or spoken words. Since the dawn of man we have used visual means to communicate with each other.

In a technical context, visual aids, drawings, charts and pictures are often used to convey information about data and spatial forms. Charts of many kinds are used for data, and you need to think about your goal when deciding which to use: does the user need to know the general shape of a curve or the actual coordinates? Visual media include the following:

- bar charts,
- line graphs,
- pie charts,
- flow charts,
- maps,
- drawings, and
- photographs.

Tables of data are also used to give information that could not be presented effectively in words.

In design, it is often necessary to convey 3D information in a 2D form and technical drawings are readily interpreted by the initiated, but people from other disciplines need a sketch, artist's impression or model to understand design concepts.

22.4   WRITTEN COMMUNICATION

Whether you use e-mail or pen and paper, messages, memos, information and instructions all have to be written down, and the way you write will determine how well the information is transferred.

It is suggested that information technology will lead to the end of literacy, but new media actually put additional demands on writing skills, because they add to the range of settings for which we need to learn appropriate writing techniques. It is true that IT gives more scope for communication in graphical ways: drawings, pictures, photographs, maps, animation, video, 3-D simulations etc. It is also true that IT can assist people with literacy problems to communicate, e.g. technology can help people with dyslexia to be integrated in society, rather than excluded, and they often have extraordinary abilities with spatial awareness, 3-D thinking and other design skills.

In the commercial setting, sending memos and instructions by e-mail or fax (rather than by 'phone or conversation) requires the writer to take much more care to communicate clearly and fully because feedback and confirmation are not immediately elicited.

In industry report writing is a particular way of recording work done and informing others of work required. Reports can also set objectives, and communicate from one to many people. The biggest problem most people say they have with reports, is finding time to write and read them. Time is one thing money can't buy, but it can be saved, and you should cultivate the skill of writing short and succinct reports in which every word counts. Table 22.2 shows some differences between an industrial report and an intellectual essay: the former is required urgently and the latter may be written at leisure.

The response to written communications is often coloured by the reader's assumptions about the writer: what does the reader know or think about the writer, are they acquainted, what was their last contact? If the author is unknown to the reader, such as the author of a book or academic paper, a photo and brief resume may be supplied to give the reader a mind-set to start with.

Readers look for hidden meanings, whether intended or not. If a report is critical or threatening to the reader, great care must be taken to convey positive messages. When writing, try to put yourself in the place of the reader as their perspective may be very different from yours.

When a report writing yourself, have these objectives.

- Clarity: use straightforward sentences with short bursts of information.
- Accuracy: be specific, do not leave anything out or open to speculation.
- Simplicity: never assume the reader has your level of knowledge, explain if necessary to ensure no confusion.
- Effectiveness: what is the core of your message? Put this at the beginning and again at the end.
- Structure: work out a rational structure and stick to it without digression.

To assist you, consider the following headings.

- Summary: short appraisal of the work done.
- Introduction: explain structure of the report and why it was written.
- Information: background, prior knowledge required, other documents referred to.
- Methods: how the work was carried out.
- Findings: the results or outcome.
- Discussion: elaborate and explain.
- Conclusion: recommendations if applicable.

Table 22.3 lists report requirements; these will not apply to all reports but are an aide memoir.

Table 22.2 Comparison of style requirements

Business report	Academic essay
Limited specific audience	Large readership (potentially)
Action request or instigator	No set goal or requirement
Style secondary	Style is critical
Specific facts, details	Overall generalisations
Timescale tight, probably requiring actions immediately in response	Open-ended timescale allowing editing and re-writes
Tone not important	Tone highly valued

Commercial security of reports should be clearly understood. Who is responsible for confidentiality: the writer, the recipient or the secretary? Four categories are widely used.

1. No restriction: such a report comprises simple instructions or information that is not sensitive and may be read by anyone.
2. Commercially restricted: these reports are circulated to a defined list of people, either internally or externally. The main reason for the restriction is to limit the information to those who need to know. Normally verbal permission from the author is enough to allow handing on to extra recipients.
3. Commercially confidential: normally this means limited internal circulation to named people, with the distribution recorded and signed for. Written permission would be required to pass on details contained within the report.
4. Commercially secret: these reports are severely restricted, copies are only issued to named people who should confirm receipt and safe-keeping. Normally copies are returned to the author once read.

Sometimes reports are too long and detailed for easy understanding. The author may be asked to prepare a summary (or a report may be given to

Table 22.3 Report writing requirements

1. Clarify the objective.
   What are you attempting to do?
2. Try to know your potential readers.
   Think about their requirements.
   Find out the circumstances in which the report will be read.
3. Collect your material.
   Check the accuracy and validity of your information.
4. Arrange the material correctly.
   Give the report a logical structure.
5. Write the report as it flows, quick and easy. The report should read like a book, informative and with a conclusion. Decide on the style and use illustrations, facts, analysis, conclusions and recommendations.
6. Edit and polish.
7. Use a check list for final review

you with the request that you simplify it and prepare a summary for a meeting). Table 22.4 gives an easy six step procedure to follow for writing report summaries.

The style of a report also affects how it is received and understood. The art of good communication is how you present the report: layout, content, structure and development all contribute to a successful transfer of information. Table 22.5 lists points regarding facts, presentation and style to enhance your report. Table 22.6 gives examples of how to improve writing style. Table 22.7 lists a number of points as a checklist to ensure a good outcome.

Table 22.4 Writing report summaries

---

1. Read the report fully first and obtain a good understanding: read it again if necessary.
2. Mark or underscore salient points and pointers.
3. Make notes. Use them to write the summary but use your own words and not just a repetition or copy of the original work.
4. Write a draft from the notes, do not use the original.
5. Read the draft, edit it, check the length, check if it does represent the original.
6. Have you completed the summary as required? Check the brief.

Table 22.5 Potential errors of fact, presentation and style

Facts
Do not make
- Misstatements, exaggerations, misinterpretation or omission of facts
- Notes which distinguish between fact and opinion
- Contradictions and inconsistencies
- Conclusions that are unwarranted by the evidence
- Vague descriptions where accurate figures could be used

Presentation
Beware of
- Items left out which are important to the train of thought
- Addition of information in the wrong section or paragraph
- The inclusion of irrelevant or tedious details
- Long and complicated paragraphs
- Failure to distinguish between new information and what is already known.

Style
Things best avoided
- Long sentences (more say, than 18–20 words or two or three typewritten lines) and complicated grammar
- Lack of clarity. Sentences that require re-reading before their meaning can be grasped
- Statements that suggest an unintended relationship
- Wordiness and padding, failure to come to the point
- Needlessly technical language and sentences overloaded with unfamiliar words (to the reader)
- Clichés: use simple words and statements

Table 22.6 Avoiding wordiness

Overstatements	Better style
. . . in establishments of a workshop rather than factory character . . .	. . . in a workshop rather than a factory . . .
. . . an increased appetite was manifested by all the rats . . .	. . . all the rats had an increased appetite . . .
. . . How we speak depends on what speech communities we are actually operating in at the time . . .	. . . how we speak depends on where we are . . .
. . . it consists essentially of two parts . . .	. . . there are two parts . . .
. . . we are in the process of making . . .	. . . we are making . . .
. . . at the present moment in time . . .	. . . now . . .
. . . degree courses are in the process of development . . .	. . . degree courses are being developed . . .
. . . experiments are in progress to assess the possibility of using . . .	. . . experiments are being used to assess . . .
. . . it was observed in the course of the demonstration that . . .	. . . it was noted during the demonstration . . .
. . . there is really somewhat of an obligation upon us . . .	. . . we are obliged . . .
. . . the committee was obviously cognisant of the problem . . .	. . . the committee was aware of the problem . . .
. . . an account of the methods used and the results obtained has been given by . . .	. . . a record of the methods used and results obtained was given . . .

22.7 Guidelines for success of a technical report

Do's	Don'ts
Summarise	Assume prior knowledge
Structure the report	Talk down
Match readability to the readership	Assume agreement
Obtain knowledge of readers	Assume the outcome
Justify	Assume understanding from the reader
List comparisons (open options)	Assume acceptance of your conclusions
Make conclusions or recommendations	
Be truthful	
Provide a feedback loop for discussion	
Try to make the report look like a management idea	
Allow time for the reader to consider the information provided	

23
Product Liability

In July 1985 the EC Directive on product liability (85/374/EEC) was adopted by the European Community, with the effect that legislation regarding manufacturers liability for defective goods was to be introduced. These laws would enable member states to work to a standardised level of actions, goods would have access to the open market and manufacturers would be answerable to the legal systems of all member states. This was the intention, but a decade later these goals have still not been reached.

It was considered essential that the laws of all the member states be harmonised regarding product liability so that manufacturers in different countries did not have a competitive advantage, or disadvantage, over others. But standardisation of national laws has still not been achieved, and it is now accepted that this is not possible. The UK, along with Germany, Denmark, Ireland, Italy and The Netherlands, has argued that manufacturers should be allowed the defence of 'development' risk. This has been proposed mainly for the reason that otherwise innovative work could not occur and product development would stagnate. Consumer organisations opposed this, arguing that the development defence would significantly weaken public protection. When the EEC put forward the original Directive, they stated that 'All consumers should have the same protection as that enjoyed by the direct purchaser. The manufacturer reaps benefit if the product is a success and so he should also accept losses if the product fails and injures people. Strict liability would encourage higher safety standards, with the manufacturer in the best position to arrange insurance cover.' This was the trend in Europe at the time, as member countries moved towards stricter controls.

This philosophy was aimed at products from all industries. In the area of medical devices it has a special significance, since the majority of such products are either life threatening or detrimental to the patient if a fault occurs. The development defence highlights the dilemma that medical device products cannot be sold until clinical trials are completed, and clinical trials can't be undertaken until safety has been established, but how do you establish safety before a clinical trial?

23.1   THE EC PRODUCT LIABILITY DIRECTIVE

The Directive has 22 sections called 'articles'; I wish here to discuss four of the most important ones.

23.1.1   ARTICLE 3

The definition of producer is very wide and includes manufacturers of finished goods, producer of raw materials or component parts used in products, importers, distributors and anyone who puts their name or trademark on the product. The medical profession gets a separate mention in this article as requiring particular consideration because they are the 'last link between the medical device or medicine supply and the patient'. The mention is because doctors and health care personnel may be liable under this particular article when a manufacturer of a defective product cannot be identified. In the UK, and for NHS staff, the supplier is considered to be the relevant health authority and not a particular person. Fund holding GPs and dental practitioners are not NHS employees but are self-employed and under contract, so they should ensure full traceability of product supply to cover themselves.

It should be pointed out that the clinical judgement used to select and use one particular medical device over another will not create a situation of liability on the part of the medical practitioner should damage be caused by that product, device or drug.

23.1.2   ARTICLE 6

A product is defective when it does not provide the safety that a person is entitled to expect, taking all circumstances into consideration including presentation, instructions, labelling (new legislation introduced in 1996), and the use to which it could reasonably be put at the time the device was distributed. A product should not be considered unsafe simply because a safer product is subsequently developed. A good example is safety devices introduced into the latest model of a car: models from previous years are not considered unsafe to drive.

Medical products raise particular problems in respect of reactions to invasive and implantable devices. Establishing a defect in a device or medicine already administered to a patient is highly complex for many reasons, including the body's defence mechanisms and the pathological condition of the patient. The more benefit the patient derives from the treatment, the more likely it is that there may be an adverse effect. The directive expects a greater degree of safety corresponding to the complexity of the device.

The Directive states that 'an inferior quality product is not considered "defective" for the purposes of the Directive, unless it actually introduces a risk of injury'. The risk of injury can be estimated by the technique called FMEA, which is described in detail in Chapter 25. FMEA should be carried out as early as possible in product development, and revised at several stages. There is also a new European Standard on Risk Assessment of Medical Devices which has been drafted and is being circulated for comment prior to implementation. The resulting legislation will be mandatory and the draft standard is discussed in detail later in this chapter.

23.1.3 ARTICLE 7

Article 7 provides six exemptions from liability for the manufacturer.

1. 'The manufacturer will not be liable if he proves that he did not put the product into circulation.' This is understood to mean when a product is delivered to a second person in the course of business or when it has been incorporated into an immovable (this definition is explained in better detail in Article 2). Medical materials and devices used in trials before marketing will therefore generally be exempt under this provision, but beware because of the conflicting clause in Article 6: 'provide a product fit for use'.

2. 'The manufacturer or producer will not be liable if he proves that the defect which caused the damage did not exist when the product was placed in circulation.' This refers to the shelf-life of products, damage or modification by a final supplier or distributor, or where labels or instructions for use are defaced or removed by a distributor.

3. 'The producer also has a defence if he can show that he did not manufacture the product for an economic purpose, nor distribute it in the course of business.' This applies to private transactions and supply.

4. 'The producer will not be liable if he can prove that the defect is due to the compliance of the product with mandatory regulations issued by national public authorities.' However, compliance with a regulation will not necessarily discharge a manufacturer from liability, it must be shown that the defect was the inevitable result of compliance with that regulation. For example, that it was impossible for the product to be manufactured to the regulations without the finished product being defective. 'Mandatory regulations' means those imposed by the law, not contractual obligations. For example, beer brewed in Germany must comply with purity laws regardless of contracts between companies.

5. The Development Risk Defence (as described earlier) is to allow the evolution of new and innovative products, as well as the development of existing products.

6. 'A manufacturer of a component will not be held liable if it is proven that the defect is attributable to the design of the product into which the component is fitted or to the instructions given by the manufacturer

of the finished product.' If you are following instructions, drawings or specifications from the final assembler or distributor, then the responsibility and liability is theirs.

Here is a timely reminder from Article 3: if you sell, pack or assemble a product with your name on, then you are liable, not the manufacturer. If you manufacture a device, but a second or third party places their name or logo on it, the liability is then theirs.

23.1.4 ARTICLE 17

'The Directive shall not apply to products put into circulation before the implementing legislation comes into force.' This means that the Directive will not be retrospective.

These Articles show the extent and viability of the Directive, even though it is not yet fully implemented in all member states, it is on the statute books and the framework is there for all to work within. As existing and potential designers you need to be aware of the law.

The Directive is phrased in such a way so that it is not possible to contract out of liability. There is no maximum liability set (although to discourage trivial claims individual items worth less than 500 ECU are excluded) and a defendant has a right to place a claim on co-producers or others 'with responsibility'. This could be the manufacturer, the head company of a group, individuals concerned with the production or the designer.

It should also be noted that, apart from this Directive, there is a growing trend now for 'no win, no fee' contracts with lawyers. At present some claimants do not carry on with a case for fear of costs, but this is changing and Europe is beginning to follow the USA.

Finally, concerning the Directive. If a product is defective the defendant does not have to allocate blame or prove negligence or incompetence, they only have to prove that the product is defective, being unsuitable for its purpose. Then compensation is decided by the court.

Table 23.1 is the Directive 85/373/EEC as presented in 1985.

Table 23.2 is notes on the Articles of the Directive.

23.2 LIABILITY AND QUALITY ASSURANCE

Increasingly, quality managers need to be aware of the legislation affecting their company's products. The quality department should, in effect, be the eyes and ears of the company, reporting and informing relevant people of statutory requirements and enforcing compliance via the quality control personnel. Effective quality control and management, records, procedures and policies provide an ideal framework by which products, components, raw materials and even processes of manufacture can be controlled to ensure conformity with the specification. The department has to be able to demonstrate that the products are safe to use, safe to sell and safe once distributed. No matter how good a product is, it is only the quality department which actually has the ability to demonstrate compliance with the statutory regulations and mandatory standards. The quality department needs to be involved in the design, development, manufacture and sale of a product, in order to demonstrate compliance and minimise liability. Liability is minimised by the following measures:

- reduce the number of defective products produced,
- increase the number of defective products detected,
- reduce the possible consequences of an error or fault, minimise the number of defective products distributed,
- record additional information which will aid a defence, showing that you as the end supplier were not at fault,
- reduce the financial and economical penalties which may occur following any accident by prompt investigation of complaints,
- instigate a recall procedure if necessary, and
- provide all members within the company with up-to-date guidance and advice on legislation.

To accomplish these measures the quality assurance department must effect seven policies:

- use test and probability systems,
- be involved in design justification, from start to finish,
- be aware of and contribute to live testing,
- verify suppliers of materials, components and sub-assemblies,
- control quality during manufacture and assembly,
- control the marketing and documentation of products,
- check that QA systems are water tight.

These prompts are for quick reference: Table 23.3 elaborates on each heading.

You may sometimes come across the phrase 'closing the loop'. This simply refers to the actions that must be undertaken to ensure that any outstanding problems or quality aspects are progressed to a satisfactory conclusion. It means get a decision and make sure it is recorded and acted upon. Even if the decision is 'no action', get it recorded with the reasons why. If there are actions to do then make sure there is a record of who will do what and when.

The following tables provide points for quick reference.

Table 23.4 shows those liable.
Table 23.5 lists defences.
Table 23.6 – documents: destroy or keep?

Table 23.1 Directive 85/374/EEC © European Communities, 1985 (Official Journal of the EC, L210, 25.7.1985, p. 29)

COUNCIL DIRECTIVE

of 25 July 1985

on the approximation of the laws, regulations and administrative provisions of the Member States concerning liability for defective products

(85/374/EEC)

THE COUNCIL OF THE EUROPEAN COMMUNITIES,

Having regard to the Treaty establishing the European Economic Community, and in particular Article 100 thereof,

Having regard to the proposal from the Commission (¹),

Having regard to the opinion of the European Parliament (²),

Having regard to the opinion of the Economic and Social Committee (³),

Whereas approximation of the laws of the Member States concerning the liability of the producer for damage caused by the defectiveness of his products is necessary because the existing divergences may distort competition and affect the movement of goods within the common market and entail a differing degree of protection of the consumer against damage caused by a defective product to his health or property;

Whereas liability without fault on the part of the producer is the sole means of adequately solving the problem, peculiar to our age of increasing technicality, of a fair apportionment of the risks inherent in modern technological production;

Whereas liability without fault should apply only to movables which have been industrially produced; whereas, as a result, it is appropriate to exclude liability for agricultural products and game, except where they have undergone a processing of an industrial nature

which could cause a defect in these products; whereas the liability provided for in this Directive should also apply to movables which are used in the construction of immovables or are installed in immovables;

Whereas protection of the consumer requires that all producers involved in the production process should be made liable, in so far as their finished product, component part or any raw material supplied by them was defective; whereas, for the same reason, liability should extend to importers of products into the Community and to persons who present themselves as producers by affixing their name, trade mark or other distinguishing feature or who supply a product the producer of which cannot be identified;

Whereas, in situations where several persons are liable for the same damage, the protection of the consumer requires that the injured person should be able to claim full compensation for the damage from any one of them;

whereas, to protect the physical well-being and property of the consumer, the defectiveness of the product should be determined by reference not to its fitness for use but to the lack of the safety which the public at large is entitled to expect; whereas the safety is assessed by excluding any misuse of the product not reasonable under the circumstances;

Whereas a fair apportionment of risk between the injured person and the producer implies that the producer should be able to free himself from liability if he furnishes proof as to the existence of certain exonerating circumstances;

Whereas the protection of the consumer requires that the liability of the producer remains unaffected by acts or omissions of other persons have contributed to cause the

(¹) OJ No C 241, 14.10.1976, p. 9 and OJ No C 271, 26.10.1979, p. 3.
(²) OJ No C 127, 21.5.1979, p. 61.
(³) OJ No C 114, 7.5.1979, p. 15.

Table 23.1 *(continued)*

---

damage; whereas, however, the contributory negligence of the injured person may be taken into account to reduce or disallow such liability;

Whereas the protection of the consumer requires compensation for death and personal injury as well as compensation for damage to property; whereas the latter should nevertheless be limited to goods for private use of consumption and be subject to a deduction of a lower threshold of a fixed amount in order to avoid litigation in an excessive number of cases; whereas this Directive should not prejudice compensation for pain and suffering and other non-material damages payable, where appropriate, under the law applicable to the case;

Whereas a uniform period of limitation for the bringing of action for compensation is in the interests both of the injured person and of the producer;

Whereas products age in the course of time, higher safety standards are developed and the state of science and technology progresses; whereas, therefore, it would not be reasonable to make the producer liable for an unlimited period for the defectiveness of his product; whereas, therefore, liability should expire after a reasonable length of time, without prejudice to claims pending at law;

Whereas, to achieve effective protection of consumers, no contractual derogation should be permitted as regards the liability of the producer in relation to the injured person;

Whereas under the legal systems of the Member States an injured party may have a claim for damages based on grounds of contractual liability or on grounds of non-contractual liability other than that provided for in this Directive; in so far as these provisions also serve to attain the objective of effective protection of consumers, they should remain unaffected by this Directive; whereas, in so far as effective protection of consumers in the sector of pharmaceutical products is already also attained in a Member State under a special liability system, claims based on this system should similarly remain possible;

Whereas, to the extent that liability for nuclear injury or damage is already covered in all Member States by adequate special rules, it has been possible to exclude damage of this type from the scope of this Directive;

Whereas, since the exclusion of primary agricultural products and game from the scope of this Directive may be felt, in certain Member States, in view of what is expected for the protection of consumers, to restrict unduly such protection, it should be possible for a Member State to extend liability to such products;

Whereas, for similar reasons, the possibility offered to a producer to free himself from liability if he proves that the state of scientific and technical knowledge at the time when he put the product into circulation was not such as to enable the existence of a defect to be discovered may be felt in certain Member States to restrict unduly the protection of the consumer; whereas it should therefore be possible for a Member State to maintain in its legislation or to provide by new legislation that this exonerating circumstance is not admitted; whereas, in the case of new legislation, making use of the derogation should, however, be subject to a Community standstill procedure, in order to raise, if possible, the level of protection in a uniform manner throughout the Community;

Whereas, taking into account the legal traditions in most of the Member States, it is inappropriate to set any financial ceiling on the producer's liability without fault; whereas, in so far as there are, however, differing traditions, it seems possible to admit that a Member State may derogate from the principle of unlimited liability by providing a limit for the total liability of the producer for damage resulting from a death or personal injury and caused by identical items with the same defect, provided that this limit is established at a level sufficiently high to guarantee adequate protection of the consumer and the correct functioning of the common market;

Whereas the harmonization resulting from this cannot be total at the present stage, but opens the way towards greater harmonization; whereas it is therefore necessary that the Council receive at regular intervals, reports from the Commission on the application of this Directive, accompanied, as the case may be, by appropriate proposals;

Table 23.1   *(continued)*

Whereas it is particularly important in this respect that a re-examination be carried out of those parts of the Directive relating to the derogations open to the Member States, at the expiry of a period of sufficient length to gather practical experience on the effects of these derogations on the protection of consumers and on the functioning of the common market,

HAS ADOPTED THIS DIRECTIVE:

Article 1

The producer shall be liable for damage caused by a defect in his product.

Article 2

For the purpose of this Directive 'product' means all movables, with the exception of primary agricultural products and game, even though incorporated into another movable or into an immovable. 'Primary agricultural products' means the products of the soil, of stock-farming and of fisheries, excluding products which have undergone initial processing. 'Product' includes electricity.

Article 3

1. 'Producer' means the manufacturer of a finished product, the producer of any raw material or the manufacturer of a component part and any person who, by putting his name, trade mark or other distinguishing feature on the product presents himself as its producer.

2. Without prejudice to the liability of the producer, any person who imports into the Community a product for sale, hire, leasing or any form of distribution in the course of his business shall be deemed to be a producer within the meaning of this Directive and shall be responsible as a producer.

3. Where the producer of the product cannot be identified, each supplier of the product shall be treated as its producer unless he informs the injured person, within a reasonable time, of the identity of the producer or of the person who supplied him with the product. The same shall apply, in the case of an imported product, if this product does not indicate the identity of the importer referred to in paragraph 2, even if the name of the producer is indicated.

Article 4

The injured person shall be required to prove the damage, the defect and the causal relationship between defect and damage.

Article 5

Where, as a result of the provisions of this Directive, two or more persons are liable for the same damage, they shall be liable jointly and severally, without prejudice to the provisions of national law concerning the rights of contribution or recourse.

Article 6

1. A product is defective when it does not provide the safety which a person is entitled to expect, taking all circumstances into account, including:

(a) the presentation of the product;

(b) the use to which it could reasonably be expected that the product would be put;

(c) the time when the product was put into circulation.

2. A product shall not be considered defective for the sole reason that a better product is subsequently put into circulation.

Article 7

The producer shall not be liable as a result of this Directive if he proves:

(a) that he did not put the product into circulation; or

(b) that, having regard to the circumstances, it is probable that the defect which caused the damage did not exist at the time when the product was put into circulation by him or that this defect came into being afterwards; or

(c) that the product was neither manufactured by him for sale or any form of distribution for economic purpose nor manufactured or distributed by him in the course of his business; or

(d) that the defect is due to compliance of the product with mandatory regulations issued by the public authorities; or

Table 23.1 *(continued)*

(e) that the state of scientific and technical knowledge at the time when he put the product into circulation was not such as to enable the existence of the defect to be discovered; or

(f) in the case of a manufacturer of a component, that the defect is attributable to the design of the product in which the component has been fitted or to the instructions given by the manufacturer of the product.

Article 8

1. Without prejudice to the provisions of national law concerning the right of contribution or recourse, the liability of the producer shall not be reduced when the damage is caused both by a defect in product and by the act or omission of a third party.

2. The liability of the producer may be reduced or disallowed when, having regard to all the circumstances, the damage is caused both by a defect in the product and by the fault of the injured person or any person for whom the injured person is responsible.

Article 9

For the purpose of Article 1, 'damage' means:

(a) damage caused by death or by personal injuries;

(b) damage to, or destruction of, any item of property other than the defective product itself, with a lower threshold of 500 ECU, provided that the item of property:

(i) is of a type ordinarily intended for private use or consumption, and

(ii) was used by the injured person mainly for his own private use or consumption.

This Article shall be without prejudice to national provisions relating to non-material damage.

Article 10

1. Member States shall provide in their legislation that a limitation period of three years shall apply to proceedings for the recovery of damages as provided for in this Directive. The limitation period shall begin to run from the day on which the plaintiff became aware, or should reasonably have become aware, of the damage, the defect and the identity of the producer.

2. The laws of Member States regulating suspension or interruption of the limitation period shall not be affected by this Directive.

Article 11

Member States shall provide in their legislation that the rights conferred upon the injured person pursuant to this Directive shall be extinguished upon the expiry of a period of 10 years from the date on which the producer put into circulation the actual product which caused the damage, unless the injured person has in the meantime instituted proceedings against the producer.

Article 12

The liability of the producer arising from this Directive may not, in relation to the injured person, be limited or excluded by a provision limiting his liability or exempting him from liability.

Article 13

This Directive shall not affect any rights which an injured person may have according to the rules of the law of contractual or non-contractual liability or a special liability system existing at the moment when this Directive is notified.

Article 14

This Directive shall not apply to injury or damage arising from nuclear accidents and covered by international conventions ratified by the Member States.

Article 15

1. Each Member State may:

(a) by way of derogation from Article 2, provide in its legislation that within the meaning of Article 1 of this Directive 'product' also means primary agricultural products and game;

Table 23.1 *(continued)*

(b) by way of derogation from Article 7 (e), maintain or, subject to the procedure set out in paragraph 2 of this Article, provide in this legislation that the producer shall be liable even if he proves that the state of scientific and technical knowledge at the time when he put the product into circulation was not such as to enable the existence of a defect to be discovered.

2. A Member State wishing to introduce the measure specified in paragraph 1 (b) shall communicate the text of the proposed measure to the Commission. The Commission shall inform the other Member States thereof.

The Member State concerned shall hold the proposed measure in abeyance for nine months after the Commission is informed and provided that in the meantime the Commission has not submitted to the Council a proposal amending this Directive on the relevant matter. However, if within three months of receiving the said information, the Commission does not advise the Member State concerned that it intends submitting such a proposal to the Council, the Member State may take the proposed measure immediately.

If the Commission does submit to the Council such a proposal amending this Directive within the aforementioned nine months, the Member State concerned shall hold the proposed measure in abeyance for a further period of 18 months from the date on which the proposal is submitted.

3. Ten years after the date of notification of this Directive, the Commission shall submit to the Council a report on the effect that rulings by the courts as to the application of Article 7 (e) and of paragraph 1 (b) of this Article have on consumer protection and the functioning of the common market. In the light of this report the Council, acting on a proposal from the Commission and pursuant to the terms of Article 100 of the Treaty, shall decide whether to repeal Article 7 (e).

Article 16

1. Any Member State may provide that a producer's total liability for damage resulting from a death or personal injury and caused by identical items with the same defect shall be limited to an amount which may not be less than 70 million ECU.

2. Ten years after the date of notification of this Directive, the Commission shall submit to the Council a report on the effect on consumer protection and the functioning of the common market of the implementation of the financial limit on liability by those Member States which have used the option provided for in paragraph 1. In the light of this report the Council, acting on a proposal from the Commission and pursuant to the terms of Article 100 of the Treaty, shall decide whether to repeal paragraph 1.

Article 17

This Directive shall not apply to products put into circulation before the date on which the provisions referred to in Article 19 enter into force.

Article 18

1. For the purposes of this Directive, the ECU shall be that defined by Regulation (EEC) No 3180/78([1]), as amended by Regulation (EEC) No 2626/84([2]). The equivalent in national currency shall initially be calculated at the rate obtaining on the date of adoption of this Directive.

2. Every five years the Council, acting on a proposal from the Commission, shall examine and, if need be, revise the amounts in this Directive, in the light of economic and monetary trends in the Community.

Article 19

1. Member States shall bring into force, not later than three years from the date of notification of this Directive, the laws, regulations and administrative provisions necessary to comply with this Directive. They shall forthwith inform the Commission thereof([3]).

2. The procedure set out in Article 15 (2) shall apply from the date of notification of this Directive.

([1]) OJ No L 379, 30.12.1978, p. 1.
([2]) OJ No L 247, 16.9.1984, p. 1.
([3]) This Directive was notified to the Member States on 30 July 1985.

Table 23.1 *(continued)*

Article 20

Member States shall communicate to the Commission the texts of the main provisions of national law which they subsequently adopt in the field governed by this Directive.

Article 21

Every five years the Commission shall present a report to the Council on the application of this Directive and, if necessary, shall submit appropriate proposals to it.

Article 22

This Directive is addressed to the Member States.

Done at Brussels, 25 July 1985.

For the Council

The President

J. POOS

Table 23.2 Notes on European Directive 85/374/EEC

Article 1	Lays down the principles of strict liability
Article 2	Defines products as all movables (tangible property other than land or buildings) with the exception of primary agricultural products and game
Article 3	Defines the scope of the word 'producer' for the purpose of establishing who is liable under the directive With particular consideration and mention concerning pharmacists, doctors, nurses and others operating in the health sector.
Article 4	Provides that the injured person must prove the damage, the defect and the causal relationship between them The injured person is not required to prove any fault on the part of the product supplier
Article 5	Provides that where two or more persons are liable for the same damage, they shall be liable jointly and severally Existing rights of contribution or recourse are not affected
Article 6	States that a product is deemed defective when 'it does not provide the safety which a person is entitled to expect, taking all circumstances into account' It also expands upon the actual definition of defective and reportable faults
Article 7	Provides six exemptions from liability for the producer
Article 8	Provides that a producer cannot avoid or reduce his liability under the directive when the damage is caused both by a defect in his product and by an act or omission of a third party
Article 9	Defines the types of damage for which compensation may be claimed under the terms of the Directive
Article 10	Provides for a limitation period of three years for the bringing of proceedings, counting from the day on which the plaintiff became aware, or should reasonably have become aware, of the defect, the damage and the identity of the producer
Article 11	Provides that, notwithstanding the limitation period in Article 10, no action can be commenced under the Directive after a period of ten years from the date on which the actual product was put into circulation
Article 12	Provides that liability of the producer to the insured person may not be limited or excluded by contract or any other form of agreement
Article 13	Provides that the rights of an injured person under the laws of contract and tort (and delict) of Member States remain unaffected by the Directive
Article 14	Provides that the directive does not apply to damage arising from nuclear accidents covered by international conventions
Article 15	Allows Member States to derogate from Article 2 by extending strict liability to primary agricultural products and game, and/or to derogate from Article 7 (e) by extending strict liability to development risks

Table 23.2 *(continued)*

Article 16	Provides that Member States may introduce a financial limit on liability, resulting from the same defect in identical items, of not less than 70 m ECU
Article 17	Provides that the Directive shall not be applied retrospectively to products put into circulation before the date of entry into force of the directive in individual member states
Article 18	Concerns the definition of the ECU for the purposes of the optional financial limit and of the threshold limit to private property claims: reviewed every 5 years
Article 19	Requires the Directive to be implemented by July 1988
Article 20	Requires Member States to inform the commission of measures they have taken to implement the Directive
Article 21	Requires the commission to report to the Council every 5 years on the application of the Directive. The Commission is, of course, free at any time to make fresh proposals to the Council.

Table 23.3 Departmental requirements for liability reduction

Department	Requirement
QA	• Obtain regular updates on legislation, standards, regulations and codes of practice. If you fail the GMP audit, then it does not matter how good your other systems are. • Update and upgrade test equipment, control systems and safety techniques: a continually changing subject as materials and processes come and go in fashions, or are removed completely. • Complete Failure Mode and Effects Analysis on all products as soon as possible in the design cycle, update at least three times before launch. There are other systems available all with the same end result: to spot the problems before they occur and eliminate then before manufacturing even begins.
Design	• Ensure sufficient information obtained from the end user. Review the application and modify instructions to ensure safe handling. • Complete a critical index for each part of the design. • Instigate design reviews from concept through to final format. • Implement and control a check list of agreed stages for the life of the product through design to development. • Post launch checks required to monitor devices once introduced to batch manufacture. • Discuss early on the testing requirements and the methods to match/confirm/exceed the design brief requirements.
Development	• What effect will the final finished product have on the patient, area of use, environment? You may manufacture an ideal sought after device but if in 10 years people still cannot dispose of it then your company may end up with a substantial reclaim bill.

Table 23.3 (*continued*)

Department	Requirement
	• What test programmes are necessary for 'live' appraisal? What's required to ensure the finished item is safe to use on a patient? • In-house testing, are your staff safe? What level of testing is statistically required? Short or long term use? • Or use an outside test house, if independent certification of the correct equipment is not available on your own site. But beware using outside house because this will not remove any of the liability, but it will add a certain level of confidence by way of an independent assessment of components and assembled product.
Pre-production	• Verify and vet suppliers of materials and components. An audit on their record keeping and paperwork system is essential, traceability of the raw materials used. Also check their quality control. • Verify contracts and specified supply of goods. • Verify instruction sheets and manuals, control changes and any safety information required. • Verify system in place to inform and record authorised suppliers. Any changes or additions to be agreed in writing.
Production	• Install a control system to monitor manufacture, methods, instructions and changes or concessions necessary. • Maintain QC inspection system to check the production complies with the instructions for assembly. Same applies for specifications and record sheets. • Train QC staff up to and above required levels to ensure they are adequate at and aware of the full product use. • Traceability must be maintained on all materials, component parts and sub-assemblies. Record sheets of delivery, storage and issue. • Ensure any changes in the method of manufacture must be documented and authorised before implementation. • Maintain calibrated equipment for reference and regularly re-calibrate test gear.
Marketing and sales	• All statements to be verified and accepted before product launch. • Safety considerations to be paramount and no product issued without authorised agreement in writing. • Maintain full records of batch dates, sizes, quantities dispatched and to whom. Recall of product must be done efficiently and quickly.
QA	• Are the department's record systems audited internally on a regular basis and are these audits monitored by an off-site director or agency? (To ensure retrospective action) • Install system of audits on all departments to ensure controls are maintained. • Management reviews should be regularly held and minuted to ensure the efficient transfer of information.

Table 23.4 Those liable

- Can suppliers be identified? Is the fault due directly to their error or non-compliance to specifications?
- Putting own name or logo on a product a wise policy? Once a product is claimed as your own, full liability is yours.
- Producer's name clearly shown? Credit and liability go hand in hand.
- Contractual recourse? Legal commitment between manufacturers and distributor may reduce your financial outlay.
- Contractual limitation period. As before, commitment within groups can be limited by a set time.
- Joint and several liability. Can co-producers pay their share? If agreement can be written into the contract, sub-assemblies manufactured outside can be made accountable.

Table 23.5 Defences

- Compliance with mandatory requirements.
- Defect did not exist at the relevant time.
- State of the art.
- Product comprised in another product, defect attributable to design of other product or to compliance with instructions.
- Article 7 of the Directive: six specific points.

Table 23.6 Documents: destroy or keep?

- Criminal offence: if during a case there is evidence that documents had been destroyed, the court will allocate blame automatically.
- All copies destroyed? There is always a rogue copy somewhere.
- Cross-references: even if all copies have been destroyed, there may well be references which are just as incriminating.
- Other evidence reveals content, or policy of destruction.
- Missing documents assume enormous significance: guilt by omission, assumption that there was something to hide.
- Evidence of deliberate destruction could lose a case, incur costs, exemplary damages.
- Effect on reputation of cover-up campaign: once accused, rightly or wrongly, your company will always be regarded suspiciously.

Table 23.7 Documents: reasons to keep copies

- Anything written or recorded is likely to be discovered.
- It is not possible to destroy, alter or hide later.
- A smart lawyer will use any documents to their advantage.

Some readers may still be confused about the actual liability and who is responsible. Figure 23.1 shows four examples of the route to determine who is liable. Importers and exporters may think that they are exempt from any claims if they did not actually manufacture the finished item, but they have the same or similar liability to the producer, perhaps even more so if the goods were made outside the EC.

Supposing a person 'A' buys a car from a dealer 'B' in the UK, who had originally obtained it from a distributor 'C'. The car had been produced in Germany by company 'D' using components from company 'E' in Belgium. Unfortunately 'A' had an accident while on holiday in Denmark, owing to a fault in one of the components: who is liable? Well, under Articles 1, 3 and 5 of the Directive, 'A' can sue 'D' and 'E' separately or jointly, he can also sue 'B' or 'C' if the original manufacturer can not be identified. The case could be heard in the UK, Germany or Denmark, whichever 'A' feels would be to his advantage.

There are methods used by some big companies to limit their eventual liability in cases like this. Figure 23.2 shows one such method which is quite legal, at present.

Table 23.8   Documents: do's and don'ts

Do	Don't
State facts: clear, true and to the point	Exaggerate or assume: no conjecture.

Give full information to enable action to be taken and prevent repeated requests for additional information.	Speculate about
	   Causes
	   Consequences

Request action: state even the obvious.	Solutions
Seek feedback: do not leave the request open, clarify the objective.	Give unqualified opinions
Be conservative in conclusions and remarks	Set unrealistic objectives or standards for timescales or test results.

Justify actions take or instigated	Criticise,
	   The product
	   Other staff or departments

	Imply cost or resource constraints take priority over safety
	Admit unreasonable risks are being taken
	Admit defects are bound to occur

Table 23.9 Incriminating evidence

- The company was aware of the risk but failed to take effective action.
- A safety-related modification was proposed but rejected on unjustifiable grounds.
- A potentially safer alternative was not considered.
- Procedures for overcoming safety-related problems are inadequate.
- Procedures are not adhered to.
- The company is prepared to take risks on safety and quality.
- There is insufficient proof that problems were resolved.

Table 23.10 Procedures

1. Raise them: controlled by the QA department.
2. Check they are workable: signed-off by at least the production, marketing/sales, design and QA departments.
3. Review and update: management review, design review etc.
4. Ensure familiarisation among staff: adequate training for all, plus documented proof.
5. Work to them: written confirmation, all changes or concessions to be agreed before implementation.
6. Insist that others work to them: ensure it is mandatory to confirm to all specifications and manufacturing procedures.

Table 23.11 Potential engineering problems

- Inadequate testing, especially for concessions. All concessions must be justified and authorised (in writing) signed-off by at least three independent people.
- Rejecting a safety-related proposal on cost/resource grounds alone: this should never be allowed.
- Not assessing a potential safety improvement: all options should be considered.
- Lack of documentation on design and test work, especially on reasons for rejecting a proposed safety feature. All test results should be recorded and assessed.
- Exaggeration of the dangers: 'crying wolf' would prevent others from taking the problems seriously.
- Denigrating existing designs: never dismiss other options or designs out of hand.

23.3 RISK

Identification of the risks presented by a product or device is the first step to minimising liability. If there are risks, what potential is there to cause injury to anyone, damage to property, loss of property, or monetary loss to a person or company?

There can also be problems with 'perceived risk'. This is something which the customer may think might go wrong, without any rational proof. Perceived risks can limit sales and consequently profits. There are standard

Table 23.12 Sales policy

- Give accurate information.
- If unsure; check, don't guess.
- Do not imply suitability for non-approved applications, modifications or accessories.
- Give realistic tolerances on any specifications.
- Ensure the customer is aware of the limitations and potential (if any) dangers of your device.
- Do not understate the dangers.
- Do not suggest that other models are unsafe.
- Do not suggest an optional safety feature is essential.

Table 23.13 Handling complaints: do's and don'ts

Do	Don't

• Get all the facts
    from the customer or dealer
    from the production department
    from the design and engineering
    departments
    about the injury or danger identified
• Communicate full details
    to your personnel
    instigate necessary action
    immediately
    to the customer who raised
    the complaint
    to the MDA if necessary
• Do not hide or understate the problem
• Avoid the words 'defect', 'neglect',
  'blame' or 'fault' (or preface with
  'alleged')
• Use words like 'difficulty', 'problem'
  'breakdown'
• Keep to procedures
• Retain correspondence
• Ensure the documents 'close the loop'
	• Exaggerate
	• Speculate or give opinion about
	    cause
	    consequences
	    solutions
	• Admit the complaint is justified
	• Admit liability
	• Suggest that optional safety features
	  should have been fitted as standard

Table 23.14 QA rules

- Those conducting in-house audits or evaluating risks should not be misled by simple 'paper qualifications'.
- Certificates do not necessarily demonstrate real competence.
- Quantitative evidence must also be available to show that effective control does exist.

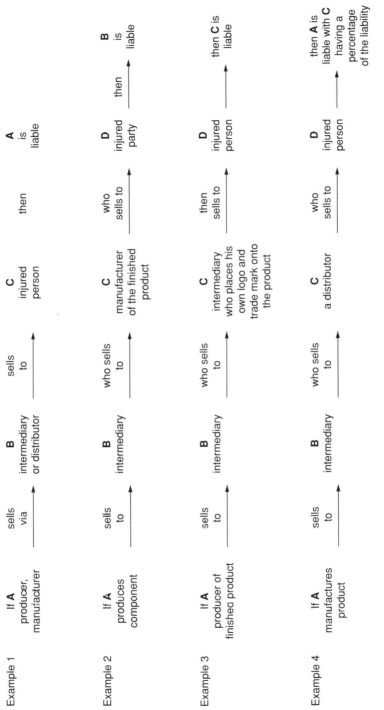

Figure 23.1 Who is the liable body?

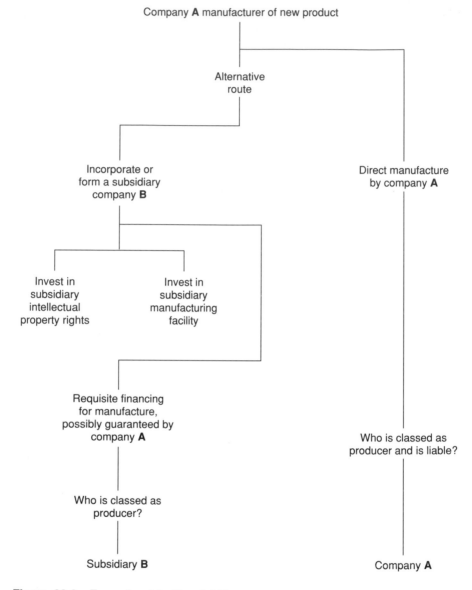

Figure 23.2   Example of limiting liability.

safety limits that all design and development departments build into new devices, but there must always be reviews and assessments of the potential risks as well.

One method is a continuous review of the product's development via a formal design audit, as previously described. Another method is a rolling

FMEA, meaning continuous updates and reassessments. I would suggest at least three over the course of the design cycle for any device.

In October 1994 a draft European Standard, pr EN1441, was put forward for the Risk Analysis of Medical Devices. This is still under discussion but could well be introduced as a full European Standard. If so, there would be another level of control.

23.4 PRODUCT RECALL

If a product is found to be faulty after distribution, then the company may reduce its liability by recalling the relevant products as promptly as possible. Even though this is a virtual admission of guilt, it also shows an awareness and responsibility on behalf of the company and can be described as a precautionary measure. Recall can reduce punitive payments at a later date of settlement.

A recommendation to conduct a full recall should be able to be made at any level, but the final decision should be at board level since the implications are so great. There should be a system of control with one person designated as the overall coordinator. Once started a recall should be quick, quiet and thorough. Remedial action for the defect should be investigated at the same time as recall.

23.5 SUMMARY

- Strict liability will be introduced in due course. It will apply to manufacturers and importers and suppliers who claim the product as their own or fail to identify the source.
- Any distributor or company which assembles kits or uses component parts which eventually prove faulty will be liable.
- Liability applies throughout the EC to the advantage of the plaintiff and not the manufacturer. You may have to defend your product in another country, in another language and in a possibly hostile court.
- The product need not 'fail' in the usual sense. It is defective if it does not provide the safety that a person is entitled to expect, having regard to all the circumstances including the presentation of the product. This is stated in Article 4 of the Directive and is in accordance with Article 2 of the Strasbourg Convention.
- Product liability will run for ten years after a product or device has been placed in general circulation.
- A company can be liable as the manufacturer or producer. Named individuals can also be liable if the courts decide to narrow down responsibility. This could include designers, production managers, and quality assurance managers.

24
Patents and Registration

Sometimes the best protection for your ideas is 'say nowt, tell no one, lose nothing'. This is sometimes effective, but only sometimes. Mostly other ways of protecting your ideas are necessary to ensure a competitive edge on your rivals in the market.

Often competing firms are working to satisfy similar market needs at the same time. The firm that launches first and has ample manufacturing capacity can monopolise the market: even if someone else had the idea first. In a competitive world staff may move from one employer to another taking knowledge and ideas with them.

I will not be setting out hard and fast rules for idea, concept or innovative device protection, nor do I intend to advise you on which route to follow. What I will do is go through the various methods of obtaining limited protection for your idea. How limited it is depends on three factors.

- Money – how much are you prepared to spend?
- Time – how much do you have available to ensure that a fully documented claim is filed?
- Return – is it really worth the commitment and resources to protect this gem of an idea?

Even a full patent provides intellectual protection for a maximum period of 20 years and only in the countries which agree to work within the 'rules'.

24.1 PATENTS

Patents are granted to individuals or companies who can prove or claim a new process, product, component or improvement on existing processes or products.

A patent allows the individual a monopoly on the idea, either to manufacture or licence or sell for a set period. In exchange for the protection of the idea the details of the invention are publicly disclosed.

Patent application follows a set formal pattern from initial application to final granting and registration, Figure 24.1 shows the UK procedure along with approximate timing and cost (based on 1996 information).

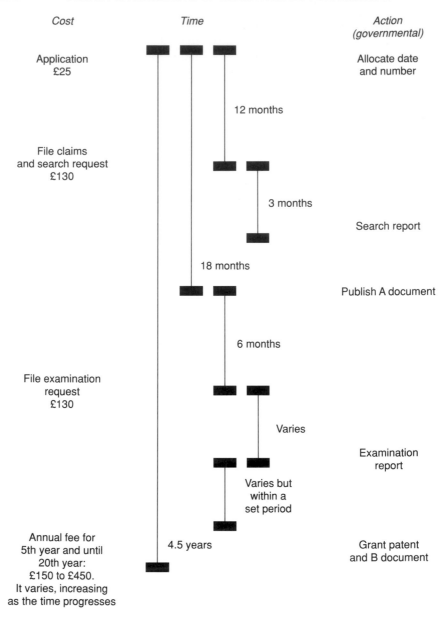

Cost   *Time*   *Action*
                                                                        (governmental)

Application   Allocate date
£25   and number

                                                    12 months

File claims
and search request
£130

                                                     3 months

                                                                         Search report

                                     18 months

                                                                         Publish A document

                                                     6 months

File examination
request
£130

                                                     Varies

                                                                         Examination
                                                                         report

                                                  Varies but
                                                  within a
                                                  set period

Annual fee for   4.5 years   Grant patent
5th year and until   and B document
20th year:
£150 to £450.
It varies, increasing
as the time progresses

Figure 24.1   Patent application procedure (1996).

There are three essential criteria for a formal application to meet before an invention can be protected: it must be new, it must be an innovative step (not obvious), and it must be capable of industrial application. These three requirements should be explained more fully but I had better slip in one item here before I proceed any further: to whom is the patent granted?

An inventor is normally granted a patent unless the inventor is employed and the invention was conceived as part of their normal duties or as a direct result of a specific contract, in which case the invention belongs to the employer. The named 'inventor' must by law be indicated on the application (recent developments within the UK have prompted additional payments to employees if the invention makes 'excessive' profits for a company and the inventor is only receiving normal salary and no other financial rewards).

24.1.1 NEW

New means not just a modification or evolution of an existing process or product, but something 'not state of the art' at the time of the application. A patent will not be granted if the invention was prior knowledge, even if it was never used. One of the best known examples of 'prior knowledge' is the patent application for a windsurfer. It was decided that the application was invalid since years before a 12-year-old boy had built a crude version and sailed for two years near a caravan site in full view of anyone on the cliff tops: admittedly a limited audience, but never the less in full public view. So all inventions should be kept secret until applications have been filed: a presentation, paper or demonstration might be sufficient to prevent obtaining a patent.

24.1.2 INNOVATIVE

Innovative means an original idea, not an obvious progression or development of a product or process which could be undertaken or evolved by another 'skilled person' in the same field of work.

24.1.3 INDUSTRIAL APPLICATION

Simply put, this means can it be made? The idea must be able to take a physical form. The word industrial is only used as a general term and covers all useful and practical activities.

24.1.4 COST

As shown in Figure 24.1, the basic costs are not too expensive but there are a number of other factors to be considered. First, a badly constructed or worded application will afford little or no protection from those wishing to profit from your efforts. So professional advice is necessary to draft and formally present an application. Table 24.1 shows the cost of obtaining patents under various procedures.

Second, there are more costs when you start to consider protection further afield and wish to have either European cover or international patents. Table 24.2 shows the member countries of the European Patent Convention (EPC) and the international Patent Cooperation Treaty (PCT).

Table 24.1 Patent application costs (1996)

Action	Via UK agent	UK Patent Office	EPC procedure	PCT procedure
Filing initial application	£350–600	£25	£260	£350 + £55 on transmittal
Search	£400 min	£130	£815	£1030
Designation, per state	–	–	£150	£85
Substantive examination	£400 min	£130	£1200	National fee £130 per state International Examination fee Request system via EPO £1300
Granting of patent	£400–1000	£150–£450	£600	National fee

Note that EPC and PCT search fees are payable on filing
EPC = European Patent Convention
PCT = Patent Cooperation Treaty
EPO = European Patent Office

Table 24.2 Member countries of European Patent Convention (EPC) and Patent Cooperation Treaty (PCT)

EPC Contracting Countries
Austria, Belgium, Denmark, Eire (Ireland), France, Germany, Italy, Liechtenstein, Luxembourg, Monaco, Netherlands, Portugal, Spain, Sweden, Switzerland, United Kingdom.

PCT Contracting Countries
Armenia, Australia, Austria, Barbados, Belarus, Belgium, Benin, Brazil, Burkina Faso, Cameroon, Canada, Central African Republic, Chad, Congo, Côte d'Ivoire, Czech Republic, Denmark, Estonia, Georgia, Kirghizia, Democratic People's Republic of Korea, Finland, France, Gabon, Germany, Greece, Guinea, Hungary, Iceland, Ireland, Italy, Japan, Kazakhstan, Kenya, Latvia, Liberia, Liechtenstein, Lithuania, Luxembourg, Madagascar, Malawi, Mali, Mauritania, Mexico, Monaco, Mongolia, Netherlands, New Zealand, Nigeria, Norway, Poland, Portugal, Republic of Korea, Republic of Moldova, Romania, Russian Federation, Senegal, Singapore, Slovakia, Spain, Sri Lanka, Sudan, Swaziland, Sweden, Switzerland, Tajikistan, Togo, Trinidad and Tobago, Uganda, Ukraine, United Kingdom, United States of America, Uzbekistan, Vietnam.

A normal British application to final granting (using an agent to compile, progress and monitor) will cost a minimum of £2000 over a period of three to four years. This will be much greater for complex subject matter and any subsequent objections raised which require answering. Taking out a European patent to cover, say, ten countries is likely to cost in excess of £9000 over the same three to four year period. Then there is the additional cost of obtaining patents in other countries would be approximately £2500 per country.

Before applying for a patent it is important to assess the rewards gained from holding a monopoly for the designated time. Normally an employee can expect no additional payments if an invention is part of his or her job, say that of a Design Engineer. But if the patent granted is deemed to provide an employer 'outstanding benefit' then the Patent Act 1993 states that the employee should be appropriately rewarded. Unfortunately the definition of 'outstanding benefit' has yet to be quantified, to date there have been no court cases to set a precedent, but this also indicates that employers are recognising the need for rewards and that no one as yet has a major complaint. If an employee makes an invention, independently of the company and then sells the invention to an employer for an agreed single payment, then if the benefit to the company is deemed to be 'considerable' in relationship to the original payment, the Patent Act says the employee should be allowed another payment or reward.

Remember that Patents are in the public domain, and you could find therein information and assistance you might need to solve problems on different projects. It has been estimated that 75% of the information in patents is not available elsewhere. If used correctly they can show how a solution from the past can give the information or key to unlock your creative concept. All UK Patent Offices offer services for searches, abstracts, classifications etc., and can be contacted to clarify their charges and the exact information that can be supplied.

To end this section here is an anecdote: the inventor of the non-intrusive method of riveting ring pulls to the tops of drinks cans arranged a royalty of one tenth of a penny (£0.001) per can from the manufacturers. Since Coca Cola alone sold over 150 million cans worldwide per day, it shows that glory is very nice but the money is better.

24.2 DESIGNRIGHT

Patents are the ultimate in design protection but they are not the only way of looking after your interests. Anything you produce which is new, not necessarily of technical or scientific merit, but because of its function or shape is 'intellectual property'. Any product with an original or definitive shape is automatically protected by designright. No documentation or

Table 24.3 Information protection: applies to the UK only, additional protection required for other countries

Method	Example of product or idea	How to apply	Length of protection	Action if copied or counterfeited	Approx. cost (fee)
Patent	New ideas, concept or process: must be novel with no prior knowledge.	Apply to Patent Office: specifications, abstract and fee on one form.	20 years.	Civil action brought by the patent holder.	Between £450 to £750 over a 4–5 year period, then an annual fee over the next 15 years, varied.
Copyright ©	Records, films, literary, musical or artistic work, visual or audio broadcasts, computer software.	Automatic: no applications required but proof of original ownership may be necessary.	50 years for records and films. 50 years after the death of an author for musical, artistic and literary work, also software, 15 years for industrial designs, 25 years for published editions.	Civil actions claiming damages and halting further infringements. Actual trade infringement is a criminal offence and can/is controlled via the Customs office.	None
Designright	Product shapes or external configuration which enhances or aids the function.	Similar to copyright and is automatic when the design is created, again keep records of design and when first available for sale.	10 years from first placed on sale (15 years from concept).	Similar to copyright.	None

Table 24.3 *(continued)*

Method	Example of product or idea	How to apply	Length of protection	Action if copied or counterfeited	Approx. cost (fee)
Design registration ®	New and original designs, patterns or ornaments not directly effective to the function.	Apply to the Patent Office with form and fee.	Initially for five years then reapply every five years to a maximum period of 25 years.	Civil action by the registration holder.	Initial payment of £60 on application with £130 each succeeding 5 years for the maximum 25 year term.
Trade mark ™	Symbols or letters to identify products and companies. (Subject at the moment to change, wider classification to come 1996).	Apply to the Patent Office with form and fee.	Indefinitely, once registered (for initial ten years) the trade mark can be renewed continuously every 10 years thereafter.	Civil action by the holder although the Customs do have the power to impound and/or seize infringing items.	Initial £225 on application then £250 each 10 year interval.

bureaucratic approval is required; there is no registration but you need good in-house records of the design concept and a drawing. Designright protects a 'shape' for ten years from the date of the first saleable item, although for the last five years of the ten anybody can obtain a licence from the design-right owner (i.e. a licence must be given whether the owner likes it or not).

Other methods of protecting designs are: copyright, Trade Marks, and Registered Designs: Table 24.3 gives a quick breakdown.

24.3 COPYRIGHT

Copyright protection is automatic and applies to the actual production or presentation in printed, visual, audio or data forms, of ideas, concepts or drawings. As the name implies it is only to stop others from 'copying' the original, which is why the majority of legal cases come from literary, artistic and musical areas. In recent years the computer world has been in the news since software programs cannot be patented and are only protected by the copyright laws. Copyright gives certain rights to the original creators (or their descendants) and allows them to control the actual use of the finished article for up to:

- 25 years for published editions,
- 50 years after death of the author of musical, dramatic, literary or artistic work (including photographs) whether published or unpublished,
- 50 years for films, sound recordings and broadcasts (visual or audio), and
- 50 years after the death of compiler for computer programs.

As mentioned before the protection is automatic once published. It is now standard practice internationally to mark all work with © followed by a date and the owners name. Provided your record keeping is accurate (and it should be to obtain the CE mark) then ownership should not present any problem. Even so, sometimes as an individual (not as a company employee) it would be wise to deposit a signed and dated copy of your work with a bank or solicitor if you think there may be potential problems is the future.

Very soon there will be an European Copyright Duration Directive introduced, whereby the time scales have been changed, for example literary works will be protected for 70 years after the death of author. So it is worth checking regularly on the state of the law.

24.4 TRADEMARKS

Trademarks identify goods or product groups: consumers then come to identify these symbols or words. This is useful for sales and marketing, but trademarks can sometimes become more protective than patents or registered designs, because the ™ designation entitles the owner to the exclusive use of the symbol and prevents anyone else using or copying it. With the increasing commercial importance of the 'brand' rather than the product, buying and selling trademarks has become big business.

Trademark registration takes place simply after a single payment and application presentation: the registration process may take up to 1.5 years because of the cross-checking and notices of intent that have to be advertised (to allow for any objections from other companies and to prevent duplication of symbols). Designing the actual shape and form of trademarks can become a very complex process which may involve negotiations with other manufacturers. Sometimes professional advice may be needed to avoid conflict with other trademarks. Owners of unregistered trademarks can obtain similar rights under common law, though this is certainly more difficult (and expensive) than for registered ones. Once registered, the trademark is protected for 10 years and this protection is renewable indefinitely at regular intervals for a fee (presently £250 for 10 years).

Until mid-1994 trademarks could only be a word or logo or some combination of the two, but now the mark can be 'anything that is distinctive of a company or product', which means shapes, slogans – even jingles can be registered. However, there are some restrictions, the main one being that the trademark should not be a description of the product as this would limit other companies.

European Community Trade Mark Registration has been available throughout the EC from April 1996, reducing the cost of applying for trademarks from £750–900 for each of the 15 countries to a single £3000 for a full EC application. If an existing trademark registration exists in a member country, then that filing date will carry 'seniority' for the Community Trade Mark (CTM).

24.6 REGISTERED DESIGN

With designright, shapes and product configuration have automatic protection. If a certain shape, like a turbine blade, has a specific benefit then additional protection can be obtained by registering it with the Design Registry as a 'registered design'. Even surface textures qualify, as would any similar modification designed as decoration.

The original registration lasts for 5 years and it is renewable every 5 years up to a maximum period of 25 years. The main reason for design registration is for protection of a design drawing or concept, but it is increasingly being applied to a wide range of products because of their appearance. This applies to items like pens, cases, car bodies, cameras, even computers; but the biggest number of applications over the last few years has been for toys. With toys the main method of attracting customers is by visual appearance: whether the toy functions satisfactorily, or even at all, seems not to matter.

24.6   INTERNATIONAL COVER

There is no automatic cover or protection outside the UK for any of the above methods, but agreements are available with the majority of countries (shown in Table 24.2). All require addition documentation and paperwork, plus the inevitable costs.

Making use of this extra protection is a decision you or your company must make on a commercial basis. Consider the following.

- Where are your target markets – home only or export?
- Which countries?
- Would legal protection be an advantage or is the product complex enough to dissuade copying?
- Will someone manufacture and import copies into your own home market?
- Is the product's life span short or long? Compare design registration with patent cover.

These factors will determine if one, several or no methods are adopted.

24.7   ENFORCEMENT

Obviously this chapter has only been able to scratch the surface of design protection but you will now be slightly more informed and able to form an opinion. To obtain up-to-date information and further guidance contact the Patent Office. There is a complete confidentiality and the advice they provide could protect your invention fully. The Patent Office can also advise on methods of presentation, requirements for complete cover, potential pitfalls and patent agents. Also, for a nominal fee they will conduct an initial search, something which may shatter your dreams but save you money in the long run. If there is a prior application, obtain a copy and compare; see if your original idea can be improved upon and then be accepted as a novel concept.

Finally litigation: here are a few comments on legal actions for protecting what's yours. It is commonly thought that patents, trademarks, copyright and design registrations are policed by the countries involved in issuing the documents, but this is not true. The law is there to provide judgement and implementation of that protection, but it does not keep a check on its use.

Patentees or holders have to uphold their own interests and so it is their own responsibility to use the law. You have to monitor any infringements, log the full details and then seek advice on proceeding with civil action.

If there is a possible infringement under no circumstances either speak, contact or write to the people involved; you should immediately contact the patent agent or solicitor. In the eyes of the law it is unlawful to issue an unjustified threat against an alleged infringer, and what is actually classed as a threat is never easy to decide upon and so a simple contact could affect the result of any claim.

If the reverse happens and someone threatens you with the law courts, the same applies: do not speak or contact direct, leave that to your professional advisers.

25
Quality Assurance

Quality control via total quality assurance is hard to describe without going into complex details of QA systems. I intend only to discuss three main areas: should you wish to go deeper into quality assurance there are quite a few excellent books available.

The three subjects I intend to describe are Quality Control Audit, the Design Dossier, and Failure Modes and Effects Analysis (FMEA). All of these need to be addressed at some stage in the design and development of your product. These three quality issues are linked, of course, and are likely to involve the same personnel. The regulatory authorities require these topics to be dealt with and correctly documented, otherwise your product could fail to earn approval or, worse, have to be withdrawn.

I shall not discuss retrospective quality analysis, because I think this is counter productive. But you can be sure that if the MDA, FDA or other national regulatory body does require information about past products, they will let you know.

25.1 DESIGN AUDIT

Design audit is an independent review or assessment of a design or completed project. Independence is guaranteed by the Quality Assurance department. The audit should normally be stringent, objective and open-minded. The overall objective of the audit is to provide assurance that the design meets all requirements laid down in the brief, is safe to manufacture and use, and does not present any danger to the patient or the doctor using it. These three qualities should apply not only during any testing or initial assessment but for the full duration of the product's working life. Points specifically to consider are:

- quantity produced, batch to batch and overall,
- quality limits (for acceptance/rejection),
- manufacturing costs and profit,
- manufacturing methods,
- COSHH implications,

- method of use,
- environmental effects, during and after manufacture, and
- regulatory requirements for home markets and abroad.

Particular attention is needed when the design has incorporated a new type of material, a new technique for manufacture, a new type of application or is intended for a new form of treatment.

All audits should be split into two defined sections: the component audit and the finished product audit.

Evaluation of a component is critical since the assessment of individual items for suitability can prevent failure during use which would not so easily be spotted in the complete assembly. Also endurance tests, specific requirements and target limits are more easily carried out at this level.

The finished product is considered from the point of view of its function. Does it present the correct edge, provide the necessary strength, allow easy manipulation? Do not forget that an audit also has to consider production needs, equipment manufacture, and operator training.

Normally the design audit does not result in major changes, but any change will cost money and should not have happened. However, it is acknowledged it is still better than customers finding fault and reactive measures being necessary.

Each design audit should be considered as a risk reducer, a precaution against errors being incorporated or allowed to continue, a low cost method of controlling or reducing manufacturing expenses. To this end the audit should be carried out at the earliest convenient time before finalising the design, and two or three times during the development stages. Not all assessments need be formal with every aspect noted and recorded; some can be an informal information gathering exercise for the Quality department, so they have a greater understanding of the product when a formal audit is carried out. Any prior assessments should, however, be noted on the audit documentation for reference.

Quality auditing should involve more than just viewing materials in use or how component parts fit together. It should encompass the whole process of design and development, verify the calculations, question selections, methods of assembly etc. It should involve more than one discipline or department as a joint effort from all concerned is far better. All queries should be answered fully to everyone's satisfaction, or the process should stop until problems are resolved. Personnel attending such audits should comprise members from Design, Production, Quality and Sales departments. Design representatives should:

- describe aspects of the design,
- explain reasons for particular actions,
- give background information on use, and
- provide documented records and justification notes if required.

Production representatives should:

- explain equipment required and why,
- give capital budget requirements,
- describe assembly methods, and
- state component supply.

Quality staff should:

- state test methods and initial results,
- explain manufacturing QC test methods,
- give documental records, and
- quote staged inspection level.

Sales or marketing staff should:

- verify the Design department's interpretation of use,
- quantify production numbers required, and
- confirm market sales forecast.

Table 25.1 should be used as a check list before design audit, regardless of whether it is internal, external or part of a customers request before purchase.

As more and more documented evidence is being called for by various regulating bodies a design audit is virtually becoming mandatory. The EC mark, FDA Information Declaration, the MDA Medical Device Directives, and the Design Dossier: all specify an audit at one or more stages. So you must get used to it, have your answers ready, anticipate queries and have the paperwork, calculations, test results etc., to prove it.

Resulting actions necessary from the audit report should be documented and returned to the original committee for reassessment. These actions should tie up exactly with the reported problem to ensure that the fault cannot be repeated.

Table 25.1 Quality audit checklist

---

1. Any external auditor offering a pre-assessment? Make use of them.
2. Prior to any external audit carry out an in-house version, with all non-compliance rectified immediately.
3. Construct an audit team with members from each department, and ensure adequate training.
4. Compile a structured procedure: the same for internal or external audits.
5. Adopt a no blame policy. This will eliminate automatic defences of a concept/method/idea and allow progress to a more constructive solution.
6. Penalise anyone using the audit system to score points or gain advantage within the company.
7. Publish all audit findings, encourage all staff to assist.

25.2 THE DESIGN DOSSIER

One aspect of any design audit should be to examine and comment on the contents and depth of detail contained in the Design Dossier. This document is a detailed specific file (separate from the normal development file in a design office which contains all correspondence, quotes, references, etc.) which is maintained by a designated responsible person within the company and must provide evidence or documented proof of a design, in such detail that the manufacture, performance and function of a product can be evaluated. This is required to comply with the MDD 93/42/EEC but there may be other requirements for CE work, manufacturing regulations, or international export/import regulations. Table 25.2 shows the general requirements necessary of a design dossier but specific details vary depending upon the finished application. Obviously a Class I device does not need to be so closely monitored as a Class III device. Always check with the relevant authority or regulating body as to the specific requirements. As an indication of the level of detail required the *Interpretation of Technical Documentation Required for Class I, IIa, IIb and III Devices by MDD* is fourteen pages long. This collection of detailed information on the design and development of a medical device is governed by the Medical Device Directive 93/42/EEC article 11.1a

Table 25.2 Basic requirements for a design dossier

1. Product title and any references
2. Drawings of the finished product plus detail drawings of component parts
3. Any users' manual or reference book containing instructions on use
4. Description of the product and its intended use plus details of any necessary additional equipment used in conjunction with or for the actual use
5. Fully detailed documentation, specifications and performance information
6. Details of any future planned modifications
7. Failure Modes and Effects Analysis (FMEA) or risk control methods
8. Information of mandatory and voluntary regulations which apply and simple informative responses to each point
9. All data needed to safely operate the product or equipment
10. Results of all clinical assessments or trials. Details of acceptance of FMEA analysis on risk(s)
11. QC audit report and validation of the function against set test requirements. Full listing of the test criteria
12. Interface details where the product must conform to other equipment to aid or allow its use
13. Label format conforming to latest regulations. Details of packaging and sterility indication
14. Production record sheets or details of assembly sequences, including QC inspection stages
15. Full material justification and acceptance
16. Proof of sterilisation method (validation)
17. Director's signature exonerating design team from any blame!

for Class III (an alternative route for Class III is set out in 11.1b) these also require conformance to QA requirements EN ISO 9001/46001.

Table 25.3 sets these issues out in a simpler format. More simply still: you are required to justify your selection, method, design aspect, then prove it and document the calculations and acceptance then save it, continue this through the development period of the project and place copies of these documents into a folder. Looked at like this, the Design Dossier then becomes an easy procedure and not a frantic paper chase to satisfy an auditor or regulatory visit.

25.3 RISK ANALYSIS

The Medical Device Directive (MDD) is now well established and is used by medical device manufacturers as a yardstick for the minimum standard of quality required. During manufacture faults can occur. It is understood that some manufacturing faults are inevitable, but they must be detected and

Table 25.3 Design dossier minimum contents

Directive 93/42/EEC provides the following information on what must be included in the Design Dossier.

1. Description of the actual design, its manufacture and end use performance, plus details and documents which conform to the Directive, Annex II, 4.2, namely those referred to in Annex II 3.2c.
2. Details of any planned changes or developments that will change the product
3. Design brief plus all functioning requirements, the FMEA and actions implemented as a result
4. Methods of control and design verification, plus how the design's progress was checked and measured during development
5. Proof of conformity to additional regulations if connected to other equipment to aid, increase or allow its use
6. Specific statement relating to substances referred to in Section 7.4 of Annex I of the Directive, plus any applicable data in connection with testing carried out
7. Label copy and operating instructions (if any)
8. All clinical data which was compiled during the development stage
9. Details of the manufacturer, the group or type the device falls within
10. Device classification and the justification regarding its selection
11. Details of any similar devices already in circulation
12. Full device description and technical features
13. Catalogue details, numbers and descriptions
14. Material data for all component assemblies
15. Specific manufacturing methods
16. Sterilisation, bioburden and microbiological testing information where applicable.

The Design Dossier should be retained by the manufacturer for a minimum of five years after the last device has been produced. Annex II, 6.1.

eliminated in products which effect the health and welfare of patients. Some faults are considered critical and life threatening.

These faults are described by the MDD as risks which may occur in manufacture, sterilisation and use. If they can be measured, they can be analysed and predicted statistically in order to reduce their incidence.

Acceptance of a level of risk is a decision made by the manufacturer after consultation with the regulatory bodies and the medical profession. All assessments (and recommendations to proceed) should be made after weighing the benefits gained by the patient against the overall effect of the risk occurring. These assessments should be recorded and retained in case of any possible legal action resulting.

To this end all devices are grouped into four different classes and the rules regarding risks are 'based on the vulnerability of the human body taking account of the potential risks associated with the technical design and manufacture of the devices'. This just means the onus or responsibility is set down by the MDD, Table 25.4 puts this classification simply. Table 25.5 shows the regulations from June 1998.

Risk analysis is a rolling requirement for any product at any stage in its evolution, and should be updated regularly depending on the information gained during development. The MDD is quite explicit about this as the revaluation does not depend on the classification of the device. To provide guidelines (presently voluntary) a standard has been issued. This is EN 1441 which sets out procedures and recommended methods of assessment. This is necessary because most companies and still using their own methods of analysis, e.g.

- market analysis,
- FMEA,
- analysis of complaints, returns and reject levels, or
- QA assessment and hazard identification.

In EN 1441 there is a flow diagram which shows the simplest steps needed to reduce the level of risk: Figure 25.1 shows the diagram with these component steps.

1. Compile documents.
2. List main characteristics of the product.

Table 25.4 Risk assessment classfication

Class I	The assessment and decision to proceed is sole responsibility of the manufacturer.
Class IIa	Notified bodies should be contacted at the production stage.
IIb	Inspection of the product should be at the development and manufacturing stage, it should also be mandatory.
Class III	Same as with IIa but additional critical assessment needed as well as authorisation to proceed before manufacture.

Table 25.5   Device classification guide

From June 1998 products must conform to the Medical Device Directive 93/42/EEC before they may be sold on the European market.

Devices are classified into four groups; Class I, IIa, IIb and III. Class I is for low risk and Class III for those whose failure presents the highest risk to health and safety.

Class I   General unpowered devices which do not penetrate the body.
Class IIa   Diagnostic instruments, body fluid storage, surgically invasive devices for transient use.
Class IIb   Surgically invasive devices for short term use, contraceptives, radio-therapy devices, implantable or long-term invasive devices.
Class III   Devices which contact the central nervous system or heart or are absorbed by the body, or which include a pharmaceutical substance.

To demonstrate a product's conformity to the directive the product will be marked by affixing the 'CE mark'.

The Directive specifies specifies essential requirements which are the minimum necessary for the design and manufacture of medical devices to ensure the protection of patients, users and third parties. This principle of safety should be integral to the design of the product, and it should be suitable for its intended purpose.

Manufacturers are given a choice of routes for conforming to the directive and these routes are determined by the product classification. The conformity procedure covers two stages; design and manufacture.

For the design stage documented proof of how the product meets the essential requirements is required. This information should be held in a technical file or 'Design Dossier'.

During manufacture, to ensure that products comply with the essential require-ments and are consistent with the information in the technical file, a documented QA system must be in place.

3. Select and identify potential hazards.
4. Quantify and place a value on the risk of each hazard.
5. Decide which risks are acceptable and which are not.
6. Can the risk be reduced or removed?
7. Are any complications or potential hazards added by changing the design?
8. Have all potential risks been identified?
9. Make a decision about the acceptability of the device. If no, re-examine and assess. If yes, document the decision and record.

It should be noted that the MDD Annexes II, III and VII all require that the results of risk analysis should be documented, implying that no matter what the product or device classification or method of assessment made there should still be a form of risk analysis.

All the previous statements on risk assessment assume that the product is well into the development programme and well on in commitment. It is, of

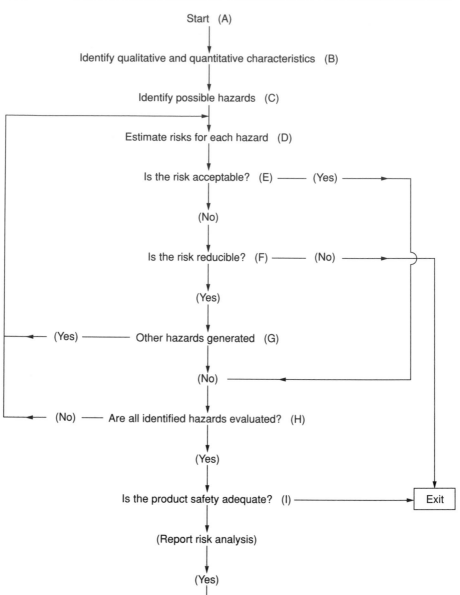

Start   (A)

Identify qualitative and quantitative characteristics   (B)

Identify possible hazards   (C)

Estimate risks for each hazard   (D)

Is the risk acceptable?   (E) ——— (Yes) ———→

(No)

Is the risk reducible?   (F) ——— (No) ———→

(Yes)

←— (Yes) ——— Other hazards generated   (G)

(No)

←— (No) — Are all identified hazards evaluated?   (H)

(Yes)

Is the product safety adequate?   (I) ———————→ Exit

(Report risk analysis)

(Yes)

Finish

Figure 25.1   Flow diagram for EN1441 risk analysis.

course, important that a preliminary risk analysis is conducted to screen out 'no hopers' before there has been much investment in their design. A diagram of the recommended assessment shown in Figure 25.2

The level of risk and the methods used to assess these risks are the basis of the quality audit in an attempt to ensure the safety of the product, but do not overlook other relevant factors.

- The intended use of the product, assembly or device: confirmation with the marketing and sales department and by contact with medical staff.
- Potential misuse of the product: not only the foreseeable but also the incredibly unlikely ones. (Never be surprised at the ingenuity of idiots.)
- Regulatory standards or codes of practice. Industrial or practical physical restrictions.
- The lifetime of the finished product, and of individual components.

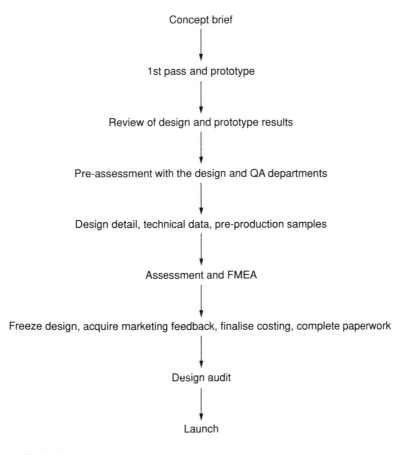

Concept brief

↓

1st pass and prototype

↓

Review of design and prototype results

↓

Pre-assessment with the design and QA departments

↓

Design detail, technical data, pre-production samples

↓

Assessment and FMEA

↓

Freeze design, acquire marketing feedback, finalise costing, complete paperwork

↓

Design audit

↓

Launch

Figure 25.2 Assessment schedule.

- The environment in which the product will be used and the possibility of contamination of the product as well as from it.
- The level of training and education that the end user will actually have before using the product or equipment.

25.3.1 FAILURE MODES AND EFFECTS ANALYSIS (FMEA)

With so many safety factors to consider we need a method of assessment which is easy, simple, explicit and suitable for a wide range of product groups or types. A formalised approach to this problem is Failure Modes and Effect Analysis (FMEA) a systematic method that considers the potential failures of each component, sub-assembly and final product assembly. This is done by breaking down the finished product into a number of functional items. The actual analysis starts by considering the effect of failures on the output of one level and the resultant influence on higher levels. It is considered a bottom-to-top analysis working from a possible failure to the possible consequence.

FMEA is an established design technique for assessing the suitability of a design in matching the requirement brief. The resulting information provides a basis for any or all of the following.

- Planning a quality improvement program.
- Assessing the design and implementing necessary changes.
- Planning a development program.
- Documenting proof of the design's suitability.

The technique's method is set out in Table 25.6 but is dependent on the level at which the analysis is completed. Table 25.7 explains the rating values (see also Figure 25.3).

Table 25.6   FMEA operating method

---

1. Identify the level at which the assessment should start.
2. Start at each level, lowest first and list all failure modes.
3. Assess the frequency of modes determined in a set period of time.
4. Examine the effects of all the failure modes at lower level on the next level up. The resulting failures at that level are then examined for their effect at the next higher level and so on.
5. Allocate a value to each effect logged: normally valued between 1 and 10 with 1 representing the minimum and 10 the maximum effect.
6. Derive a criticality (frequency × effect rating) for each primary failure mode.
7. As a final assessment or value, assign a value determining the detection rate during manufacture (or QC). Normally 1 for detection before sales and customer input and 10 representing unlikely to be detected.
8. A final risk priority value can then be calculated from (frequency × effect rating × detection rating) to provide an accurate in-field assessment prediction.

Table 25.7 FMEA ratings

Rating	Severity	Occurrence	Detection
1	Better than the specification unnoticed by the customer	Never	Very high, any deviation will be detected
2	Noticed by the customer but will not have any detrimental effect on the product function	Rarely	High, very likely any defects detected
3	Minor effect on product's function but accepted by the customer	Very occasionally	Slightly lower detection rate than 2
4	Function affected and noticed by the customer	Occasionally	Medium, failures may be detected
5	Significant effect on the product function	Occasionally and rising	Same detection frequency as 4
6	Customer inconvenienced and may reject product on quality	Frequently	Low, failures unlikely to be detected
7	Customer annoyed at quality and function failure	Frequently	Majority of failures pass the inspection stage
8	Reluctance by customers to use product	Very frequently	Odd failure actually found
9	Customer refuses to use product	Regularly	Rarely detected
10	Product will not function at all	Very regularly	Never detected

Although each FMEA chart should be individually compiled and completed for a specific product, they will contain the same data:

1. part name,
2. description of part function,
3. list all potential failure modes,
4. estimate potential effect of failure,
5. score the severity of the effect,
6. consider the probable causes of failure,
7. assign probability of the cause occurring and part value,
8. list method(s) of detection,
9. mark a detection rate,
10. calculate an overall risk priority value,
11. recommend remedial action to correct potential failures.

The FMEA can be regarded as a form of risk identification for all new products. If you wish to you can assess the safety of a product by this method alone. Table 25.8 sets out to present formally the questions that need to be answered.

Table 25.8 Product risk identification. © 1978 Breham Press Ltd. First published in *Product Liability* by James Tye and Bowes Egan

---

1   Is product risk analysis made of each new or modified product including, as appropriate, investigation and assessment of test results, design considerations, materials and parts, production process, packaging, storage, transport distribution, installation and maintenance, and do analyses adequately co-ordinate information and opinions of specialists from these areas of activity and take account of the views of legal and marketing specialists?

2   Are product risk analyses documented, and are identified risks classified and evaluated?

3   Where a product has been identified as carrying an inherent danger, has consideration been given to:
(a) identification through the chain of supply;
(b) substitution and related financial considerations;
(c) promotion and warnings;
(d) the state of the art;
(e) special factors?

4   Where an initially unobjectionable product may become dangerous because of physical or chemical deterioration or exposure to ordinary or unusual elements, or through prolonged use, has attention been directed to:
(a) identification of risks to those who hold and use the goods;
(b) identification through the chains of supply;
(c) substitution and related financial considerations;
(d) promotion claims and carrier and user warnings;
(e) the state of the art;
(f) special factors?

5   Where a product can conceivably be used in an improper manner which may render it inherently dangerous in future use, or immediately though temporarily dangerous for the duration of such improper application, has attention been directed to:
(a) steps to inhibit creation of inherent risk;
(b) identification of proper use and hazard through the chain of supply;
(c) substitution and related financial considerations;
(d) promotion, instructions, training and warnings;
(e) the state of the art;
(f) special factors?

6   Where a product must be used with particular skill and knowledge, or is likely to be used in an activity which is dangerous, has attention been directed to:
(a) measures to secure that it is used only by appropriate persons;
(b) identification of hazard and proper use through the chain of supply;
(c) substitution and related financial considerations;
(d) promotion and warnings;
(e) the state of the art;
(f) special factors?

7   Where a product is hidden or is not readily accessible after installation or erection, and danger may develop with product deterioration, has attention been directed to:
(a) provision of adequate, lasting and separately located hazard identification and guidance;
(b) identification of intermediate responsibilities in the chain of supply;
(c) substitution and related financial problems;
(d) promotion and warnings at installation and purchase stages;
(e) the state of the art;
(f) special factors?

Table 25.8 *(continued)*

8   Where unreliable product performance can develop through heavy use, long service or periods of non-use or incorrect storage, has attention been directed to:
(a) provision of hazard history to initial users in a form designed to co-exist with the danger;
(b) provision of an information service for subsequent users;
(c) substitution and related financial considerations;
(d) promotional claims and warnings;
(e) the state of the art;
(f) special factors?
9   Where defective design or manufacture is dangerous, has attention been directed to:
(a) design reconciliation;
(b) hazard identification to all involved in the chain of supply;
(c) substitution and related financial considerations;
(d) promotion and warnings;
(e) the state of the art;
(f) special factors?
10   Where faulty or incompetent installation of a product can create dangers, has attention been directed to:
(a) information, instruction, training or supervision of installers, as appropriate;
(b) guidance on tests, hazards and proper use as required under s. 6 of the HASAWA;
(c) identification of the last-mentioned matters through the chain of supply;
(d) substitution and related financial considerations;
(e) promotion and warnings;
(f) the state of the art;
(g) special factors?
11   Where faulty or incompetent handling or treatment of products at any subsequent link in the chain of supply can introduce hazard, has attention been directed to:
(a) information, instruction, training or supervision of operatives, either directly or under control or direction;
(b) identification of these possible problems through the chain of purchase, supply and installation;
(c) substitution and related financial considerations;
(d) promotion and instruction;
(e) the state of the art;
(f) special factors?
12   Where inadequate or insufficient maintenance of a product can lead to danger, has attention been directed to:
(a) maintenance instructions and the producer position;
(b) information, instruction, training and supervision;
(c) identification through the chain of supply;
(d) substitution and related financial considerations;
(e) promotion and instruction;
(f) the state of the art;
(g) special factors?
13   Have systems been established to ensure effective monitoring of product user complaints, problems and experience, so that this information can be used in periodic and continuous product risk identification:
14   Has responsibility been clearly identified for ensuring that knowledge of risks is accumulated and passed for assessment and guidance by relevant key specialists?

Failure Mode and Effects analysis

Catalogue Number: Description: Present: Date: Sheet of

No	Part No.	Function	How can it fail	What is the effect of failure	Current controls	Severity	Detection	Risk	Recommended corrective action	Action by	Action taken	Severity	Detection	Risk

Figure 25.3   Example of a Failure Modes and Effects Analysis (FMEA) sheet. © Reproduced by permission of Rocket Medical Plc.

Finally, whether you are considering reliability, product life, faults or the effect of environmental conditions, these need to be statistically calculated. These calculations depend on the concepts of random variables and probability distributions, so a quick refresher course on statistical analysis might be a good idea.

26
Manufacturing Methods

This is a short chapter listing the various methods of manufacturing, material manipulation or surface treatment. Although it may appear very basic to set down these processes, considering all the options can prompt an alternative train of thought leading to another manufacturing route which may save you time, cost less or provide a better, safer device.

The processes and methods described may apply to a single component or final assemblies, the examples may suggest certain actions or directions in which materials may be handled. Do not just accept and think in straight lines, speculate on alternatives, ignore the obvious method and deliberately select an alternative (or two) and compare the advantages and disadvantages. If you later return to your original selection then there is a justification for that selection, and proof of some form of planned assessment of other manufacturing processes.

With the new documentation requirements, EC marking audits and the Design Dossier, all actions and methods of manufacture will need to be justified. Company directors will want to know why a component is five times more costly than first thought if you choose to have it machined from solid and not sintered.

An example of the complexity of selecting a method of production, which in turn influences the components required and their manufacture, can be seen in Figure 26.1, illustrating a requirement for a mechanism to produce a loud sound.

The final selection often comes down to a matter of cost, but within these limitations there can still be scope for choices. When selecting a manufacturing process the end use should be fully understood since secondary needs may well force a design over and away from the 'best' choice.

In Chapter 15 the case of a contact aerial electrode is described, when the best manufacturing method depended on the volume of production. If there was demand for 10 000 items per year, the best option would be plastic moulding and metal coating giving a unit cost of 25p. But with the actual demand for 100 items per year, a stainless steel fabrication at a unit cost of £5 was the best choice, and this had been the method for prototypes. This is illustrated in Table 26.1.

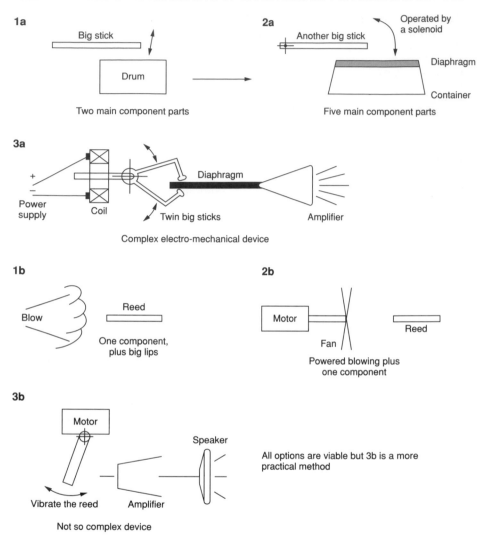

Figure 26.1 Selection options for construction of a device to make a loud sound.

Manufacturing methods provide for assembly, component production and surface texture. Choosing a surface finish not only influences the cost, fabrication and assembly of the final product but may enhance the appearance too.

Figure 26.2 shows machining and manufacturing marks for surfaces.

Figure 26.3 shows surface roughness from different manufacturing methods.

Table 26.1   Manufacture of transmitter tip

Requirements
- Finite shape
- Transmit signal
- Must attach to an extension shaft
- Non-toxic
- Quantity of 100 per year

Materials options
- Metal
- Plastic
- Ceramic

Coating options
- Uncoated
- Paint it
- Plate it
- Encase it

Manufacturing options
- Fabricate
- Mould
- Cast (investment type)
- Machine from solid
- Pressure cast

The cheapest option is to injection mould the tip shape (in ABS or similar) with an external thread, then plate the outer surface, base copper flash first. But this method would require capital investment in tooling of approx. £10 000 and use of injection moulding machine. Best for quantities over 20 000, giving a product at £0.20 each.

A second option is stainless steel rod turned, bent, machined and then polished, suitable for one off and the required 100. No capital investment. Product cost £5.00 each.

Table 26.2 shows surface coatings.

Table 26.3 shows surface treatments.

Table 26.4 shows a classification of surface treatments.

I think the next step in this set of options is to list the manufacturing methods and divide them into groups. If you have a manufacturing problem, ponder the lists and seek inspiration.

Table 26.5 shows main manufacturing groups.

Table 26.6 lists casting methods.

Table 26.7 lists moulding methods.

Table 26.8 lists fabrication techniques.

Table 26.9 lists machining methods.

Table 26.10 lists assembly methods.

Table 26.11 lists extrusion methods.

Table 26.2 Coatings applied to dies, moulds, tools and cutting instruments

Method	Effect	Comment
Electroless plating or electroplating or tumble	Creates an extra 'skin' over the original material by depositing selected coatings.	Commonly used materials are nickel, zinc, tin, chrome, silver, gold.
Anodise	Chemically modifies the surface to provide a hard, abrasive and corrosion resistant skin.	Normally used on aluminium and its alloys. Also used as a purely decorative coating. Some limited use on steel parts in marine environments.
Phosphating	Provides protection to steel parts by way of a phosplate coat, three main types: zinc, iron and manganese phosphate.	The coating provides a base for painting or as a lubricant.
Vapour deposition	Thin coating applied in 'line of sight'. Corrosion resistant and cosmetic variations. Applies to virtually any material.	Three methods: vacuum, sputtering and ion plating.
Spraying: thermal or plasma	Provides a comparatively thick coating to the substrate. Normally applied to metals.	Provides wear, corrosion and high-temperature resistance.
Toyota diffusion (TD)	Compound layers of alloyed carbides to low-cost steel components.	Increases working life of tools especially hot/cold forging, dies and moulding tools.
Ion implantation	Ions penetrate the surface and enhance physical properties.	Provides increased wear, chemical and corrosion resistance. No effect on the original dimensions. Sometimes argued a surface modification not a coating.

Symbol	Meaning	Example	
=	Parallel to the line representing the direction of symbol		
⊥	90° to the line representing the direction of the symbol		
×	Diangular: in two directions from the symbol		
M	No defined or fixed direction, multi-directional		
C	Circular from the centre point		
R	Radial markings from the centre point		
P	Non-directioned, particulate		

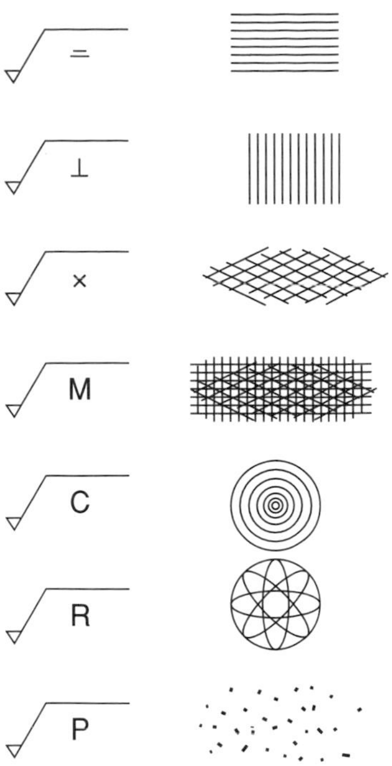

Figure 26.2 Machined surface textures.

Table 26.3 Common surface treatments

Method	Effect	Comment
Heat treatment (hardening and tempering)	Increases strength and wear resistance. Will require tempering to provide best results.	Oldest and most widely used method, easy to control and do, method of applying heat varies: flame, induction, r.f., oven.
Carburising	Heat and chemical process which increases the carbon content in the outer skin of an item. Hardening and tempering then required. Also carbonitriding to absorb nitrogen.	Increases the wear and corrosion resistance cheaply.
Laser	Treats a selected area and transforms it into a harder wear-resistant surface. Minimum distortion or effect on surrounding areas.	Best suited to cast iron, low carbon and alloy steels. Cooling times fast.
Plasma nitriding and carburising	Forms hard nitrides or carbides in the surface. Similar process to carburising by creating a hard layer: thickness variable on demand.	Minimal distortion to items. More control and selection than the gas system.
Oxygen enhanced nitriding	Increases wear, fatigue and corrosion resistance. Low to medium alloy steels.	Also provides a self-lubricating 'skin'. Normally produces a black finish.
Shot peening	Modifies the surface by inducing compressive stresses. A 'cold' method of surface treatment.	Improves fatigue strength in most metals and alloys.
Shot blasting	Cleans and prepares surfaces, normally for a secondary and final finish.	Forceful application of small abrasive particles against the surface.

Table 26.4 Classification of surface treatments

Gas system	Liquid system	Heat system	Mechanical system	Chemical system
Nitriding	Painting	Thermal spraying	Flame hardening	Anodising
Carburising	Dipping	Plasma spraying	Laser treatment	Electroplating
Plasma carburising	Salt bath	Explosive detonation	Electron beam	Electroless plating
Chemical vapour deposition	Enamel	Powder coating	r.f. treatment	Chemical dipping
Plasma vapour deposition		Flow coating	Plating	Phosphating
Ion plating			Shot blasting	
			Shot peening	

Table 26.5 Main manufacturing method groups

Casting	Moulding	Fabrication	Machining	Assembly	Extrusion
Sand	Injection	Sheet metal	Horizontal	Bonding	Impact
Investment	Compression	Welding	Vertical	Ultrasonic	Compression
Pressure	Rotational	Pressing	Grinding	Vibration	Drawing
Shell	Blow	Forging	Broaching	Spin weld	Continuous
Die	Vacuum	Electroforming	Sparking (EDM)	Mechanical	
Rotary	Dip	Spinning	Acid etching	Welding	
Ceramic		Deep drawing	Chemical	Snap fit	
		Thermoforming	Water Jet	Screws	
		Upsetting	Laser	Solder	
		Super-plastic forming	Ultrasonic	Brazing	
				Rivetting	
				Potting	
				Friction	

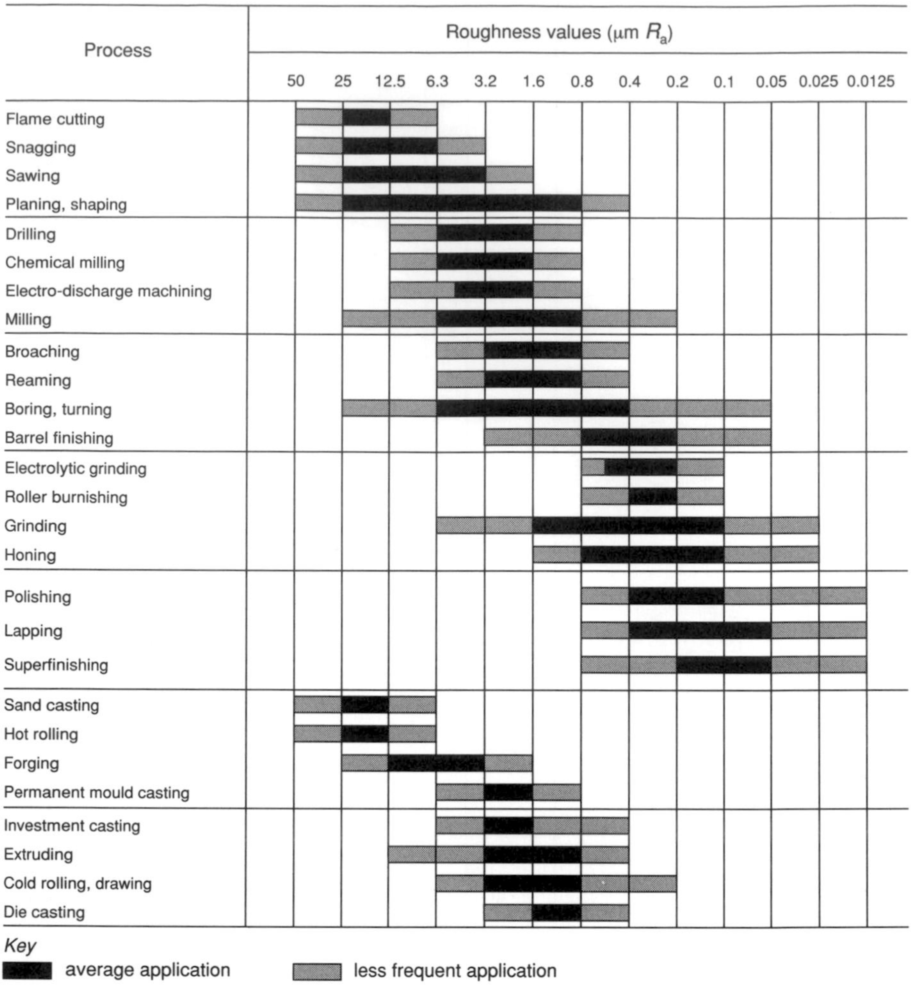

Process	Roughness values (µm R_a)												
	50	25	12.5	6.3	3.2	1.6	0.8	0.4	0.2	0.1	0.05	0.025	0.0125
Flame cutting	░	█	█										
Snagging	░	█	█										
Sawing	░	█	█	░									
Planing, shaping	░	█	█	█	█	█	░						
Drilling				░	█	█	░						
Chemical milling				░	█	█	░						
Electro-discharge machining				░	█	░							
Milling		░	░	█	█	█	█	░					
Broaching					░	█	█	░					
Reaming					░	█	█	░					
Boring, turning		░	░	█	█	█	█	█	░	░			
Barrel finishing						░	█	█	█	░			
Electrolytic grinding							░	█	░				
Roller burnishing							░	█	░				
Grinding						░	█	█	█	█	░	░	
Honing							░	█	█	█	░	░	
Polishing								░	█	█	█	░	
Lapping								░	░	█	█	█	░
Superfinishing									░	█	█	█	░
Sand casting	░	█	█	░									
Hot rolling	░	█	█										
Forging		░	█	█	░								
Permanent mould casting				░	█	█	░						
Investment casting				░	█	█	░						
Extruding			░	█	█	█	░						
Cold rolling, drawing				░	█	█	█	░					
Die casting					░	█	█	░					

Key

█ average application   ░ less frequent application

Note: The ranges shown above are typical of the processes listed. Higher or lower values may be obtained under special conditions.

Figure 26.3 Roughness of finish and method of manufacture.

Table 26.6 Casting, methods

Sand casting	Basic, cheap and somewhat rough finish, the most frequently used system.
Investment casting	Good surface finish and detail. Lost wax method.
Pressure casting	High pressure Low pressure Vertical high pressure All based on a variation of injecting molten metal into a die (or multi-cavities). Uses either 'hot or cold' pre-chambers. Produces accurate, cheap good quality components.
Gravity die casting	Generally a two part metal die, used for large items. Good quality dense structures.
Shell casting	Thin form (shell) made up against a pattern and molten metal poured in, requires external support.
Rotary casting	End results have a good surface, seam free appearance. Normally closed and hollow, also used widely for large plastic containers.
Ceramic	Used to produce cast tooling for fine detail and good surface finish. An alternative to investment casting.
Slip casting	Material poured into closed mould, 'skin' set and the still-liquid inner poured off.
Vacuum casting	Hitchiner process, vacuum sucks liquid metal into pre-formed porous mould. 'V' process, vacuum forms in plastic sheet over male mould and supported with sand, vacuum applied.
Squeeze casting	Used on aluminium, liquid forced within heated cavity pressure held until metal solidifies.
Rheocasting/ thixocasting	Semi-solid ingots heated and placed on slide then pressed into die.

Table 26.7 Moulding methods

Injection moulding	Plastics and some metal alloys (die casting). Common method now, cheap component manufacturing system, but tooling comparatively expensive. Tooling may be made from steel or aluminium depending upon the final quantities required for production.
Compression moulding	Heated mould plus pressure to form components. Similar tooling and quantity advantages/disadvantages as above. Metal compression moulding – see sintering.

Table 26.7 *(continued)*

Rotary moulding	Sealed, hollow, seamless components. Large cost consumer items. Molten plastic (pre-measured amount) squirted into cavity and the die rotated in all directions coating all of the cavities inner surfaces, until the polymer is set. Sets from the outside first.
Blow moulding	Similar process for plastic or glass. Measured material sealed at one entry point in a cavity, air pressure applied which blows the material into a type of balloon which takes the shape of the inner surfaces of the cavity. Cools, tool splits and the finished item is removed.
Vacuum moulding	Pre-heated plastic sheet is pulled down over a cavity of male forming die, the edges sealed and vacuum applied. The sheet conforms to the die shape and cools/sets.
Dip moulding	Pre-formed mandrels are dipped into molten plastic/latex/rubber lifted out and allowed to cool/set. Once solid and strong enough the component is stripped from the mandrel and if necessary heat treated to 'fix' the finished shape.

Table 26.8 Fabrication techniques

Sheetmetal
Welding
   Metal inert gas/tungsten inert gas (MIG/TIG)
   Metal active gas (MAG)
   Electric arc
   Resistance
   Laser
   Electron beam
   Oxyacetylene flame
   Brazing
   Plasma arc
   Friction
Pressing
   Coining
   Blanking
   Piercing
   Fine blanking
   Multi-stage pressing
Forging
Electroforming
Metal spinning
Deep drawing
Thermoforming
Upsetting
Super-plastic forming
Rubber die forming

Table 26.9 Machining methods

Horizontal
Vertical
  Single and multipoint
  Turning
  Milling
  Broaching
  Drilling
  Sawing
    Machine
    Hand
  Grinding
  Boring

All the above may be either manual, semi-automatic or fully NC/CNC controlled.

Sparking, electrical discharge machining (EDM)
  Electrical discharge grinding (EDG)
  Electrical discharge sawing (EDS)
  Electrical discharge wire cutting (EDWC)
Acid etching
Chemical machining
  Electrochemical grinding (ECG)
  Electrochemical machining (ECM)
Water jet
Laser
Ultrasonic
Oxyacetylene cutting
Photofabrication
Abrasive jet

Table 26.10 Assembly methods

Bonding
  Solvent
  Adhesives
  Chemical
Ultrasonic
Welding
  Various methods
Soldering
Brazing
Mechanical fixtures
  Screws
  Nuts and bolts
  Clips
    Spring clip
    Circlips
    Clamps
Vibration

Table 26.10   *(continued)*

Spin weld
Snap fit
  Permanent
  Temporary
Potting
Rivetting
Friction
  Push fit
  Spring
  Cryo (freezing)

Table 26.11   Extrusion methods

Impact
  Horizontal
  Vertical
  Reverse
Compression
Drawing
Continuous hot

Part Three

Future Trends

27
Future Trends

I suppose I could try to emulate Jules Verne or Issac Assimov and write an elaborate imaginary view of the future: possibly a series of speculative predictions for the medical device industry on the trends and methods that will be adopted. Fortunately this has already been done many times by far better writers than me, so I shall just write down my personal observations.

My views about medical devices presently in use are probably well known by now either through articles or discussions held. The next generation of devices clamouring to be released, new materials and techniques await their first practical application and opening of the floodgates. Some have not yet been tapped, and applications somewhat radical last year are accepted as possible today and tomorrow.

Drug delivery systems were once restricted to oral or direct injection; now even capsules are being described as 'intelligent' because the drugs are released not only on a time delay basis but also in response to a need or demand within the body. Drug delivery methods are evolving particularly rapidly.

Do feel free to use any concept or idea described here: anything I speculate on is yours to follow up. I would advise you to read this chapter thoroughly, form your own opinions and allow a few radical thoughts to be generated. If you keep an open mind you will be well placed to optimise your future device designs.

27.1 SLS AND SLA

SLS (selective laser sintering) and SLA (stereolithography) are poised for medical exploitation. Normally an engineering process has a limited application within the medical device industry, but these techniques will be used to produce implants, replacement parts, duplicated joints etc., directly from anatomical information compiled within a computer from imaging systems (section 27.9 below). The methods are restricted at present by the properties of the available polymers and resins but new materials for specific applications are being developed. Work here in the UK and in the USA is well on the way to providing metal models using SLS, although the strength is comparable at the moment with aluminium and could be classed as 'soft'; future improvements will produce 'hard', safe metal components.

27.2 SENSORS

Sensors at the forefront of current development are biosensors and fibre optic systems. The first includes either an enzyme or an antibody coupled with an electrode: the most well-known form being based on an enzyme, glucose oxidase, that indicates glucose and used by diabetic patients as 'glucometers' (a device to measure directly the concentration of glucose in the blood). This type of monitoring can be developed so that the chemical or 'bio' component of the finished sensor identifies a single compound or medical entity. Testing for many deficiencies or diseases will in future be carried out by using only a blood or urine sample.

Fibre optic sensors work differently and can be classed as a single physical sensor. This is a far cry from just transmitting light for illumination or as a method of data transport. Fibre optic methods of monitoring can be applied to changes in pressure, temperature and stress. Basically the fibre acts as a simple send-and-return cable with the tip being a form of mirror. As changes occur on and around the tip the signal is modified and this modification is calibrated and translated into the information required. Potential future uses include heart monitoring during an operation, both core temperature and blood pressure, and moisture increase or decrease within selected organs: remember that a single fibre can be as small as 0.1 mm diameter, ideal for use in veins.

Another technique not yet fully exploited uses hydrogels. Hydrogels are compounds which respond to external aqueous stimuli and/or biological molecules such as glucose, urea or morphine. These can trigger swelling of the gel and the increase in size can be used to monitor the change. One example would be an activation device switched on by dehydration which caused a hydrogel membrane to reduce in size, allowing liquid to pass a valve. The membrane could press against two valves, for inlet and outlet. Once the liquid saturated the area, the hydrogel would swell again, closing the valve and stopping the flow. A further extension of this for the future is an unpowered system which could control anything from temperature to moisture content.

A combination of the above ideas is to use hydrogels and fibre optics together. The assembly could be a hydrogel membrane wrapped around a fibre optic cable (spiral configuration): as moisture caused the gel to swell the fibre could bend in a pre-determined way thus modifying the return signal. Applications could be internal catheterisation monitor or skin check.

27.3 DRUG DELIVERY

There are presently several modes of drug delivery.

- Injection: syringe plus needle, single application.
- Mouth: direct liquid, solid tablet, time delayed, acid reaction.
- Patch: skin, moisture, cream.
- Pellet: implanted.
- Aerosol: by mouth, by nose, under pressure.
- Gas: direct or indirect.

Trends exist towards a needle-less form of pneumatic syringe, similar to the famous Star Trek version. There will probably be a commercial product within the next five years because of high profile requirements for a non-contact, non-invasive unit.

Look at microdevices later on in the text for another form of drug delivery.

27.3 MINIMALLY INVASIVE HEART SURGERY

In late 1996, USSC of the USA introduced a set of instruments for minimally invasive coronary bypass graft surgery, enabling surgeons to operate on a heart through a 75 mm incision. The entire set, apart from the clamp, has been cleared by the FDA for market sales and was launched in Europe and the UK in 1997. The set includes a retraction base, a site stabiliser to control the heart's movement, a clamp to stop the blood flow through the target artery and the Arthoscw Suturing Device and Surgistich designed to sew vessels together in a confined space. These are made by United States Surgical Corporation, Norwalk, CT, USA.

This type of 'key-hole' surgery is on the increase with instruments being designed to suit individual procedures. But teaching methods must be established and standards set and checked regularly. Future use may eliminate the need for barbaric open surgery which is time consuming, traumatic for the patient and costly.

27.4 MATERIALS

Material developments can be of several types: new applications for old materials, new materials for old problems, and evolutionary changes. These combine to create a large materials base from which designers can select. In the future there will be 'intelligent' materials and components which can change to suit the application or requirement placed upon them. Some of the advances known about now are as follows.

- A composite of a polyethylene and hydroxyaptite (HAPEX) has been developed, which forms a ceramic similar to the structural component of bone. This material has already found a commercial application as a major company intend to use it to manufacture tiny ear implants (see Figure 16.18).
- Fibre optic monitors of temperature and pressure can be embedded in the walls of dams during construction. The same devices placed under airport runways monitor the concrete and provide warning of freezing to a central control. Used as strain gauges in large structures such monitors provide constant checks on stress within the building or fabrication. A reduction in size could allow introduction to medical applications.
- An inert, impervious hydrocarbon film can be produced by ionising a hydrocarbon polymer coating, resulting in a substance with properties resembling those of diamond. These attributes arise from the molecular structure of the diamond-like carbon (which is tetrahedral) but with hydrogen atoms substituted for some of the carbon atoms. It is hard, impervious, chemically inert and has a low coefficient of friction. There are many industrial applications, but for medical device use biocompatibility needed to be confirmed to allow progress. This advance occurred early in the 1990s when both in vitro and in vivo trials were carried out and established that the 'diamond like' carbon coating caused no adverse effects on cell cultures. JRA Technology, a member of Spacelink Europe Gie, is now actively promoting this material, offering biocompatability, protection and impermeability, as a coating for orthopaedic implants and prosthetic devices. It can also be used for dental instrument tips allowing easy removal from 'new' types of filling compounds. Future applications will exploit the wear and fatigue resistance of this material.

27.5 MICRODEVICES

In addition to the information given in Chapter 16, I will only mention here that nanotechnology or microengineering will evolve as the fastest growing method of manufacturing medical devices.

Another application of nanotechnology is the development of drug delivery using nanoparticles. Such particles, < 100 nm diameter, can carry a drug through the bloodstream to a specific target. One way of making them is to dissolve a drug and a suitable biodegradable polymer in the same solvent and then bring the two out of solution together. The skill will be in manipulating the surface of the particle so that it will deliver the therapeutic substance to the target tissue.

Two more potential uses would be attaching DNA to assist gene therapy and targeted delivery of iron-bearing particles so that an enhanced MRI scan could be produced.

27.6 GENE THERAPY

Dr Isner, Professor of Medicine at Tufts University and Head of Cardio-vascular Research at St Elizabeth Medical Centre, Boston, is promoting a method of depositing DNA near to obstructed arteries thus generating new blood vessels bypassing the original blockage. This occurs because the gene used controls the production of a protein called VEGF, the same protein which triggers the growth of new blood vessels. The major problem at the moment is the self-destruction or 'switching off' of the gene that occurs after approximately 30 days, before the new vessels are fully mature. Research continues to establish the correct dosage, placement and control, and it is hoped that the need for surgery may be eliminated if this new technique can provide a way of circumventing serious blockages in the arteries before the onset of heart attacks or strokes.

27.7 ORGANS FOR TRANSPLANTATION

The idea of growing your own spare parts from a 'soup' of donor cells, biodegradable supports and nutrients, is being pursued by Dr Vacanti in Boston, USA. This may sound far-fetched, but any form of donor part or transplant suffers from rejection, so if the new replacement is grown from the patient's own cells the body does not consider it a threat and actually encourages acceptance. There is potential for replacement organs, recon-structive surgery after accidents, growth of skin for plastic surgery or repair to worn out parts. The most impressive demonstration of the method to date was a 'living ear': cartilage cells were taken from a patient who had lost an ear and grown on a biodegradable material used to construct a frame in the required shape. The framework mesh fibres dissolve gradually over a pre-determined time which can be modified to suit the tissue or organ desired. This particular example took only 4 weeks to grow and no rejection occurred once surgically transplanted.

27.8 CARDIOMYOPLASTY

This is a technique to assist a failing heart. A muscle is removed from the patient's back and placed in the chest cavity wrapped around the ventricles of the heart. A stimulator is then implanted to make the newly transplanted muscle contract in time with the heart, thus providing extra muscle power.

Unfortunately, as with all new ideas, there are drawbacks, the main one for this technique is the 're-education' or conditioning of the grafted muscle so that it acts more like a cardiac muscle. The procedure was first performed in the UK in 1992 and has been carried out successfully on 600 patients worldwide. Implantable neuromuscular stimulators can contain 16 programs and be selectable remotely, they are about 20 mm diameter × 2 mm thick. Their placement is as critical as that of the donor muscle. In 1995, 1.9 million people worldwide required some form of heart surgery: it is to be hoped that some of the innovations described here will reduce the numbers in future.

27.9   MAGNETIC RESONANCE IMAGING (MRI)

MRI presently gives a cross-sectional view of the body allowing close and accurate examination of the head, brain, back and joints. Existing systems can create 3D representations (sliced version registered then overlayered with a second view at 90°, repeated many times) of certain areas of the body.

The 3D views provide the surgeon with valuable information before an operation; the next step is to link this information to a computer so that solid rapid prototype models can be created (SLA, SLS and LOM used at the moment). The end result is a replica of the patient's anatomy where the surgery is planned, and a model on which the surgical staff can safely plan and practice.

The logical extension of this process is the manufacture of an implant from the data scanned. Modifications could be suggested, tried, and then removed for evaluation: all without a cut being made. Finally the implant is produced in one piece from virgin materials: no machining is required so no internal stresses are created. The area to receive the implant is prepared as rehearsed on the computer and model, so there is less time in theatre, less trauma and a greater probability of success.

The MRI system should not be confused with virtual reality (VR) and imaging visits inside the body, even if the patient's details and anatomical data would be obtained the same way. VR is suitable for look–see and examination but not the physical surgery – or at least, not yet.

An additional application for MRI is in non-invasive sampling and less stressful assessment of cardiovascular function. No more blood samples, tread-mills or catheters inserted, just a set of MRI scans allowing the consultant to access the whole picture.

27.10   TRANSMYOCARDIAL LASER REVASCULARISATION (TMR)

This is a technique put forward by surgeons in the USA, in which they drill small holes into the left ventricle of the heart. The laser used actually cuts holes while the heart is still beating (eliminating the risks associated with stopping and re-starting the heart) and the end result is an improved blood supply to the area treated. This is initially intended for angina patients but a similar system is hoped to achieve ventricular remodelling.

27.11   HEART REMODELLING

Heart tissue, although designed by nature to constantly contract and pump blood, is very susceptible to damage if stretched. When enlarged by trauma or heart failure the stretched tissue will not return to its original shape and blood supply to the body is restricted. Randas Batista remodels the left ventricle by cutting out a triangular section and rejoining the edges, effectively reducing the surface area of the inner chamber. As with TMR these techniques are very new and controversial, but indicate a possible method of heart surgery for the future and medical devices will be needed to assist.

27.12   MICROMACHINES

A few years ago I wrote a tongue-in-cheek article describing a miniature pre-programmed device which could be injected into an artery and scour the walls of clots, plaques etc, to create a better blood flow.

A few years on, although there are differences and it is not exactly as I speculated, something is now on the market. In the USA a stent is used to enter an artery, the tip rotates at a formidable rate (90 000 r.p.m.) and removes obstructions. Now imagine allowing the tip to run free, powered by the blood flow, add a memory and return system to prevent it from ending up in the heart and you have a true micromachine. With added computer power its journey could be programmed to visit several locations. This may be out of reach now, but the next generation may well have the problems ironed out and working units to ensuring trouble free blood supply, or ease prostate problems, or remove stones early from the gall bladder or kidneys.

27.13   DIATHERMY

At present diathermy current is applied by having a large contact pad stuck to the patient's leg, and the other contact linked to an instrument: a hook, loop or probe, which requires a good contact to the plate electrode and easy access to the area of operation. There is the potential for mis-directed current to burn anywhere the hand-held electrode may be placed. Imagine the advantages of a bio-polar instrument, one which had both the electrodes connected internally, no external patient plate and a guarantee of energy transfer only at the point of contact. Figure 27.1 shows a tip profile concept which may be useful for future applications. There may be a fair sized crater created but only at the site selected by the surgeon.

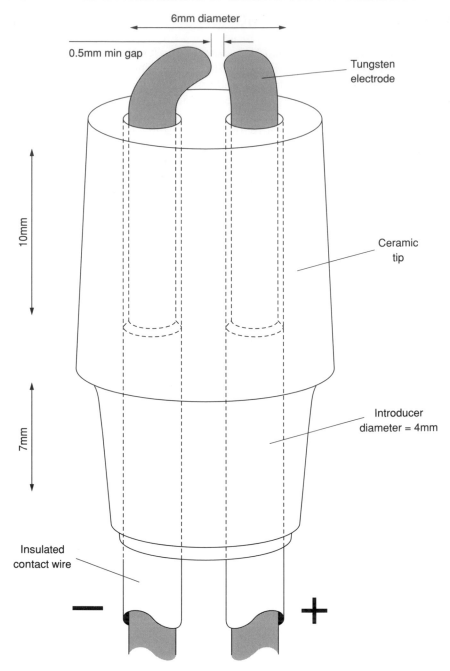

Figure 27.1   Bipolar diathermy tip profile concept.

27.14 DISPOSABLE LASER

Purchasing normal laser systems costs between £50 000 and £70 000, with the additional fittings and instruments costing £200 each day they are used.

Fibre optics and acrylic sheets now have a feature of outer surface catchment and transfer of light (energy) to the edge. Imagine an extension of this feature where metres of optical fibre (equivalent to a surface catchment area of 8000 mm^2) are wrapped around a high intensity light source and transferred to a single exit point for use as optical ablation. The whole unit can be disposable and because of the small diameter of the fibres $\approx$1 mm diameter, the tip could reach nearly every part of the body.

Figure 27.2 is a sketch of the idea: a possible application could be in neurosurgery with a fibre threaded into the brain, monitored by ultrasound and controlled by magnets, able to clear areas of clots deep within the brain without the present unavoidable damage from open surgery.

27.15 MAGNETIC PROPULSION

Imaging using the MRI system suggests a speculative method of propulsion which could in future allow access to parts of the body and brain which are presently out of reach. During the development of MRI it was noted the huge magnetic field used pulled hard against metal objects. If this power could be applied and directed there would be huge potential to manoeuvre metallic devices around the body.

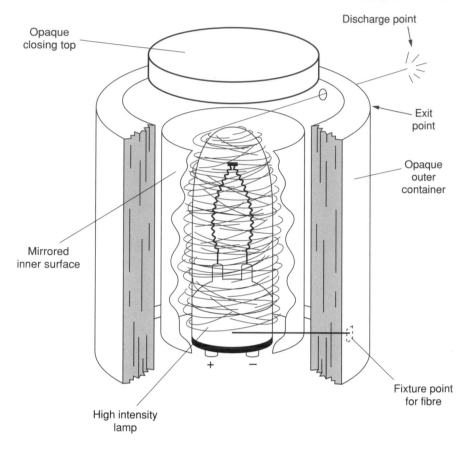

The high intensity lamp provides the initial energy which is captured and transmitted along the fibre. Collection is the fibres' outer surface, transferred to the edge and tip. The mirrored inner skin prevents any loss of energy and returns it towards the centre.

Figure 27.2   Design concept for a disposable laser (HILTYR).

28
Environmental Issues

Depending on your personal preference this may be the most important chapter in the book. It will not provide all the answers and may not be to your own liking but it is an attempt on my part to promote a concept for the future.

Many things have been written concerning the environment, the effects of manufacturing, disposal of waste and recycling. Environmental issues affect our own lives and future generations. I wish to comment on these issues without actually entering the debate. It is my intention to present factual information and let you, the reader, form your own conclusions.

Sterilisation, for example, raises many environmental concerns.

- Gamma sterilisation: radioactive contamination and problems of isotope disposal.
- ETO: ozone depletion, contamination of personnel, waste product disposal, extended timescales.
- Cold fluid: contamination of user, effectiveness of the system, carcinogenic effects.
- Steam: energy use, safety to user, excessive protective packaging.

Similarly, there are other issues with medical devices.

- Recycled or reusable metal instruments: time and cost of manufacture, raw materials, energy conversion costs, lost resource. Also resterilisation time, effort and cost; possibility of infection transfer.
- Disposable plastic parts: waste disposal, raw material processing, consumption of finite resources.

I mention these subjects as examples of some of the questions that must be addressed soon.

28.1 DESIGN FOR THE ENVIRONMENT

The global issues of oil pollution, damage to the ozone layer, global warming and potential loss of fossil fuels are familiar. In the context of medical device engineering the most significant issue is the manufacture and use of plastics for disposable devices. If plastic materials were to run out or become impossibly expensive, then many medical treatments would not be available. To work towards sustainability, there are three options.

1. Design for reuse: re-engineer the product, allow for different methods of sterilisation, and the product can be reused. This has the consequence of expanding the choice of materials.
2. Design for recyclability: if reuse doesn't seem feasible, or uses too much energy, then recycle as much of the product as is possible and create a design policy that more than 50% of material used should be reclaimed.
3. Failing 1. and 2., the third option is to design for easy and safe disposal.

Here are examples of these three approaches.

1. Consider a disposable ABS tube fitting which is bonded to the tube with adhesive and is held in place by a clip. If the material was changed to polycarbonate or polysulphone, the joint changed to a screw thread and the area entering the tube changed to a tapered single barb, then the assembly could be stripped down and autoclaved, not disposed of after a single use. The disadvantages of this approach include the extra cost of the base materials and assembly time. Also there is nursing staff time to disassemble, clean, sterilise and reassemble not to mention repackaging and sealing for storage. Finally the ever present worry of cross-infection if the product is incorrectly cleaned must be considered.
2. Often with disposables the final item is finished, checked and has an ID or instruction label stuck on, it is packed and sealed then sold. To remove any potential contamination from the label or adhesive when the item is broken down and recycled, the information could be moulded into the packaging. This could also save some money on paper and printing. Arguments against this approach are that potential changes in the ID or instructions would be more costly and time consuming and space might not be available for all the text needed.
3. If a glass collection bottle becomes chipped or broken and is dumped in a landfill, it will still be there 200 years on. Glass recycling is possible but uses as much energy as virgin glass manufacture. Consider a change to a biodegradable polymer; once disposed of with suitable exposure to UV or H_2O the material degrades over a number of years to a safe molecular product which can be used in compost. The disadvantages are a higher initial cost of raw material, and the present unfamiliarity of such biodegradable materials. This is discussed in more detail further on.

28.2 SERVICE LIFE

Materials respond to their environment as well as having an effect on the environment. These reactions can be duplicated and accelerated to a certain extent in the laboratory and every effort should be made to collect sufficient data to be able to predict how a product will respond during use. It is also necessary to predict performance during and after storage to determine both shelf life and service life. Deterioration of packaging could perhaps occur and jeopardise sterility. Figure 28.1 shows interlinking tests which should be considered as a fundamental part of the design and development cycle. Table 28.1 lists potential causes of failure.

28.3 ENVIRONMENTAL EFFECTS

External conditions can adversely affect a product before it is even used. These effects need to be considered, allowed for or in some instances used to your own advantage. Table 28.2 lists environmental conditions to consider, with Table 28.3 highlighting temperature variants in different environments.

Biological contamination can cause problems. The US government conducted an investigation when it became known that a mould was growing inside the fuel tanks of aircraft: the resulting moisture retention and contaminated fuel caused great concern. Biological contamination can come from anything: bacteria, moulds and fungi as well as insects and animals. When assessing the effects on your product Table 28.4 lists some areas which can act as indicators.

Table 28.1 Potential causes of product failure

Direct	Indirect
Creep	External packing seal
Melting	Temperature variants
Impact failure	Time
Brittle fracture	Storage
Ductile yield	Stacking damage
Ductile fracture	
Fatigue	
Corrosion	
Solvent stress	
Wear	
Legal (retrospectively introduced legislation)	
Heat	
Mechanical/electrical/chemical constraints	
Upgraded performance requirements	
New processes	
New materials, compounds, alloys	

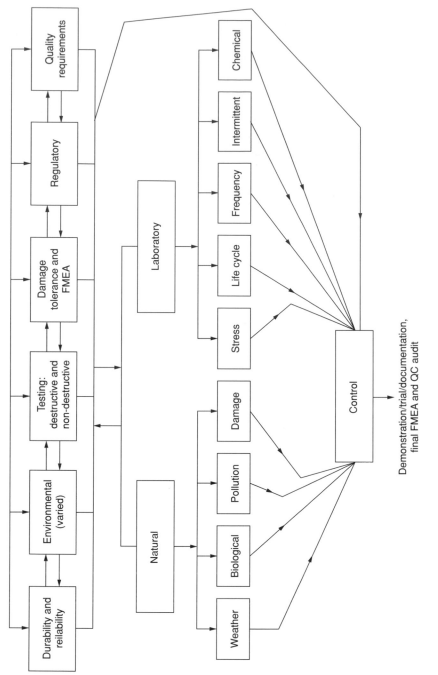

Figure 28.1 Environmental testing considerations.

Table 28.2 Environmental conditions to be considered in design

Factor	Effect or cause
Radiation	Sterilisation method. Solar, nuclear, thermal
Temperature	Increase/decrease. Cycle frequency
Chemical	Solvents, acids, alkalis, vapour corrosion, induced stress, weakened joints
Stress	Cycle, compressive, continued loading
Mechanical/electrical	Tracking, tensile strength, loadings, misuse, insulation, physical abuse
Biological	Fungi, bacteria, animals, insects, micro-organisms
Atmospheric	Dust, water vapour, pollution, oxides, ozone
Air	Aerosols, salts, alkalis, sulphur dioxide, halogen compounds
Wind	Physical damage, sand, grit particles
Water	Snow, ice, water, stream, humidity, hail
Other	When the item is not used as designed. Patient or doctor wear and tear.

Table 28.3 Temperature variants in different climates

Tropical	Desert	Temperate	Arctic
Temperatures vary between 20°C and 50°C. Direct UV and sunlight result in exposed surfaces reaching 70°C. Relative humidity in excess of 90% at night.	Temperature ranges from –10°C to 60°C. With exposed areas reaching 75°C in the daytime. Humidity varies between 5% and 10% inland.	Varies between the arctic and tropical but never in excess. Rainfall predictable.	Worst case area can vary between –40°C and 70°C.

28.4 NEW DEVELOPMENTS

Some companies have taken up environmental concerns and introduced 'greener' products before legislation comes along. Or maybe they are keen to scoop the market – but perhaps I am too cynical.

Disposal of hazardous chemical and toxic waste is being tightened up by continued legislation. In the case of batteries manufacturers are not only working to the letter of the law, but are even pre-empting future legislation and implementation of an EC Directive, see Table 28.5. One major change which looks likely to be introduced is a returns facility for 'spent' batteries. This cleans up waste disposal but also raises the question of who pays.

Table 28.4   Effect indicators

Factor	Indicators
Mechanical/electrical	Insulation. Tracking. Surface receptivity. Tensile/compressive strength. Dielectric breakdown. Arc resistance. Creep. Stress.
Strength	Elongation. Notch strength. Impact strength. Tear. Shear. Flexibility.
Appearance	Colour. Surface roughness. Erasing. Transparency. Gloss. Biological attack.
Dimensions	Warping. Delimitation. Changes in mass. Thickness. L × W.
Volume	Thermal conductivity. Moisture retention.
Permeability	Porosity. Bond strength. Swelling.

Table 28.5   Hazardous chemicals in batteries

System	Notes
Mercury (various cells)	Reduction of mercury to below 0.025% of a standard cell. Performance levels will change but even now 'mercury free' batteries are on sale.
Nickel–cadmium (rechargeable)	Contain potassium hydroxide which is corrosive. Cadmium, cadmium hydroxide and nickel hydroxide are toxic, and long-term heavy metal poisoning sometimes goes unnoticed.
Mercuric oxide (button cells)	Sometimes considered the worst because of the 30%, by cell, weight of mercuric oxide.
Alkaline manganese (varied cell sizes)	Potassium hydroxide which is the electrolyte used is not only corrosive but also strongly alkaline. Additional chemical toxic cocktail is amalgamated zinc powder and manganese dioxide.
Zinc–carbon, Zinc–chloride (varied sizes)	An acidic electrolyte coupled with manganese dioxide.
Lead–acid (rechargeable)	Common car battery containing lead oxide, sulphuric acid and lead plates. If ignited the vapours are also toxic, corrosive and flammable.
Lithium (varied sizes and systems)	Lithium is a very flammable metal which will ignite in air, water or so called safe areas. The electrolyte contains inorganic salts with some oxidising agents dissolved in organic salts. Other systems contain corrosive and toxic liquids like sulphur dioxide. At present there are six different lithium systems in use.
Zinc–air	Amalgamated zinc powder suspended in potassium hydroxide.

In Chapter 7 details were given about a range of new products being marketed by a company called Zeneca Bio Products. A new generation of novel polymers is being produced from natural, plant-based resources in a process which uses sunlight as the primary energy source. Normally stable, durable and moisture resistant in use, these polymers are capable of being processed by conventional methods and techniques. The special feature is that the base resin is fully biodegradable upon disposal in a wide range of microbially active environments and is particularly suited for composting with the biodegradable fraction of household waste. Alternatively the resin can be reused, recycled or cleanly incinerated, see Table 28.6 and Table 28.7. Products already in production are:

- packaging for cosmetics and toiletries;
- food packaging, cups and forks;
- agricultural and horticultural containers (plant pots);
- marine fishing nets, seaweed nets; and
- waste collection bags.

Table 28.6 Biodegradation of Biopol polymer. Reproduced by permission of Monsanto Company

Environment	Demonstrated by
Anaerobic sewage	ICI (Brixham)
Aerobic sewage	PIRA International Chemicals Inspection and Testing Institute, Japan ICI (Brixham)
Estuarine marine sediment	University of Newcastle upon Tyne, UK ICI (Brixham)
Lake pond water	Gent University, Belgium University of Stuttgart, Germany
Sea water	Gent University, Belgium Tokyo Institute of Technology, Japan ICI (Brixham)
Soil	University of Newcastle upon Tyne, UK Minnesota University, USA Gent University, Belgium ICI (Ag Division & Plant Protection)
Compost	Gent University, Belgium University of Stuttgart, Germany Hechingen Compost Works, Germany
Simulated managed landfill	University of Stuttgart, Germany

NOTE: Gent University have isolated 270 bacteria, 120 streptomycetes and 100 moulds which degrade Biopol resin. The Biopol business was developed by Zeneca but is now owned by Monsanto.

Table 28.7 Physical properties of Biopol resin. Reproduced by permission of Monsanto Company

Property		D300G	D310G	D400G	D410G	D600G	D610G
Melting point	(°C)	162	151	153	144	144	136
Melt flow index (ASTM method No. 1238-906/2.16 kg load at 190°C)	9/10 mins	8	–	9	–	12	–
Melt flow index (ASTM method No. 1238-906/5 kg load at 170°C)	9/10 mins	–	5	–	7	–	8
Young's modulus	(GPa)	1.0	0.8	0.9	0.7	0.5	0.4
Tensile strength	(MPa)	31	28	28	25	23	20
Elongation at break	(%)	8	16	15	20	35	42
Flexural modulus	(GPa)	2.7	1.8	2	1.0	1.4	0.8
Izod impact strength	(J m^{-1})	60	161	98	198	200	360
Specific gravity	g cm^{-3}	1.25	1.25	1.25	1.25	1.25	1.25
Thermal conductivity	W m^{-1}°C^{-1}	0.156	0.156	0.156	0.156	0.156	0.156
Specific heat	J g^{-1}@80°C	1.97	1.97	1.97	1.97	1.97	1.97

This is only the beginning of a new market with potential limited only by the ideas for applications.

In contrast an old material commonly in use is still being discussed to determine if it is one of the good guys or not – PVC. Poly(vinyl chloride) has caused environmental controversy for a long time, but because of all the public interest it is probably one of the most thoroughly researched materials used in medical devices today. A more detailed assessment of PVC and its applications is given in Chapter 6.

The controversy is two fold: firstly, environmental damage from PVC manufacture, and secondly the long term problem of disposal. PVC has attracted the particular attention of the environmentalists because it contains chlorine.

- Chlorine was within herbicides used as defoliating agents in Vietnam which contained dioxins.
- Older chlorine production plants caused severe pollution.
- DDT, a banned insecticide, contains chlorine.
- CFCs compounded from chlorine contribute to destroying the ozone layer and the greenhouse effect.

- When incinerated incorrectly chlorine can lead to the formation of dioxins in the gases generated.

As a result of all this publicity PVC became a central part of the environmentalists' arguments against plastics and disposables in particular. The above points manifested themselves as concerns about emissions during production, the potential toxicity of heavy metal stabilisers, degradation during use and recycling. Because of this concern, changes have occurred in the PVC industry and the issues have now gone full circle. Chlorine and chlorine by-products are now employed in numerous beneficial products and PVC is recognised as providing actual benefits. Advantages of PVC products include the following.

- It is considerably lighter than metal counter parts, giving benefits in transport.
- Less energy is used to manufacture and process PVC than many other materials available for the same application.
- PVC is durable and weather resistant.
- It will not rot or rust.
- It is self-colouring.
- No external coating is necessary and it is easily cleaned.
- It is one of the best available thermal and electrical insulators.

The debate is still going on but with changes in production processes, technical improvements in disposal and selective applications, a balance can be arrived at which is acceptable on price, performance and the environment.

28.5 SUMMARY

Environmental changes are happening in product design with recycling being actively promoted, renewable power sources introduced into more and more equipment and the public's awareness increased. Examples of some of the 'green' products recently put onto the market are shown in Table 28.8. No matter what ideas designers try to introduce, environmental protection can only be achieved by public demand. Unless purchasers favour environmentally friendly products, there will be little progress, and this is only likely to come about when economic systems are modified to meet long-term objectives.

Table 28.8   Green products

Fuel Cell Car Mercedes-Benz have unveiled an advanced fuel cell powered car which is claimed to be the world's most environmentally friendly vehicle. The fuel cell uses oxygen and hydrogen gases to produce electrical energy powerful enough to drive a family sized saloon at more than 60 m.p.h., with a range of 150 miles between refuelling. Even though progress has been extremely quick in its development it still will not be ready for domestic use until approximately the turn of the century. Now the fuel cell is technically viable with future development finance virtually guaranteed it offers superb prospects not only for automotive applications, but other units requiring safe, powerful, portable power with low toxicity.

Drinking Water A leading environmental engineering company has designed a unit to extract salt from sea water making it drinkable. By means of a unique reverse osmosis mechanism it is possible to produce over 3 m^3 of pure water per day (enough for nearly 200 people) using solar energy as the power source and operating unsupervised. Dules, the company involved, specialises in the design and implementation of renewable energy systems among other consultancy services.

Energy Saving A motor controller called the 'supermizer' is claimed to save between 35% to 50% energy by using microcomputer technology to match voltage supply to current load on AC induction motors. Designed for use on fans, pumps, compressors and any type of production machinery. The end result is a desired reduction on energy use/required and the long term environmental effect.

Packaging A simple packing system using double skin pouch which when inflated surrounds the product with a resilient cushion of air. Fully protected but still visible, even bar codes can be read through the skin. Known as the 'airbox' and claiming to save as much as 40% over the cost of conventional packing using bubble wrap, foam or polystyrene. Made by Persuasion Resources Ltd., it has the added advantage of being tidier, easier to handle and takes less volume for disposal than normal packaging – by over 90% of the volume.

Part Four

Information

29
Sourcing

Some may say it's buying, networking or just making the right contacts at the right time, but any information obtained regarding a product, or that aids the development of that product or which will reduce the costs, is to your advantage. Some people make their living by sourcing information, materials and contacts, and set up companies to provide this service to you. But there is no great skill or secret involved; the details, information, and contacts are all freely available and easily obtained.

Sourcing starts by one-to-one contact; discussions with colleagues on how best to do a certain job or apply a process. Then you look for a supplier by leafing through books, catalogues and guides. Your first, second or third try may be unsuccessful but by talking and asking questions a possible option you can follow will be offered. The first contact is then made.

Over the years you create your own network, but imagine expanding it a hundredfold in a fraction of the time: how much more successful and easier your next project would be. So how do you gain this increase?

You need to learn to use data bases, company services, published directories and selection programs. Ten minutes a day just leafing through technical trade magazines is a start.

Most people you contact will try to help, not only to sell their own products or services but to assist you to the correct solution. Many will freely discuss and suggest advice just to appear knowledgeable on their own subject, others do it to try and place you under an obligation, some to show off and a few from genuine helpfulness.

Suppose you need an electrode of fixed dimensions and limited functions. A first step is to look for a ready-made item. If none exists can you assemble one from available parts? If not, you'll have to design and manufacture: but how? Talk to everyone and anyone: promote the idea that you are seeking to make use of all resources to achieve the best result for your firm.

Everyone must admit that they are not expert in many disciplines. This is rightly so: no one expects an electronics engineer to be conversant with how to die cast aluminium or a mechanical engineer to know how to design a PCB. But engineering disciplines do overlap so there is no shame in learning from each other.

I have attempted to put together a list of information sources; some are obvious and some less so. The list is here to prompt you and show how many different methods of obtaining information there are. Once you have the technical information, you need the paths to follow for the acquisition of raw materials, component parts, assemblies, finished goods or services.

29.1   INFORMATION SOURCES

29.1.1   PUBLICATIONS

There is a wide range of publications: trade organisation magazines, academic journals, bulletins from individual firms or magazines. From highly scientific research papers to easily read data sheets specific to one item: Table 29.1 lists some of the more commonly available ones but nearly every industry, process, group etc., has its own.

29.1.2   LIBRARIES

Often overlooked, libraries contain a wealth of information. If you use the reference section cleverly most of the work will be done for you by the staff. Library networks enable information not available in one place to be obtained from elsewhere. Also a good librarian will become personally involved and not want to be beaten by a technical enquiry so they will respond to the challenge and put themselves out to answer you questions.

29.1.3   THE INTERNET

With everyone providing their own version of the 'truth' you need to be able to verify the information obtained this way. Still, there's the world at your finger tips: just post your query and await the responses.

29.1.4   DIRECTORIES

Directories are not very exciting but contain information cross-referenced, sub-divided and indexed: also addresses, services, 'phone numbers etc. for you to collect and compare. Directories are published by trade organisations, government departments, individual companies, and anyone wishing to inform you about the services available.

29.1.5   DATABASES

You can compile your own specific database and use general ones available for a small charge. Computer databases offer global coverage and experts

Table 29.1   Selected journals useful to the materials designer

Ceramics	*Glass Industry*
	British Ceramic Abstracts
	Physics and Chemistry of Glasses
Corrosion	*Corrosion Sciences*
Design	*Eureka*
	Design Engineering
	Materials and Design
	Industrial Technology
Metals	*Metal Bulletins*
	Metallurgist and Materials Technologist
	Metals and Materials
	Journal of Applied Metalworking
	Tin and its Uses
	Materials in Engineering
Miscellaneous	*The Engineer*
	Chemistry and Industry
	Materials in Engineering
	Buyer's Guide
Plastics	*Journal of Polymer Science*
	British Plastic and Rubber
	European Plastic News
	Plastic Engineering
	Plastic and Rubber International
Science	*Material Science & Engineering*
	Journal of Material Science
	Chemistry in Britain
Finishes	*Metal Finishing*
	Plating and Surface Finishing
Testing	*Non-Destructive Testing International*
Trade Directories	*Dial*
	Kelly's
	Technical Services for Industry (DTI)
	Engineering Index
	Material Information Sources (Design Council)
Medical	*Medical Device Technology*
	European Medical Device Manufacturer

who will do the searches for you (again, at a charge). Check if you have access to free services via local business support services. The technology is still in its infancy but growing fast: the professional databases must and will offer better services. Table 29.2 shows some of the databases already established.

29.1.6   RESEARCH ORGANISATIONS

Many Research Associations are based on one process or industry; they are keen to provide you with information. Sometimes they are biased towards

Table 29.2 Examples of database information

Campus	Computer Aided Material Preselection by Uniform Standards (Plastics)
Epos 90 & F	ICI plastics
Cen BASE	Thermoplastic elastomers and composite engineering materials
PAL	Permabond Adhesive Locator
ALUSELECT	Aluminium Federation's own selection program
Cambridge Material Selector	Wolfson Cambridge compilation
CHEMRES II	Rapra Technology materials program
Plascams	Plastics data base and selection program from Rapra
ORBIT	Search System via modem
IRS Dialtech	Search System via modem

certain companies (who finance their research) but they can still be very useful. The assessment of which way to proceed is up to you, but their references will point in the right direction. Research companies provide a valuable service for design, testing and technical backup, and can be an enormous source of specific information. Most offer contract use of their facilities. Table 29.3 gives examples of some such groups.

29.1.7 INSTITUTES

Most Institutes offer services only to their members, but joining is no problem and gives access to publications. Institutes carry out their own limited research, publish papers and journals for members, and supply information regarding new developments in related fields. Table 29.4 is a list of some of the more predominant institutes.

29.1.8 CONFERENCES, SEMINARS AND TRADE SHOWS

Working away in your office with everything on your own projects and processes at your fingertips, you can become insular. Attending shows and

Table 29.3 Research associations

PERA	Production Engineering Reserarch Association
RAPRA	Rubber and Plastics Research Association
ERA Technology Ltd.	
SIRA Institute Ltd.	
MRPRA	Malaysian Rubber Producers' Research Association
Spring Research and Manufacturers Association	
BHRA (Cranfield)	British Hydromechanics Research Association
PIRA	Paper Industries Research Association

Table 29.4   Professional institutes

IED	Institution of Engineering Designers
IGE	Institute of Gas Engineers
ICorr	Institute of Corrosion Science and Technology
IoM	Institute of Materials
IMfgE	Institute of Manufacturing Engineers
IEE	Institution of Electrical Engineers
IProdE	Institute of Production Engineers
IMechE	Institution of Mechanical Engincers
PRI	Plastic and Rubber Institute
TWI	The Welding Institute

meetings allows you to visit areas not necessarily directly related to your business. You can learn other aspects of industry and manufacturing, and maybe discover with surprise that equipment designed for an unrelated purpose is just what you need to solve one of your problems.

29.1.9 COMPANY REPRESENTATIVES

An honest exchange with these modern gentlemen of the road can still be achieved. Salesmen will initially, of course, be set on providing only their products but if it proves that they can't meet all your requirements they will still try to help in order to maintain good customer relationships. They hope you will remember who helped.

APPENDIX A: USEFUL ADDRESSES FOR PLASTIC INFORMATION AND ADVICE

The British Plastics Federation
6 Bath Place
Rivington Street
London EC2A 3JE
Tel: 0171 457 5000
Fax: 0171 457 5045

Composites Processing Association
Tannery Court
Westover View
Crewkerne
Somerset
TA18 7AY
Tel: 01460 72870
Fax: 01460 76697

The Institute of Materials
1 Carlton House Terrace
London SW1Y 5DB
Tel: 0171 839 4071
Fax: 0171 823 1638

Moldflow (Europe) Ltd
Central Court
Knoll Rise
Orpington
Kent BR6 0JA
Tel: 01689 878111
Fax: 01689 878678

The Materials Information Service
The Design Council
28 Haymarket
London SW1Y 4SU
Tel: 0171 839 8000
Fax: 0171 925 2130

The Polymer Engineering Group
The British Plastics Federation
6 Bath Place
Rivington Street
London EC2A 3JE
Tel: 0171 457 5012
Fax: 0171 457 5045

Rapra Technology Ltd
Shawbury
Shrewsbury
Shropshire
SY4 4NR
Tel: 01939 250383
Fax: 01939 251118

Society of Plastics Engineers
14 Fairfield Drive
Brookfield Center
CT 06805
USA
Tel: 00 1 203 775 0471
Fax: 00 1 203 775 8490

The Society of the Plastics Industry
1275 K Street NW, Suite 400
Washington
DC 20005
USA
Tel: 00 1 202 371 5200
Fax: 00 1 202 371 1022

APPENDIX B: PC-BASED MATERIALS DATABASES

Plastics	Available from	
CAMPUS	Bayer UK Ltd	*
(Computer Aided	Bayer House	
Material Preselection by	Strawberry Hill	
Uniform Standards)	Newbury	Tel: 01635 39000
	Berks RG13 1JA, UK	Fax: 01635 39822
	BASF UK Ltd	*
	PO Box 4	
	Earl Road	
	Cheadle Hulme	Tel: 0161 485 6222
	Cheshire SK8 6QG, UK	Fax: 0161 486 0891
	Dow Information Centre	*
		Tel: 0800 898487
		Fax: 00 31 206
		916418
	Du Pont (UK) Ltd	*
	Maylands Avenue	
	Hemel Hempstead	
	Hertfordshire	Tel: 01442 218500
	HP2 7DP, UK	Fax: 01442 249463
	Hoechst UK Ltd	*
	Polymers Division	
	Walton Manor	
	Walton	
	Milton Keynes	Tel: 01908 665050
	Bucks MK7 7AJ, UK	Fax: 01908 680516
	Huls (UK) Ltd	*
	Plastics & Rubber	
	Division	
	Edinburgh House	
	43–51 Windsor Road	
	Slough	Tel: 01753 571851
	Berks SL1 2HL, UK	Fax: 01753 820480

*Free of charge

Plastics	*Available from*	
	Petrochemie Danubia	*
	GmbH	
	Danubiastrasse 21–25	
	PO Box 4	
	A-2323 Schwechat-Mannsworth, Austria	
	Solvay Ltd	*
	Unit 1	
	Grovelands Business Park	
	Boundary Way	Tel: 01442 236555
	Hemel Hempstead, UK	Fax: 01442 238770
Cen BASE (Thermoplastics, Thermosets Elastomers and Composite Engineering Materials)	Infro Dex Inc 12872 Valley View St Unit 10 Garden Grove CA 92645, USA	Tel: 00 1 714 893 2471
ELASTOMER P & A	3M, 3M House, PO Box 1 Bracknell, Berks, RG12 1JU, UK	Tel: 01344 426726
International Plastics Selector	HTI Ltd Portman House 16/20 Victoria House Romford Essex, UK	Tel: 01708 746447 Fax: 01708 765709
Laminate Analysis Programme	Centre for Composite Materials Imperial College of Science & Technology London SW7 2AZ, UK	Tel: 0171 589 5111 x4003 Fax: 0171 584 8120
MORPHS	Rubber Consultants Brickendonbury Hertford, UK	Tel: 01992 554657 Fax: 01992 554837

Plastics	*Available from*	
PLASCAMS	Rapra Technology Ltd	
(Plastics Computer Aided	Shawbury	
Materials Selector)	Shrewsbury	
	Shropshire	Tel: 01939 250383
	SY4 4NR, UK	Fax: 01939 251118
CHEMRES II	Rapra Technology Ltd	
(Plastics and Rubber	Shawbury	
Chemical Resistance	Shrewsbury	
Selector)	Shropshire	Tel: 01939 250383
	SY4 4NR, UK	Fax: 01939 251118

Adhesives		
PAL	Permabond Adhesives Ltd	
(Permabond Adhesives	Woodside Road	
Locator)	Eastleigh	Tel: 01703 629628
	Hants SO5 4EX, UK	Fax: 01703 629629

Metals		
PM Selector	MPR Publishing Services	
(Powder Metallurgy)	Old Bank Buildings	
	Bellstone	Tel: 01743 364675
	Shrewsbury, UK	Fax: 01743 362968
	Copper Development	*
Copper and Copper	Association	
Alloys	Orchard House	
	Mutton Lane	
Copper-Nickel Alloys	Potters Bar	Tel: 01707 50711
	Herts EN6 2BR, UK	Fax: 01707 42769
Aluminium Bronze Alloys		
Magnesium Alloys	Magnesium Electron Ltd	*
	Regal House	
	London Road	Tel: 0161 794 2511
	Twickenham, UK	Fax: 0161 728 4842
Titanium and Alloys	Titanium Information	
	Group	
	c/o 20–30 Derby Road	
	Melbourne	Tel: 01332 864900
	Derbyshire DE7 1FE, UK	Fax: 01332 864888

Metals	*Available from*	
Aluminium	Aluminium Federation Ltd	
	Broadway House	
	Caithorpe Road	
	Five Ways	
	Birmingham	
	B15 1TN, UK	Tel: 0121 456 1103
Tin	International Tin	
	Association	Tel: 01895 272406
	Tin Information Centre	Tel: 00 1 614 424
	of North America	6200
		Fax: 00 1 614 424
		6924

General Materials		
MATUS	Engineering Information	
	15/17 Ingate Place	
	London	Tel: 0171 622 8155
	SW8 3NS, UK	Fax: 0171 627 5076
	Wolfson Cambridge	
Cambridge Materials	Industrial Unit	
Selector	20 Trumpington Street	
	Cambridge	Tel: 01223 334755
	CB2 1QA, UK	Fax: 01223 332662
	Comline Engineering	
Mat.DB	Services	
	Blakes House	
	98 Icleford Road	
	Hitchin	Tel: 01462 453211
	Herts HP2 7DP, UK	Fax: 01462 332662
CD/ROM	PDA Engineering Ltd	
M/VISION	Rowan House	
	Woodlands Business	
	Village	
	Coronation Road	
	Basingstoke	Tel: 01256 477799
	RG21 2JX, UK	Fax: 01256 840296

General materials	*Available from*	
Metadex	Dialog Europe	Tel: 01865 730275
	PO Box 188	Fax: 01865 736354
	Oxford OX1 5AX, UK	

APPENDIX C: ON-LINE MATERIALS DATABASES

Aluminium   World Aluminium Abstracts covering the worlds technical literature on aluminium, from ore processing to end uses such as transportation and building.

Available from: ESA-IRS, DIALOG

BNF Metals   BNF Non-Ferrous Metal Abstracts. Subjects covered include properties, processing and uses of non-ferrous metals together with economic and environmental information relating to the non-ferrous metals industry.

Available from: ESA-IRS, DIALOG

CETIM   On-Line version of Bulletin de la Construction Mechanique. Subjects covered include general problems of firms, materials, tests and measurements, control, regulation, metal machining and forming, surface treatments and coatings.
(In French)

Available from: ESA-IRS

Ceramic Abstracts   Covers worldwide literature on all scientific, engineering and commercial aspects of ceramics and related materials, including processing and manufacturing aspects.

Available from: ORBIT, DIALOG

COMPENDEX   Journal articles and items from engineering and technical conferences provide coverage of aerospace engineering, bioengineering, chemical engineering, civil engineering, construction materials and more.

Available from: ESA-IRS, ORBIT, DIALOG

Corrosion   Effects of over 600 agents on the most widely used metals, plastics, non-metallics, and rubbers over a temperature range of 40 to 560 degrees Fahrenheit.

Available from: ORBIT

EMIS   Provides a compilation of the latest published data on the properties of materials important in the fields of microelectronics and solid-state research.

Available from: ESA-IRS

Engineered   Provides information on technical developments in poly-
Materials   mers, ceramics and composite materials as they are
Abstracts   applied in an Engineering Environment.

Available from: ESA-IRS, ORBIT, DIALOG, STN

European Plastics   Information on Companies who specialise in the plastics
Directory   industry. This can be used to source companies that produce plastic products and also for companies that service the plastics industry.

Available from: ESA-IRS

Glassfile   Bibliographic database covering the worldwide literature related to the scientific, technological and historical aspects of glass and allied fields.

Available from: ESA-IRS

Materials Business   Contains information on technical and commerical
File   aspects of iron and steel, non-ferrous metals, and non-metallic materials such as ceramics, polymers, composites and plastics.

Available from: ESA-IRS, ORBIT, DIALOG, STN, DATA-STAR

MATUS   Contains detailed information on the properties of thousands of materials from a comprehensive range of suppliers.

Available from: Engineering Information Company

Metadex   Metals Abstracts On-Line

Available from: ESA-IRS, ORBIT, DIALOG, STN, DATA-STAR

Metals Datafile	Materials Information's bibliographically-based data-bank of numerical property information.
Available from:	ESA-IRS, ORBIT
NTIS	Covers scientific, technical, business and economic information contained in publicly-available US government reports.
Available from:	ESA-IRS, ORBIT, DATA-STAR
Packaging Science and Coatings Abstracts	Provides access to research and development literature in all aspects of packaging science, including materials, equipment, packs, transport, storage and testing.
Available from:	DIALOG
PIRA	Coverage of the world's literature on all aspects of pulp, paper, printing, publishing and packaging. Applications: company and market profiles, product and trade name searches, research and technology trends.
Available from:	DATA-STAR, ORBIT
PLASPEC	Plastics materials selection database providing detailed engineering and design data, chemical descriptions and tradenames for over 11 500 grades of plastics materials.
Available from:	DIALOG
RAPRA Abstracts	All aspects of the rubber, plastics and polymer composite industries. Topics include chemical modification, machinery and compounding properties.
Available from:	DIALOG, ORBIT
RAPRA Trade Names	Covers trademarks and tradenames used in the rubber and plastics industries including full company addresses where possible.
Available from:	ORBIT
WeldaSearch	Abstracts from publications covering the joining of metals and plastics, metals spraying, and thermal cutting.

Topics include welding design, welding metallurgy, fatigue and fracture mechanics, corrosion and more.

Available from: ORBIT

World Ceramic Abstracts   Provides coverage of the world's literature on all aspects of ceramics, including: high-tech ceramics, whitewares, vitreous enamels and refractories, clay-based building materials, glasses, cements and mortars.

Available from: ORBIT

World Surface Coatings Abstracts   Covers worldwide literature on all aspects of the paint and surface coatings industries, including synthetic resins, adhesives, corrosion, testing, polymers, hazards, solvents, storage, transport, marketing and legislation.

Available from: ORBIT

DATABASE HOST DETAILS

Data-Star
Plaza Suite
114 Jermyn Street   Tel: 0171 930 5503
London SW1Y 6HJ, UK   Fax: 0171 930 2581

Dialog Information Services
PO Box 108   Tel: 01865 326226
Oxford OX1 5AX, UK   Fax: 01865 736354

Engineering Information Co Ltd
15/17 Ingate Place   Tel: 0171 622 8155
London SW8 3NS, UK   Fax: 0171 627 5076

IRS Dialtech
British Library
SRIS
25 Southampton Building   Tel: 0171 323 7951
London WC2A 1AW, UK   Fax: 0171 323 7954

ORBIT Search Service
Achilles House
Western Avenue   Tel: 0181 992 3456
London W3 OUA, UK   Fax: 0181 993 7335

STN-International
RSC
Thomas Graham House
Science Park
Milton Road   Tel: 01223 420066
Cambridge CB4 4WF, UK   Fax: 01223 423623

Glossary

Anisotropic   Implies that properties of a material are dependent on the direction in which they are measured.

Antioxidants   Organic additives that help prevent a polymer from reacting with oxygen in hostile conditions.

Antistatic agent   Additive that helps to prevent the build-up of dust through static electric charge.

Aquatex   High-performance fabrics can be laminated with this breathable waterproof film. Unlike Gore-Tex (American) and Sympatex (German), Aquatex is British.

Architecture   The broad physical interrelationship between parts of a system.

Benchmarking   A process of comparison of different techniques, products, services to establish a hierarchy of alternatives.

Blowing agent   Additive that forms gases in the plastic during the moulding process, creating a foamed material.

Brainstorming   The uninhibited generation of ideas using group therapy. Individuals in a group environment help each other to stimulate ideas.

Compatibiliser   Additive used in alloy/blend development, and in the processing of recycled plastics. Helps in the blending of different plastics, bridging the interface between two materials that want to separate.

Computer-aided design (CAD)   The use of a computer to develop a design file and detail drawings for parts manufacture.

Control chart   A chart showing the variation of a parameter over time.

Control parameters   Those parameters that influence the functional aspects of a design. They are usually varied during experimental work.

Coolmax   Like the name says, this will give you maximum cool, especially when indulging in hot, sweaty activity. Largely used for sports and leisurewear, Coolmax by DuPont promotes evaporation while keeping the body dry and comfortable.

Copolymer A polymer made up of more than one monomer unit. The sequence of monomers may be random (–ABBABAAABAB–), in blocks (AAAAAAABBBBBAA–), or alternating (–ABABABABABA–). In graft copolymers chains of one monomer are attached to the backbone of the other.

Cordura It's tough but not rough. A long-lasting versatile fabric that can be transformed into scuff-resistant bags or super-durable biker suits. Has set industry standards for durability.

Critical parameter A design parameter that has a major influence on function and is under the control of the designer. The influence on the function is defined as major when there is a high sensitivity to the response of that function.

Critical parameter audit The checking of hardware for design intent critical parameters.

Critical parameter development The identification and optimisation of critical parameters.

Critical parameter implementation The embodiment of critical parameters into a design.

Critical parameter management The process of developing, implementing into the design and auditing the critical parameters of a system.

Density The mass per unit volume of a material at a certain temperature, usually 23°C for plastics and expressed in $g\ cm^{-3}$ (see specific gravity).

Design for assembly A process to enable a design to be assembled in the easiest and most cost-effective way.

Design quality The full and complete set of engineering activities that must be carried out to enable a product to be manufactured that meets customer's requirements.

Elasticity The ability of a material to return to its original state after deformation; that is, the material's yield point is not exceeded.

Failure mode An event in the response of a function which is unacceptable to the customer.

Failure modes and effects analysis (FMEA) A tool that identifies potential failures of a design and enables preventative actions to be put in place.

Fire/flame retardant Additive which helps to prevent ignition or the spread of flame in a plastic.

Fishbone diagram A diagram linking elemental parts to show their influence on the final effect.

Flow diagram   A diagram showing the flow of a sequence of events.

Force field diagram   A diagram showing all forces influencing a situation. It depicts those forces aiding the situation and those that are in opposition.

Functional analysis system technique (FAST)   A diagram and process that represents the functional relationships within a system, enabling an understanding of dependencies between functions and the analysis of cost and reliability for the system.

Gore-Tex   A microporous membrane that makes clothing waterproof and windproof while enabling the skin to breathe. Invented in 1976 by W.L. Gore, it can be laminated on to any traditional fabric.

Hard tooling   The tooling that will be used to make the final production parts in large quantities. Hard tooling changes are normally extremely costly and time-consuming.

Heat stabiliser   Additive which helps stop plastics from decomposing during processing.

Heterogeneous   Implies that a material's composition varies if one moves from one point to another, for example, glass reinforced thermoplastics.

Histogram   A bar diagram showing the distribution of a variable.

Homogeneous   Implies that a material's composition is constant if one moves from one point to another; unfilled thermoplastics are good examples of reasonably homogeneous materials.

Homopolymer   Polymer with only a single type of repeating unit (monomer).

Impact modifier   Additive which enables a plastic part to absorb shocks without cracking.

Isotropic   An isotropic material is one in which the properties are independent of the direction in which they are measured.

Latitude   The range of responses that are acceptable to the customer as a functional output. These are bounded by failure modes.

Light stable pigments   Help colours to last longer without fading.

Lycra   Throughout the 1980s Lycra became the most popular man-made fibre of all. It has excellent contouring and provides comfort, movement and sleek good looks. It dominated hosiery, lingerie and sportswear.

Melt   The plastic material in its molten state ready for moulding.

Microfibre   This is a generic term to describe fibres less than one decitex in diameter – 60 times finer than a human hair – and can be applied to polyester, nylon and acrylic.

Microsupplex A nylon microfibre by DuPont, this slinky fibre provides twice the wind resistance of standard nylon and greater water repellency. Durable, breathable and quick-drying, its many merits are due to its tightly formed, dense construction.

Mineral fillers Natural substances such as chalk or clay added to plastics to improve strength or electrical properties.

Monte Carlo analysis A statistical study of tolerances of parts to predict the final tolerance of the full assembly. Simulates the building of a number of assemblies to reflect the real manufacturing situation.

NASTRAN A stress analysis computer program.

Noise factor A parameter that influences function which is outside the control of the designer.

On-line quality control The practice of checking parts on the production line for their quality level.

Pareto diagram A bar chart which has bars ranked in order of importance.

Pigments Small particles, which can be organic or inorganic, added to plastics in their molten state to create decorative effects – colour, lustre.

Plasticisers Make plastics softer, more flexible and easier to mould.

Polartec This high-performance fleece is a lightweight polyester that washes and dries quickly and is warm for its weight.

Polymer alloy Combination of polymers that are mechanically entangled rather than chemically bonded. Alloys are designed to combine the optimum characteristics from each constituent that cannot be built into one polymer.

Production intent design A design that reflects as closely as possible that design which will be in the production product. For example, a production design may have a moulded part. The equivalent part in the production intent design may not be moulded but the design will have as many attributes of the moulding (radii, draft angles, intricate profiles) as possible.

QCD The measurements of quality (Q), cost (C) and time-to-market or delivery (D) of a product under development.

Quality function deployment (QFD) A tool for bringing the 'voice of the customer' to the design and manufacturing process.

Risk priority number The product of the levels of severity, occurrence and detection in the FMEA process.

Robotics   The use of automated handling machines (robots) for assembly of parts.

Soft tooling   Tooling prepared for a limited number of parts in the pre-production or early stages of production. Soft tooling is usually easier and quicker to create but can only support a small number of production parts. It is often used to develop the design of the hard tooling.

Specific gravity   The ratio of the mass of a given volume of material at 23°C, to that of an equal volume of water at the same temperature. Often used interchangeably with density, but this is not strictly accurate. Density = specific gravity × 0.99756.

Statistical process control   The control of manufacturing processes to ensure specification levels are met.

Structural foam   A plastic product having integral skins, a cellular core, and a high enough strength-to-weight ratio to be used in a load bearing application. Can be thermoset or thermoplastic.

Supplex   Launched in 1965 by DuPont, this supple sportswear nylon is soft, lightweight, durable, quick-drying and, ounce for ounce, stronger than steel. Unlike real cotton, which fades, Supplex will retain vibrant colour wash after wash.

Supplier integrated computer-aided manufacturing (SICAM)   The use of a computer to help with the manufacturing of parts from a supplier.

Sympatex   A waterproof, weather-proof, breathable membrane, but unlike Gore-Tex, this is flat, not porous, therefore less likely to become clogged with detergent and break down.

Tactel   Originally launched by ICI in 1983, it was bought out by DuPont a year later. A high-profile nylon that is fine, light and durable, it has no special needs and is silky-soft so is as popular in lingerie as the hardiest outdoorwear (it can be made wind- and water-resistant).

Tactel Aquator   A unique, two-layered construction, Tactel Aquator draws moisture away from a nylon inner layer on to a cotton (or other fabric) outer layer, keeping you dry and comfortable.

Technology   An engineering or scientific method chosen to deliver a specific function. For example, the jet engine and turboprop engine are two technologies for providing thrust for an aircraft. New technologies usually result from invention and may carry higher technical risk.

Teflon   Out of the frying pan and into your wardrobe, this chemical additive can be bonded to the fibres of any fabric without affecting feel, colour or breathability. It makes clothes weatherproof and windproof and resists stains and water.

Tencel This originates from wood pulp. A popular choice for jeans it may look like vintage denim, but it feels as soft as chamois leather.

Tolerance (design tolerance) The range over which a design parameter may vary, that is that which may be tolerated by the design.

Tooling A device to enable the consistent manufacture of a number of identical parts.

Toughness Measure of material's ability to absorb mechanical energy without fracture. The mechanical energy can be absorbed by either elastic or plastic deformation of the material.

Tyvek The paper fabric used for envelopes, Tyvek consists of tough, durable sheets of high-density polyethylene fibres bonded with heat and pressure to provide a good printing or coating surface.

UV absorbers Protect plastics against the harmful effects of ultraviolet light.

Value engineering A process during the design of a product that enables the value to be increased. For example, value may be increased by delivering the same output for less cost, with fewer parts or with higher reliability.

Variance (manufacturing variance) The range over which a manufacturing output varies. Usually this must be kept within the range for design tolerance.

Viloft A speciality viscose fibre that offers comfort, softness and warmth. Easy to care for, it takes moisture away from the body and, unlike synthetic fibres (it is made from wood pulp), does not cling to the body or attract dirt and dust.

Viscoelastic Describes materials that demonstrate both viscous and elastic behaviour under the action of an applied stress. The predominant response is determined by the magnitude, duration and rate of application of the stress or strain in addition to the temperature.

Entries in this glossary include some from a publication by Rapra Technology Limited and some from *Quality through Design* J. Fox (1993) McGraw-Hill Publishing Co., which are reproduced with permission.

Index